Emerging Topics in Statistics and Biostatistics

More information about this series at http://www.springer.com/series/16213

Xinguang Chen

Quantitative Epidemiology

Xinguang Chen
Department of Epidemiology
University of Florida
Gainesville, FL, USA

ISSN 2524-7735 ISSN 2524-7743 (electronic)
Emerging Topics in Statistics and Biostatistics

ISBN 978-3-030-83854-6 ISBN 978-3-030-83852-2 (eBook)
https://doi.org/10.1007/978-3-030-83852-2

This Springer imprint is published by the registered company Springer Nature Switzerland AG
The registered company address is: Gewerbestrasse 11, 6330 Cham, Switzerland

Preface

Epidemiology attempts to understand the health status, diseases, and health-related behaviors in the complex 3D spatiotemporal universe. Quantitative approach consists of an essential part of epidemiology. To advance epidemiology, this textbook is prepared for graduate students majored in different areas within the field of public health and medicine. It focuses on the principles, techniques, and methods essential for quantitative research to address challenging problems in the field. In addition to functioning as a textbook for faculty and students for learning in class, the book can be used for self-learning. A good mastery of the methods in this textbook will help transfer students from guided researchers to independent researchers and prepare those for more advanced training in the medicine and public health filed for a doctoral degree.

This textbook is developed based primarily on the success of the author's research and teaching since the 1990s. Different from most textbooks in the same topic area that are organized by the methods systems, this book attempts to connect different quantitative methods and skills with the actual process to carry out a research project. For example, the concepts of data and variables are introduced together with the identification of research questions and formulation of testable study hypotheses; the methods and skills for descriptive analysis are introduced together with the creation of Table 1 in published empirical studies to describe the study sample; and methods and skills for bivariate and multivariate analyses are introduced together with the association analysis for causal inference.

All concepts, principles, and methods covered in the book are demonstrated with real data from existing projects, particularly data from the National Health and Nutrition Examination Survey (NHANES). Inclusion of real data analysis will motivate students for self-learning and practicing taking the advantage of numerous existing data. New concepts, methods, and analytics are also added, including an innovative reasoning process and philosophical understanding of causal relationships; four tasks of modern epidemiology for descriptive, etiological, translational, and methodological studies; quantitative distribution study for public health diagnosis; new methods of 4-dimenional indicator system (i.e., count, population-based P rate, geographic area-based G rate, as well as PG rate) to describe a health event;

simultaneous analysis and understanding of two correlated influential factors; and geometric understanding of co-variates and interaction.

To use this book for teaching, on the first day of training, each student shall be asked to select a research question of his/her own after an introductive lecturing. Along with the lecture, students will learn to develop the question of their choice into a research project. As the class teaching proceeds, students will form testable hypothesis, find data to test the hypothesis, revise the study based on preliminary findings, interpret studying findings, and write a manuscript to report the findings. All chapters of the book are arranged step by step following the "natural" process of research study such that after each teaching session, students can immediately use what they learned to conduct their own research. The success of the training for students will be assessed by the successful completion of their own research project, plus a final paper and an oral presentation to the class.

To facilitate skills training, sample SAS programs are provided for all the quantitative methods and their applications covered in the textbook. These sample programs will greatly facilitate students to learn the analytical methods right after they learned them in class and immediately use those learned methods to analyze their own data to address the study question of their choice. For each sample analysis, the main SAS output is included with detailed interpretation of the analytical results. The commercial software SAS is used simply for convenience since the author is familiar with the software.

Despite many strengths, there are limitations to this book. The chapters and their arrangement reflect the etiological more than other types of studies; examples are prepared using primarily the 2017–18 NHANES data; and only a limited number of diseases and health-related behaviors are included. The author will appreciate comments, suggestions, and corrections from readers to improve the content for future editions.

Gainesville, FL, USA   Xinguang Chen

Acknowledgments

The author completed writing this textbook when the COVID-19 pandemic swept the world. This book would not be possible without generous support from a number of persons. My gratitude first goes to Dr. Din Chen, professor of biostatistics at the University of North Carolina. In addition to the encouragement, he generously shared with me his vision and statistical expertise that assisted me much to establish the framework, to determine chapters and to describe the analytical methods. My gratitude also goes to Dr. Stephen Kimmel, chair of the Department of Epidemiology at the University of Florida for his critical review of several chapters. His supportive comments and constructive suggestions helped me much to improve the book. Lastly, this textbook would not have been completed on time without substantial assistance from Ms. Lillian Zeman, MPH in epidemiology. As a new graduate, Lillian volunteered to review and edit all the chapters word by word. She has also made scientific contributions to the book from a student's perspective.

Contents

Chapter 1
Introduction to Quantitative Epidemiology

Numbers speak louder than words.

Epidemiology is essential for education, research, and practice in public health and medicine. As a scientific discipline, epidemiology covers four major tasks, including descriptive, etiological, translational, and methodological epidemiology. Descriptive epidemiology aims at quantifying the distribution of medical, health, or behavioral issues among people residing in a geographic area overtime; etiological epidemiology devotes to the understanding of causes and influential factors of any medical, health, or behavioral issue from onset, to progress and prognosis; translational epidemiology focuses on the transition of study findings from the descriptive and etiological epidemiology into interventions for disease prevention, treatment, and health promotion; and methodological epidemiology strives to develop new methods and innovatively use existing methods to deal with challenges in epidemiological research and practice.

A unique feature of epidemiology is that it depends heavily on quantitative analysis to extract information from raw data to address the main epidemiological tasks. First, quantitative methods are needed to describe a medical, health, or behavioral problem using numbers, tables, charts, and figures. Second, quantitative methods are essential in epidemiology to study the causes and influential factors. Third, quantitative methods are needed to aid the development and evaluation of intervention programs. Last, new analytical methods and models are needed to address emerging questions in epidemiology. In this book, we will focus on quantitative methods and skills for descriptive and etiological epidemiology. The knowledge and skills covered in this book will lay a solid foundation for further training on intervention research and methodology development.

As an introduction to quantitative epidemiology, this chapter consists of 9 sections, covering key concepts and major tasks of epidemiology, paradigm of quantitative epidemiology, population, study population, sample, and sampling methods; methods to identify a problem, frame a problem into a research

© The Author(s), under exclusive license to Springer Nature Switzerland AG 2021
X. Chen, *Quantitative Epidemiology*, Emerging Topics in Statistics and
Biostatistics, https://doi.org/10.1007/978-3-030-83852-2_1

question, defend a selected topic by considering significance, innovation, feasibility, and shape up a project after preparation. To promote research efficiency and excellence, a brief introduction to computer folders organization is added. Practices are arranged to learn how to access public domain data and use the data to conceive study projects.

1.1   Epidemiology and Quantitative Epidemiology

1.1.1   What is Epidemiology?

The term epidemiology stems from three Greek words *epi*, meaning on or upon; *demos*, meaning people; and *logos*, meaning study of. As a discipline, the definition of epidemiology varies even in textbooks well-known to many of us, including *Modern Epidemiology* by Rothman et al. (2008) and Epidemiology*: Study Design and Data Analysis* by Woodward (2014). The differences can be considered as a reflection of the development of epidemiology to meet the practical needs.

Epidemiology as a discipline was established in the early 1900s when threats of infectious diseases on the life of people were beyond the scope of clinical medicine. The first formal epidemiological study was attributed to John Snow's classic investigation of the epidemic of cholera and its transmission in London in the mid-1880s. Other historical studies often cited in epidemiology include Louis Pasteur for his contribution to theories of microorganisms and invention of the pasteurization to treat milk (Pasteur 1910), Robert Koch (Nelson and William 2014) for infectious diseases, and Richard Doll and Bradford Hill (1950) for health-risk behaviors.

Along with the epidemiological transition in the last century (Omran 2005), the threat of infectious diseases has been gradually replaced by chronic diseases, such as cancer, cardiovascular diseases, substance use, and mental health problems. Consequently, more efforts have been devoted to chronic disease epidemiology and behavioral epidemiology. Since the later twentieth century when the world entered the modern information and technological era, new health threats emerged as major problems, such as sedentary lifestyle, internet abuse, overweight and obesity, substance use, and poor quality of life. To meet these challenges, modern epidemiology advances further to include health and health-related behaviors in addition to diseases.

To date, epidemiology has expanded to include all medical, health, and behavioral problems at the population level, including personal, spatial, and temporal distribution, etiology, and interventions for disease prevention and treatment, and health promotion for better quality of life.

1.1.2 Main Tasks of Epidemiology

As described at the beginning of this chapter, despite much progress in our understanding of epidemiology, what epidemiologists have been and are working on now can be summarized into four broad categories: (i) descriptive, (ii) etiological, (iii) translational, and (iv) methodological.

Task 1: Descriptive Epidemiology. The goal is to describe the distribution of a medical, health, or behavioral event in a population in space and over time using descriptive methods, such as mean, standard deviation, rate, ratio, and proportion. Descriptive study is a necessary part of almost all epidemiological studies. The typical example is Table 1.1 in a study used to describe the characteristics of a study sample. Description of the overall status, time trend, and population/geographic differences of a medical, health, and behavioral issue can also be an independent study. For example, many reports of national surveys are in fact descriptive epidemiological studies.

Task 2: Etiological epidemiology. The goal is to investigate the causes and influential factors of a disease, health, or behavioral problem, including health risk, protective, and promotional factors. Etiological studies consist of the main part of epidemiology. Etiological epidemiology has the strongest demand on quantitative methods. In addition to bivariate methods of Student t-test, chi-square test, and analysis of variance (ANOV), advanced multivariate methods must be used, including linear and logistic regression, Poisson regression, and Cox regression, to name a few.

Task 3: Translational epidemiology. The goal is to translate research findings into interventions to prevent and treat diseases and to promote health and quality of life; these are the ultimate goal of epidemiology (Brownson et al. 2017). Consequently, translational epidemiology needs methods for randomized controlled trial design and longitudinal data analysis to evaluate the efficacy and effect of an intervention. Specialized training is needed to gain knowledge and skills for translational epidemiology.

Task 4: Epidemiological methodology. The goal of epidemiological methodology is two-fold: development of new methods and innovative application of existing methods to advance epidemiology. Conducting methodology research needs collaboration between scientists in epidemiology and other disciplines, particularly mathematics, statistics, and computation sciences.

1.1.3 Functions of and Relations Among the Four Epidemiological Tasks

Figure 1.1 summarizes the functions of the four epidemiological tasks described in the previous section and the relationship of these tasks with each other.

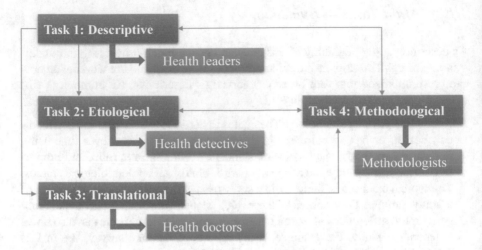

Fig. 1.1 Four tasks of epidemiology, their functions, and relationships

Functions *of* descriptive epidemiology *and its relationship with other tasks*. First, knowledge from descriptive epidemiology consists of the foundation for leadership development and decision-making. Descriptive information is essential for planners and decision makers (1) to *grasp the overall condition* of a health problem and (2) to *make a public health diagnosis* for a country, a state, a city, or a community; therefore, descriptive data are very important for health leaders (blue box). In addition, descriptive epidemiology provides data supporting research in etiological and translational epidemiology (single-arrow blue line from the task). Furthermore, descriptive epidemiology is mutually related to Task 4 on methodological epidemiology (dual-arrow blue line).

Functions *of* etiological epidemiology *and its relationship with other tasks*. Epidemiologists who conduct etiological studies are *health detectives* (blue box), functioning just like the detectives in criminology and justice. Since etiology research consists of a major part of epidemiology, many people often misunderstand epidemiology as etiological epidemiology. As shown in Fig. 1.1, conducting etiological studies requires information from descriptive epidemiology; and findings from etiological studies are the foundation supporting evidence-based precision interventions to solve problems and to promote health. Likewise, challenges in etiological studies may require novel methods while new methods can promote etiological studies (the dual-arrowed blue line).

Functions *of* translational epidemiology *and its relationship with other tasks*. With data from descriptive and etiological studies, translational epidemiology *aims at* developing intervention programs targeting specific influential factors for risk reduction and health promotion. Like doctors in clinical settings, translational epidemiology trains public health doctors (blue box) to work in the field for disease prevention and health promotion. Likewise, there is a mutual synergic relationship between translational epidemiology and epidemiological methods (the dual-arrowed blue line).

Functions *of* methodological epidemiology *and its relationship with other tasks*. Methodologists conduct research to advance epidemiology. For example, new methods are needed to draw probability samples after the landline telephone is replaced by a wireless smart phone (Chen et al. 2018), to estimate age and cohort-adjusted rates (Chen and Yu 2019), to compute geographic area-adjusted rate (Chen and Wang 2017), to quantify quantum dynamics in disease and behaviors (Chen and Chen 2015), and to analyze big data. Methodology research is thus mutually related to the other three tasks.

1.1.4   Quantitative Epidemiology

Epidemiology encompasses both qualitative and quantitative work. The goal of quantitative epidemiology is to address a medical, health, or behavioral question using numbers as evidence, no matter what it is, to describe the distribution of a medical, health, or behavioral problem, to investigate influential factors, to evaluate an intervention program. Although most of us agree that numbers can speak louder than words, we must emphasize that the numbers must be derived from reliable data using the right methods and be guided by the right theories and principles. This is the focus of this textbook.

It is worth noting that quantitative methods are powerful, but no one method alone can provide scientific answers to a problem without a sharp vision of and adequate knowledge about the problem, and appropriately framing a problem into research questions before quantitative analysis.

1.2   Paradigm for Quantitative Epidemiology

To date, epidemiology has been extended to cover almost all medical, health, and behavior-related problems. To be efficient in research, a paradigm is needed as guidance to define the boundary of a study project, to frame a medical, health, or behavioral problem into research questions, to plan and conduct quantitative research, and to recognize the strengths and limitations in result interpretation.

Figure 1.2 presents a paradigm for quantitative epidemiology, including (1) Research Question Reasoning, (2) Study Population Reasoning, and (3) Quantitative Analysis Reasoning. Different from statistics with emphasis on data driving; this *Triple-Path Paradigm* (TPP) enables us to investigate medical, health, and behavioral issues by considering both theory and data in quantitative analysis. This paradigm will be used throughout this textbook.

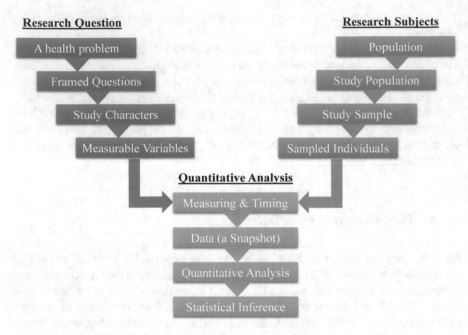

Fig. 1.2 A triple-path paradigm for quantitative epidemiology

1.2.1 Research Question Reasoning

Research question reasoning consists of four steps, starting with a problem, moving to frame several questions to address the problem, finding study characters that are directly related to the study questions, then defining a group of variables to measure the study characters (orange boxes in Fig. 1.2).

Quantitative epidemiology starts with a set of questions to address a problem, no matter if it is descriptive, etiological, or translational. The process starts with a problem with significant medical and public health impact, such as the spread of a new pathogen, increase in diabetes, obesity and overweight, increase in health disparities, etc.

A health problem consists of many aspects. To conduct research, we must frame a couple of research questions we can address with data. For example, to address overweight and obesity as an important health problem, we may think of such research questions: (i) Is the risk of overweight and obesity the same for all individuals in a country or does it differ by gender, race, and socioeconomic status? (ii) Is the relationship between physical activity and weight gain causal? (iii) Does the availability of exercise facilities in a community affect the bodyweight of community members?

To address any one of the three questions above, we need to find the characters that can be measured to describe the questions. Bodyweight is a character, overweight and obesity are two characters that can be measured and used to describe bodyweight; gender, race, and socioeconomic status are characters as well. We use these characters to frame the research question in order to address the study problem; we also use these characters to guide variable selection.

When a study character is determined and defined, study variables can be used to quantify the character. For example, height, weight, and body mass index (BMI) will be used as variables to assess the body weight status and to define overweight and obesity; male-female or more complex categories can be used to measure gender as a variable; White, Black, Hispanic, Asian, and Other can be used to measure race as another variable; distance to the closest gym can be used as a measure of accessibility to exercise facilities in a community.

1.2.2 Research Participants Reasoning

After a study question is determined, the next step would be the Study Population Reasoning process (the blue boxes in Fig. 1.2). What would be the population that is best suitable to addressing the study question? To answer this question, two factors are often considered: vulnerability and feasibility.

First, vulnerability will be the number one factor to consider. The most suitable population should be those who suffer from the problem the most. For example, for sexually-related infections, a sexually active population would be ideal; for cancers and their treatment, an older population would be ideal; for internet overuse, youth and young adults would be the best choice.

Second, feasibility is another factor that must be considered. In addition to vulnerability, we must consider feasibility to reach the population for data collection. With a population in mind, we must then assess if we can access all individuals in the population to collect research data. This consideration leads to the concept of *study population* from which a study sample can be selected. Lastly, we have to determine the number of subjects needed and methods to select the subjects.

In the next Sects. 1.3, 1.4 and 1.5, we will discuss in detail about population, study population, and sample.

1.2.3 Quantitative Analysis Reasoning

After reasoning of research question, study population, and sample, the last step is about the reasoning process for quantitative analysis (the green boxes in Fig. 1.2). This reasoning starts with measurement of study variables and timing of data collection; followed by quantitative analysis, result interpretation, and inference. Key issues in this reasoning process include understanding of the relationships between different variables for a study character, timing of data collection, data quality, selection of analytical methods and models, and expected results.

1.3   Population and Study Population

1.3.1   What is Population?

Epidemiology is a poulation science. It often frames a medical, health, or behavioral issue at the population level and the ultimate goal is to prevent disease and promote health for the population as a whole. In epidemiology, *population is defined as a collection of all individuals to whom the* findings *from a study can be generalized*. For example, if we want to estimate the mortality for people in the United States, all individuals in the country consist of the population, regardless of residential location, education, employment, marital status, and citizenship.

More examples about study population: To investigate the issue of a problem behavior or illicit drug use among youth, all individuals aged 12–17 together consist of the population. To study issues related to reproductive health among women, all females in the reproductive age (defined as 15–49) comprise the population. To study health issues related to a minority group such as Black, Asian, or Hispanic, all individuals who are identified with the group consist of the population. To study issues related to sexual minorities, all individuals who identify as lesbian, gay, bisexual, transgender, and queer (LGBTQ) consist of the population.

Heterogeneity and homogeneity of a population. In theory, a population must be homogenous to ensure valid conclusions from epidemiological research. This requirement is particularly important for etiological and intervention research to avoid bias due to population heterogeneity. Unfortunately, rarely any population in epidemiology is homogenous when survey data are used in research. This is quite different from the populations in laboratory-based studies with specially breaded strains of animals or microorganisms.

In epidemiology, we overcome this challenge of heterogeneity by including participants with certain demographic factors that are related to the research objectives, such as gender, age, race/ethnicity, and education. For example, to study aging related issues, individuals aged 65 or older are included; to study contraceptive use, females are included; to study patterns of smoking, smokers are included.

1.3.2   What is Study Population?

To carry out an epidemiological study in practice, the concept of *Study Population* is often used. Study population consists of all individuals that can be accessed practically for data collection and/or intervention delivery. As depicted in Fig. 1.3, a study population is often a large subset of the population. For example, when the landline telephone number was used for sampling, the study population consisted of only individuals in the households with a landline telephone (~95% of total population). When students in public middle and high schools are used as the adolescent population, it misses those who do not attend public schools. When conducting

Fig. 1.3 Study population and its relation to population

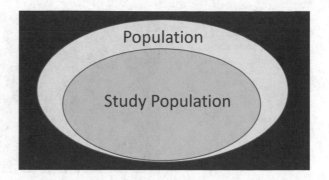

online surveys, the study population consists of only individuals who have access to the internet.

Although study population is only a subset of the population, the difference between the two must be relatively small; furthermore, the difference should be clearly delineated and justified. Focusing on the study population helps remove practical barriers; but caution must be used in result interpretation after data analysis.

1.3.3   Hidden and Hard-to-Reach Populations

This type of population consists of individuals who can be defined conceptually but are not publicly and fully identified because of legal, moral, and/or social considerations (i.e., stigma and stereotype). Typical hidden and hard-to-reach populations include illegal immigrants, homeless individuals, sex workers, drug dealers, and illicit drug users. These populations are highly vulnerable, have a lot of medical, heath, and behavioral problems, can be defined clearly, but can hardly be reached for epidemiological research.

1.4   Study Sample

1.4.1   Study Sample as a Small Subset of the Study Population

As Fig. 1.4 indicates, a study sample is a small part of the study population. Study samples must be selected carefully to represent the population with measurable sampling error. To achieve this goal, specially devised methods are used for sample selection.

The use of a study sample enhances our capability to understand an important issue of a large population with quality data collected from a small number of individuals. For example, to examine the prevalence of suicidal behavior and influential factors among youth, we may need to access several hundreds of students in middle

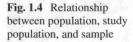

Fig. 1.4 Relationship
between population, study
population, and sample

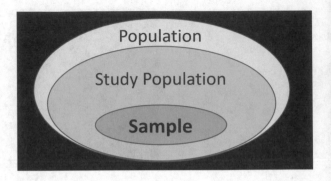

and high schools rather than the millions of all youths in a country. To estimate the
number of people who are aware of the COVID-19 epidemic in a country, we may
need to access only several thousands of individuals.

In Sect. 1.5, several sampling methods to draw individuals from a defined population will be introduced for use in practice.

1.4.2   Importance of Sample Size

Although information for a population can be generated from a small number of
individuals selected using special sampling methods, how small of a sample is adequate? This is important for quantitative epidemiology. Two approaches are commonly used in research to determine the minimum number of subjects for a sample,
known as sample size:

1. Experience-based approach: Determine sample size simply based on the experience from previously completed studies on the same or similar research questions in different populations. For new researchers, this can be achieved by
   reviewing published studies.
2. Quantitative method-based approach: Determine sample size using methods and
   software designated to determine sample size – sample size and statistical power.
   This method will be introduced in Chap. 10.

1.5   Sampling Methods

Different methods are developed to select a pre-determined number of subjects as a
sample from a study population to meet different research needs. Depending on the
objective of a research question, four types of sampling methods are often used in
epidemiology. These methods are (i) purposeful sampling, (ii) convenience sampling, (iii) simple random sampling, and (iv) complex sampling. We will briefly
introduce these methods. Other methods such as GIS/GPS-assisted sampling (Chen

et al. 2018), snowballing, and respondent-driving sampling (Heckathorn 2007) are also useful. Researchers who are interested in these methods can consult the related literature.

1.5.1   Purposeful Sampling

Purposeful sampling is also known as judgmental sampling, selective sampling, or subjective sampling. As the name indicates, this type of method allows researchers to *select a small number of typical subjects from a study population considering several main study* characters (Palinkas et al. 2015). Purposeful sampling is the method for sampling to power pilot and/or qualitative studies. Such studies are often used to test methods, procedures, concepts, and principles, and to generate study hypotheses for full-scale studies.

Purposeful sampling can be illustrated with examples. To design a survey questionnaire, a purposeful sample of individuals with different levels of education, gender, and racial/ethnic background in different age ranges will be useful to help assess the readability of all survey questions. To prepare a full-scale study on factors related to physical activity, a small purposeful sample may contain individuals who never, formerly, and are currently engaged in physical activity; for those who are currently engaged in physical activities, individuals with different types of physical activities (i.e., running, jegging, biking, playing balls) at different frequencies (i.e., occasionally, frequently and always) will be included. To support a school-based research study, a purposeful sample must include school administrators, teachers, parents, and students.

It is worth noting that data collected from a purposeful sample cannot be used to represent the study population. There is no method to determine the sampling error in hypothesis testing to draw scientific conclusions using data collected from a purposeful sample.

1.5.2   Convenience Sampling

This sampling method is also called opportunity sampling, accidental sampling, or grab sampling (Henry 1990). It is a type of non-probability method where the sample is taken from a group of people that are easy to contact or to reach. Standing at the gate of a mall or a grocery store and asking people to answer questions would be an example of a convenience sample; setting up a stand in the cafeteria and asking students who come in for a meal and recruiting them to participate in a research study would be another example; going up to and asking patients in the waiting room for doctor's visits and recruiting them to participate in a research study represents another example.

To draw a convenience sample, a key step researchers have to do is to check all potential participants against the inclusion and exclusion criteria. If a subject agrees to participate and meets the inclusion criteria and does not meet the exclusion criteria, he/she will be included. Convenience sampling has long been used in research, particularly in the field of psychology, social, and behavioral sciences due to its convenience to implement, expedited data collection, and cost-effectiveness. However, since convenience samples are not selected based on any known probabilities, sampling errors thus cannot be statistically determined. In addition, selection bias cannot be ruled out. Therefore, caution is always needed when data from convenience samples are used to address a research question.

Technically, a study with a convenience sample can be considered as an intermediate step leading toward a large-scale study with a probability sample.

1.5.3   Simple Random Sampling

Simple random sample (SRS) is the foundation of modern sampling methods (Cochran 1977). To draw a simple random sample, a complete list of all individuals in the study population will be created first. This list is termed as the sampling frame (SF). With a SF, a predetermined number of subjects will be selected from the SF using a random digits method. For example, to select 7 students from a class with a total of 45 students, a list of the 45 students is created first; a random digit is thus assigned to individual students; 7 students with the smallest (or largest) random digits will consist of a SRS.

The beauty of SRS is that individual subjects in the sample each have the same and known probability to be selected. Furthermore, all subjects in the sample are identical and independently distributed (IID). It is this character that makes the SRS method essential in quantitative epidemiology. With SRS, selection bias is minimized and errors due to sampling can be estimated using statistical methods. Consequently, parameters estimated using a statistical method and data from a SRS can be generalized to the study population.

1.5.4   Cluster Sampling

Although the SRS method is technically solid and attractive, it is highly challenging if not impossible to draw a simple random sample for population-based epidemiological studies. In such cases, it is practically not feasible to generate a SF for random sampling even for a study involving populations in a small city. New methods have been developed to overcome these challenges. Cluster sampling is one such method. Instead of individuals, a list of organizational units, called *clusters* are generated first as the SF. Typical SF for cluster exampling includes a list of all counties in a country, a list of all schools in a school district, and a list of all classes in a school. With this type of SF, a small number of clusters can be selected using SRS method; and all participants in the selected clusters will be included as the sample.

Obviously, cluster sampling is relatively easy to implement to avoid selection bias and to ensure a probability sample. However, samples selected using this method are not fully independent, this is because participants in a selected cluster are correlated with each other. Furthermore, the probability for individual subjects to be selected differs for participants in different clusters because of different cluster sizes. To overcome these limitations, sample weights are used to correct the varying sampling probabilities (Cochran 1977) and special statistical methods are used in data analysis to obtain unbiased results. We will introduce these methods in Chap. 9.

1.5.5   Multilevel Cluster Sampling

Although the cluster sampling method possesses many advantages, this method is not effective in conditions in which the cluster size is very large. For example, if schools are used as clusters, the sample size will increase rapidly as the number of randomly selected schools increases. In this case, a multi-level cluster sampling method can be use. Using school-based studies as an example, a two-level cluster sampling can be completed in three steps. Step 1, a list of all schools is created first and used as the primary sampling frame (PSF) to select schools. Step 2, for each sampled school, a list of all classes will be generated as the secondary sampling frame (SSF). Step 3, a number of classes from the SSF will then be selected using the SRS method. This method can extend further to randomly select students from the selected classes to participate in the research study.

The multilevel cluster sampling method is most commonly used in large-scale, national, and international survey studies. Similar to the cluster sampling method, sample weights and sampling deign must be considered in data analysis to obtain unbiased point and interval estimates. Likewise, we will learn some of these analytical methods in Chap. 9.

1.6   Conceive a Study Project

The content covered in the previous sections lay a foundation for quantitative epidemiology. The next step is to conceive a study project. A study project starts by finding a problem, framing the problem into research questions, and planning the research. As an introductory, we introduce four approaches to help in finding a research problem: (1) brainstorming, (2) literature review, (3) personal experiences, and (4) using the four tasks of epidemiology as guidance.

1.6.1   Brainstorming

Brainstorming has been a widely accepted approach for scientific innovation and creation, including identification of significant problems in the field of public health and medicine. Brainstorming could be very casual. A group of people get together, have a cup of coffee or tea while chatting about things of common interests. When chatting about food, it may lead to questions related to body weight control and metabolic syndromes. A group of parents who are chatting about how to raise children may bring up significant research questions related to parenting and the parent-child relationship. Free chatting with a group of friends on vacation under beautiful sunshine may lead to important research questions on sunburn and skin cancer.

In addition to the informal approaches described above, brainstorming can be organized. This is the method often used in graduate training. In organized brainstorming, a group of people with similar interests will sit together to discuss a subject. For example, there is a paradox in public health and medicine in the United States and many developed countries – there is a continuous reduction in cardiovascular diseases (CVD) along with an increase in overweight and obesity although body weight has been closely related to CVD based on laboratory and observational studies and randomized controlled trials. All participants are invited to share their opinions on the issue and propose approaches to address the issue. In small group brainstorming, a coordinator is needed. The coordinator is not necessarily an authority, but anyone who can volunteer as a coordinator.

1.6.2   Literature Review

This is the formal procedure used in academia to find research questions. Literature review is an assignment for all graduate students; and it often is the first step to develop a study project. The introduction of a research paper is essentially a literature review. Reviewing literature can serve two fundamental functions to help identify research questions: (1) learn how to find and define a research question by carefully reading the introduction part of a paper or a book; (2) directly get a research question by carefully reviewing the conclusion and limitation part of a paper and/or a book. Almost all published studies must address limitations and questions to be addressed in future studies. Findings from the published studies have already laid a solid foundation to address the new research questions, and expected findings from your research studies will contribute to the system knowledge around the subject area, enhancing the value of your efforts. In addition, your work based on the literature review is more likely to receive a fair peer review for publication.

1.6.3   Personal Experiences

Personal experience is another approach to find research questions. An individual who personally experiences a medical or health problem has often been motivated to consult many people, receive information from different sources, and think of the problem for a long time. A person who has insomnia may have a lot of thoughts about potential factors leading to sleeping problems, more than many researchers can think of. A person who is bothered by bodyweight may have a lot of personal experience and make a lot of personal observations about why it is not easy to control body weight. There are many examples of using personal experiences to find research questions.

1.6.4   Four Tasks of Epidemiology as Guidance

The four tasks of epidemiology provide useful guidance to find a problem for research. As described at the beginning of this chapter, the four primary tasks for epidemiology are (i) to describe the distribution of a disease or a health behavior among people over time and across a geographic region, (ii) to investigate the cause and/or risk factors, (iii) to develop and evaluate prevention interventions, and (iv) to develop new designs and new methods to deal with these challenging issues. Although none of these tasks are research questions, they can guide us to think of problems or research questions in any of these areas.

1.7   Shape Up a Study Project

After a problem is located and research questions are framed, a natural step next would be to shape up a study project. The key components to shape up a project include: (i) project title that reflects the research addressing the problem, (ii) study population and sample, (iii) key variables, (iv) study hypothesis, (v) plan for quantitative analysis and expected findings, and (vi) justification and defense.

1.7.1   Project Title

After a research problem is determined, a project title is needed to guide what you plan to do. A good title is simple but contains a lot of information, including the study population, key variables, and sometimes research design, source of data, and analytical methods.

For example, if you decide to address the problem of being overweight for people in a country, and have framed the problem into a research question: Is education a protective factor for overweight and obesity? With such information, you may come up with a project entitled, *"A study of the relationship between years of schooling and body* weight *for* adults *in the US – a* cross-sectional study".

If you plan to address the high prevalence of hypertension considering dietary factors and have framed the problem into a research question: drinking high-fat milk could be a risk factor for high blood pressure. A possible title for your project could be, "Associations *between fat concentration in milk and blood pressure-evidence from the 2017–18 National Health and Nutrition Examination Survey"*.

If you think prostate cancer is a major health problem and would like to challenge the widely accepted notion that high testosterone is the cause of prostate cancer. By literature review, you are attracted by the idea that testosterone declining quicker-than-normal aging could be the risk factor. A likely project title you may come up with would be: *"A* case-control *study of age-related declines in testosterone and* incidence *of* prostate cancer".

1.7.2   Study Population and Sample

With a project title, the next step is to determine study population and study sample. This can be achieved using the methods and guidance previously described in Sects. 1.3, 1.4 and 1.5. In determining the study population and sample, attention should be paid to the population vulnerability and accessibility, potential differences between the study population and the total population, sample size, and methods to select individuals from the population.

For research studies using existing data, efforts are needed to gain familiarity with original project(s) from which data are provided, including study population, sampling methods, demographics, and sample size in the original study and the sample size for your project.

1.7.3   Study Variables

With a study question, population, and sample determined, the next step will be to define the study variables. More detailed discussion about variables will be presented in Chap. 2. Three types of variables must be considered in planning a project to study risk factors: (i) outcome variables, (ii) variables for influential factors, and (iii) covariates, including demographic factors and confounders.

Study variables are dictated by study questions. For example, to study the relationship between fat concentrations in milk and high blood pressure, a potential influential factor would be different types of milk (e.g., whole, 2% and skim) and a potential outcome variable would be diagnosed hypertension. To study the relationship between age-related testosterone decline and risk of prostate cancer, an independent variable would be the differences in serum testosterone levels measured at two different times and the dependent variable would be the first diagnosis of the prostate cancer prior to the testosterone measurement.

Covariates and confounding variables are also to be considered during this planning stage. More detailed information regarding covariates and confounders will be covered in Chaps. 5, 6, 7, 8 and 9. Briefly, demographic factors (e.g., age, gender, and race) are often used as covariates; and factors that are *known to be* associated with both the influential factors and outcome variables are often included as confounders.

1.7.4   Study Hypothesis

A solid study must have at least one or two testable hypotheses. Testable hypotheses are statements composited carefully using the selected outcome variables, potential influential factors, and covariates. Using the milk intake and hypertension among US adults as an example, a testable hypothesis would be:

"Relative to skim milk with no fat, intake of whole milks with fat is associated with increased risk of hypertension among US adults."

If you plan to study if internet overuse, the the independent variable, is related to suicidality, the outcome variable, among adolescents in the United States, a possible study hypothesis would be:

"Hours of internet use is positively associated with the risk of suicidal ideation in the past 3 months."

For a study considering the interaction between internet abuse and illicit drug use on suicidal ideation, one hypothesis would be:

"The internet abuse-suicidal ideation relationship is stronger for youth who also used illicit drugs than youth who did not."

More examples of testable hypotheses will be presented in Chaps. 5, 6, 7 and 8.

1.7.5   Plan for Quantitative Analysis and Expected Findings

As a planning purpose, methods for data analysis and expected results are also to be considered. These include (1) frequency tables, rates, ratios, proportions; (2) methods for visualization such as a pie chart, histogram, bar chart, and line chart; (3) bivariate analyses (e.g., student t-test, chi-square test, simple correlation) for exploration; (4) multivariate analysis (e.g., linear, logistic regression) to verify results observed from bivariate analysis; and (5) methods for analyzing more complex causal relationships, such as interaction and mediation. These quantitative methods are the focus of this textbook and will be introduced in detail in Chaps. 4, 5, 6, 7, 8 and 9.

At this stage, we should also be able to "guess" the results from the study project. For example, for a descriptive study on time trend of obesity, we may expect a decline in the prevalence of overweight individuals over time given the sustained effort to promote a healthy lifestyle; for an etiological study on testosterone decline and occurrence of prostate cancer, we may expect a negative association (odd ratio <1.00) between speed of testosterone decline and incidence of prostate cancer.

1.7.6   Defend a Study Project

In the era of peer-reviewed research when selecting a research question, we must address questions like "So what?" "Who cares?" "How much would other like to know about the problem?" "To what extent do others (peers) agree with me that the question I proposed is a question?" "Is it worth my time and effort to conduct the research?" We often defend a project with regard to three key aspects: significance, innovation, and feasibility.

Significance   A study project would be significant if it meets any one of the three conditions: 1) addresses an important medical/health/behavioral issue; 2) expected findings add new knowledge to the literature; and 3) expected results provide support to prevention interventions for risk reduction. We can learn how to justify the significance of a study in published studies by carefully reviewing a published paper, including the first one or two sentences in the abstract, and more detailed defending in the Introduction section. As an example, to demonstrate the significance of age and cohort-adjusted rate for a study to describe trends of suicide mortality (Yu and Chen 2019), the authors described the significance using one sentence:

> Strategic planning to curb increasing suicide rate among US youths requires unbiased measures of suicide mortality, as the unadjusted suicide mortality rates conventionally used in describing time trends and sex patterns are confounded by the differences in chronological age and year of birth.

Innovation   A study project can be considered innovative if no one else has conducted the same research before, including the same question in the same population during the same time period. In this regard, an innovative study project may not be significant at the current time, but it may show its value in the future or fill in a data gap in the past. The testosterone-prostate cancer relationship is a very provocative example. The positive relationship between high testosterone and prostate cancer has been established with research by a Nobel Prize winner Dr. Higgins and colleague (Higgins and Hodges 1941). With a careful examination of the conclusion it is not hard to see that this conclusion is challenged since prostate cancer never happened in men younger than 25 or 30 years of age when testosterone is at its highest level. This observation has stimulated several innovative studies testing the alternative mechanism of quicker-than normal decline in testosterone as the risk of prostate cancer (Wang et al. 2017).

Feasibility   To defend a study project, you must demonstrate that the study you plan to do is feasible. This is also why studies with secondary data analysis are popular because such studies are highly feasible. You can conduct a secondary analysis project as long as you can have access to the data, find the variables you need, and know how to analyze the data. For studies involving data collection from study participants, feasibility justification becomes a very important issue, including sources of monetary and personal support for the project, office and laboratory facilities, and administrative, secretary and logistic support.

1.8   A Study Project Template

Repeatedly practices are needed to shape up a study project after a research question is selected. To facilitate learning, the following is a hypothetical example that can be used as a template to practice shaping up a study project.

Association Between Acculturation and Depression Among Immigrants in the United States (Title)

Name and Department (John Smith, MPH, University of Florida, Department of Epidemiology)
dd/mm/yyyy (date completed)

Research questions:	Do people become happier after they migrate to the United States and are melted into American culture to pursue their dreams?
Study population:	All immigrants in the United States
Study sample:	Subjects who participate in the study with completed data on immigration status
Study hypothesis:	Higher levels of acculturation is negatively associated with depression
Outcome variable:	Depression scores from Patient Health Questionnaire – 9
Independent variable:	Acculturation scale score
Covariates:	Demographic factors (i.e., age, gender, race) and socioeconomic status
Quantitative methods:	Linear correlation for bivariate analysis and multiple linear regression to verify results by controlling covariates.
Expected results:	Significant and negative association between acculturation and frequencies of depressive symptoms after controlling for covariates.
Significance:	Is it very important to know if immigrants achieve their dream after coming to the US? If yes, is it due to the adaption of American culture and lifestyle or something else?
Innovation:	No published study has ever examined this issue through a thorough and comprehensive literature search. Expected findings will provide data supporting interventions to reduce depressive symptoms and to promote quality of life for immigrants in the US.
Feasibility:	The study is highly feasible since we will conduct a secondary analysis of existing data using quantitative methods.

1.9   Manage Computer for Efficiency in Quantitative Epidemiology

In today's research, computers are not only the working machine but also used for information storage. We organize everything by folders in a computer instead of paper folders, cabinets, and drawers. To ensure efficiency, we recommend the concept of "folder systems".

1.9.1   A Template Folder System for Secondary Data Analysis

When conducting a secondary analysis project, we need to download the original data (usually in some format not directly analyzable by specific software) and associated documentations (technical report, questionnaire, and codebook). These data must be converted into an analyzable format. New datasets must be created by selecting variables needed for a study project, and then recoding them for use. When conducting data analysis, statistical programs will be developed. After statistical analysis, a large number of results will be generated. With the analytical results, you will start to draft manuscripts or scientific reports. When writing, a collection of references is also needed to support your writing. After a manuscript/report is completed, you may also need to reformat it for submission. In the submission, you may need to have cover letters and other materials. Figures and tables must also be prepared to support your presentation. Sometimes, additional supportive documents are used, such as a contract with others or an IRB approval of the study. Figure 1.5 depicts a folder system to organize and store all of the information described above.

Fig. 1.5 An example of a folder system for a study project

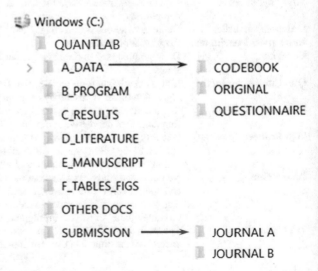

This is a four-level system with the folder QUANTLAB as level 2 immediately after level 1 Windows (C:) drive. Within the QUANTLAB, 8 sub-folders at level 3 are created, each for storing a specific type of data/documents. To make the folders in order for quick access, the letter A, B, C… are used as the first letter of the folder names. You can start with fewer folders as needed and expand the system later.

To prepare for a secondary analysis project, five folders at level 4 are created. Within the A_DATA folder, three subfolders are created with the CODEBOOK folder for storing the codebook and other technical reports of the original data, the ORIGINAL folder for storing original data downloaded from the data-sharing agency; and the QUESTIONNAIRE folder for storing the questionnaire used for data collection.

The two subfolders in the SUBMISSON folder are used to store manuscript for publication. In the case a manuscript is rejected by a journal, the manuscript must be reformatted and submitted to another journal. Using one folder for each submission will greatly facilitate the effort. This is because different versions of a paper are very similar. Separating them from each other is the best way to avoid confusion.

The folder system structure presented in Fig. 1.5 is simply a template that has been established through several decades of the author's own research experience. You are encouraged to create folder systems most suitable for you.

1.9.2   Utility of a Well-Designed Folder System

A well-organized folder system is very important. First, it provides an approach to organize a research project by putting different research related materials in different locations. With a folder system, we can easily find the materials, data, and program we created and stored at any time, thus increasing work efficiency.

Second, it creates a means by which to track completed projects for future research and for responses to inquiries from others for academic or even legal issues. As time goes on, the number of study projects will grow. With a folder system indexed by year, we can also efficiently track our own work in the past. For example, to conduct a new project for survival analysis, we can go back to the folder for statistical analysis programs of previously completed projects.

Last, all the materials saved in the folder system will be a historical record for progress reports and administration monitory.

We will use this folder system throughout this book, including data processing, statistical analysis, and reporting.

1.10   Practice

1.10.1   Data Access – the NHANES as an Example

Use the 2017–18 National Health and Nutrition Examination Survey (NHANES) as an example to practice accessing existing data. NHANES is conducted by the National Center for Health Statistics, sponsored by the Centers for Disease Control and Prevention (CDC). Archived data from different years are available online (https://www.cdc.gov/nchs/nhanes/index.htm) for use to conduct research. Targeting both children and adults, survey participants are selected using multi-level probability sampling methods to represent the entire US population. Cross-sectional biannual data have been available since 1959–62, including survey data, clinical examination and lab measurements.

Main datasets for the 2017–18 NHANES are listed below.

1. Demographic data (DEMO_J);
2. Dietary data, including nutrient intake in day 1 (DR1TOT_J) and day two (DR2TOT_J);
3. Examination data, including blood pressure (BPX_J), body measures (BMX_J), DEXA scan data for femur (DXXFEM_J), spine (DXXSPN_J), whole body (DXX_J), and liver ultrasound transient elastography (LUX_J) for chronic liver problems;
4. Laboratory data, including albumin and creatinine in urine (ALB_CR_J), cholesterol – high density lipoprotein or HDL (HDL_J), total cholesterol (TCHOL_J), chromium & cobalt (CRCO_J), complete blood count (CBC_J), cotinine and hydroxycotinine in urine (COT_J), cytomegalovirus IgG and IgM (CMV_J), fasting questionnaire (FASTQX_J), ferritin (FERTIN_J), folate – RBC (FOLATE_J), glycohemoglobin (GHB_J), hepatitis A (HEPA_J), hepatitis B (HEPBD_J), hepatitis B surface antibody (HEPB_S_J), hepatitis C (HEPC_J), hepatitis E (HEPE_J), HIV antibody test (HIV_J), standard biochemistry profile (BIOPRO_J), urine flow rate (UCFLOW_J), urine pregnancy test (UCPREG_J), and vitamin C (VIC_J);
5. Questionnaire data: A long list of data collected through questionnaire surveys are archived and listed alphabetically, including acculturation (ACQ_J), blood pressure and cholesterol (BPQ_J), cardiovascular health (CDQ_J), diabetes (DIQ_J), disability (DLQ_J), drug use (DUQ_J), access to care and hospital utilization (HUQ_J), immunization (IMQ_J), mental health (DPQ_J), osteoporosis (OSQ_J), physical activity (PAQ_J), prescription medications (RXQ_RX_J), preventive aspirin use (RXQASA_J), reproductive health (RHQ_J), sleep disorder (SLQ_J), cigarette smoking (SMQ_J), secondhand smoking (SMQSHS_J), and weight history (WHQ_J); and
6. Datasets with limited access. A large number of datasets from questionnaire surveys and lab examinations that can be accessed through a special procedure. These data include sexually transmitted infections (chlamydia, trichomonas, mycoplasma genitalium, and HSV type-1 and type-2), sexual behaviors, and reproductive health.

1.10.2   Preparation for Next Chapter

Please go to the NHANES website and do the following:

1. Take an overall review of NHANES, including its history and current status, research design, sampling, data collection, and procedure to use the data. Such background information is critical for further use of the data in quantitative research.
2. Go to the page: https://wwwn.cdc.gov/nchs/nhanes/Default.aspx, select the most recent wave of the survey, take time to review "Data, Documentation, Codebooks, SAS Code" and "Using the Data". During the review, pay attention to those data sets that may be useful for you to address a question of your interest.
3. Create a folder system on your computer following the template in Fig. 1.5. Download the relevant XPT datasets and save them in the folder named as "ORIGINAL\" and save related documents to the corresponding folders you created. These datasets and documents will be used in next chapters.

1.10.3   Study Questions

1. What are the differences between epidemiology and quantitative epidemiology?
2. What are the four tasks for modern epidemiology? How are the four tasks related to each other?
3. Describe the triple path paradigm (TPP) using your own words and use an example to show how to use the three reasoning processes to create a research project.
4. Use examples to describe the differences between population, study population, and study sample.
5. Name four sampling methods and describe each of them and use examples to illustrate their application in epidemiology.
6. Select a research topic that interests you, frame it into a research project and defend it. Be sure to include the significance, innovation, and feasibility of the research study.
7. Why are analytical methods alone and data-driving approaches inadequate for quantitative epidemiology? Discuss with examples.

References

Brownson, R.C., Samet, J.M., Bensyl, D.M.: Applied epidemiology and public health: are we training the future generations appropriately? Ann. Epidemiol. **27**(2), 77–82 (2017)

Chen, X., Chen, D.: Cusp catastrophe modeling in medical and health research. In: Chen, Wilson (eds.) Innovative Statistical Methods for Public Health Data, pp. 265–290. Springer (2015)

Chen, X., Wang, K.: Geographic area-based rate as a novel indicator to enhance research and precision intervention for more effective HIV/AIDS control. Prev. Med. Rep. **5**, 301–307 (2017)

Chen, X., Yu, B.: Age and birth cohort-adjusted rates of suicide mortality among US male and female youth aged 10-19 years from 1999 to 2017. JAMA Netw. Open. **2**(9), e1911383 (2019)

Chen, X., Hu, H., Xu, X., Gong, J., Yan, Y., Li, F.: Probability sampling by connecting space with households using GIS/GPS technologies. J. Surv. Stud. Methodol. **6**, 149–168 (2018)

Cochran, W.G.: Sampling Techniques, 3rd edn. John Willey & Sons, New York (1977)

Doll, R., Hill, A.B.: Smoking and carcinoma of the lung. Br. Med. J. **2**(4682), 739–748 (1950)

Heckathorn, D.: Extensions of respondent-driven sampling: analyzing continuous variables and controlling for differential recruitment. Sociol. Methodol. **37**(1), 152–208 (2007)

Henry, G.T.: Practical Sampling. Sage Publications, Newbury Park (1990)

Higgins, C., Hodges, C.: Studies on prostatic cancer. 1. The effect of castration, of estrogen and of androgen injection on serum phosphatases in metastatic carcinoma of the prostate. Cancer Res. **1**, 293–297 (1941)

Nelson, K.E., William, C.M.: Infectious Disease Epidemiology, 3rd edn. Jones & Bartlett Learning (2014)

Omran, A.R.: The epidemiological transition: a theory of the epidemiology of population change. Milkbank Q. **83**(4), 731–751 (2005)

Palinkas, et al.: Purposeful sampling for qualitative data collection and analysis in mixed method implantation research. Admin. Pol. Ment. Health. **42**(5), 533–544 (2015)

Pasteur, L.: The Physiological Theory of Fermentation and the Germ Theory and its Application to Medicine and Surgery Kessinger Legacy Reprint in 2010. Kessinger Publishing, LLC (1910)

Rothman, J., Greenland, S., Lash, T.L.: Modern Epidemiology, 3rd edn. Wolters Kluwer Health/Lippincott/Williams & Wilkins (2008)

Wang, K., Chen, X., Bird, V.Y., Gerke, T.A., Manini, T.M., Prosperi, M.: Association between age-related reductions in testosterone and risk of prostate cancer – an analysis of patient data with prostate diseases. Int. J. Cancer. **141**(9), 1783–1793 (2017)

Woodward, M.: Epidemiology: Study Design and Data Analysis, 3rd edn. CRC Press (2014)

Yu, B., Chen, X.: Age and birth cohort-adjusted rates of suicide mortality among US male and female youths aged 10 to 19 years from 1999 to 2017. JAMA Netw. Open. **2**(9), e1911383 (2019)

Chapter 2
Characters, Variables, Data, and Information

There will be no quantitative epidemiology without quality data.

Following Chap. 1, after a research question is framed to address a health problem in the real world, an immediate next step is to collect data and prepare to extract information from the data to address the research question. Data are a collection of numbers, text, and symbols for a set of variables obtained from a sample of individuals. These data are thus used to approximate the characters that are related to the research question in the real world. It is therefore essential to have (i) adequate understanding of study characters, variables, data, and information and (ii) competent database skills for quantitative epidemiology. In this chapter, we will cover these topics, including an introduction to the key concepts, skills to access and recode data to construct a database, and practice using a constructed dataset to create tables.

2.1 Study Characters and Study Variables

To date, few people in epidemiology explicitly distinguish a study variable from a study character in research and teaching. For example, when we used blood pressures measured on the left arm to investigate factors related to hypertension, we often treat the measured blood pressure, a variable as the character of a person, i.e., the blood pressure of a person as a whole. However, the measured blood pressure is simply an approximate of the character-true blood pressure at a specific location during a specific period. Another example, when the reported days of smoking in the past 30 days are used as a variable to describe the prevalence of tobacco use, these reported data are treated as the character of tobacco use of a study population in general. Despite the close proximity in most cases, a study variable differs much from a study character conceptually and practically. Understanding the connection and difference is of great significance for quantitative epidemiology to design and conduct research, interpret research findings, and draw scientific conclusions.

© The Author(s), under exclusive license to Springer Nature Switzerland AG 2021
X. Chen, *Quantitative Epidemiology*, Emerging Topics in Statistics and
Biostatistics, https://doi.org/10.1007/978-3-030-83852-2_2

2.1.1 Study Characters

A study character is a concept of the object we would like to gain knowledge about. This is why we often use a study character to describe a research question when introducing a research problem and to draw conclusions based on the research findings. For example, when discussing heart disease as a problem, we often start with a wholesome understanding that the heart is sick (Fig. 2.1). Few will move further to ask questions like: What is heart disease? Are there different types of heart disease? What part of the heart is sick? When did the heart disease start? What is the current status of the heart disease? How can we measure heart disease? What would be the consequences if not treated? The whole understanding of a study character is essential for people in both the general population and the scientific community while the detailed questions are primarily for researchers.

Fig. 2.1 We consider "heart disease" as a character

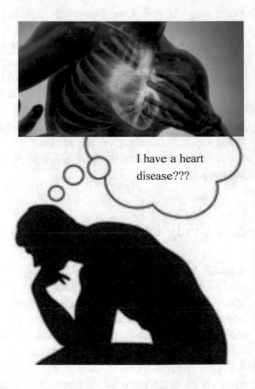

I have a heart disease???

The same is true for almost all medical, health, and behavioral problems, such as cancer, diabetes, metabolic syndrome, influenza, COVID-19, malaria, nutrition, depression, suicidality, overweight, obesity, sleep problems, substance use, internet abuse, sedentary lifestyle, physical activity, and quality of life. It is important to start with a *wholesome understanding* of a study character. This understanding functions as the foundation and guides one toward the study problem, including brainstorming, obtaining input from both professionals and experts, systematic literature search, formation of research strategy, and selection of study variables. In addition, a wholesome understanding of a study character at the beginning gives us the confidence to investigate the problem by ignoring the small details.

2.1.2   Study Variables

A study variable is a label or name of a measurement used to describe the study character. As described in the previous section, a wholesome understanding of a study character sets up the stage for research. What follows is to measure the character to obtain data. As a very simple example, to investigate the area of a rectangle – a character, we need to measure lengths of the two sides – two variables. To investigate the volume of a cube – a character, we need to measure the height, length, and width of the object – three variables. In medical, health, and behavioral studies, the relationships between the study character and study variables are often more complex than in geometry to study area size and volumes; however, the principle is the same.

To illustrate the relationship between study characters and study variables, blood pressure can again be used as an example. When talking about blood pressure, few of us have detailed understanding of blood pressure except a general understanding that blood pressure is the pressure generated by the blood in our body. However, blood pressure is a very complex character as shown in Fig. 2.2. It varies in different

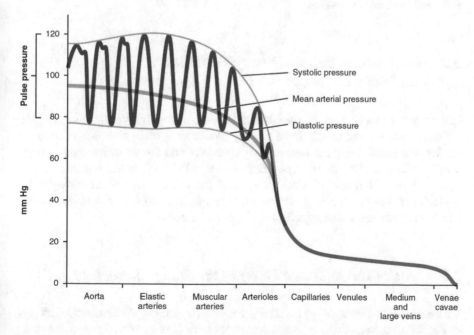

Fig. 2.2 Blood pressure varies in different parts of the body. (Source: Anatomy and Physiology II Module 4, Simple Book Production)

types of blood vessels in different parts of our body, starting at the aorta near the heart to different types of arteries, further to capillaries across the whole body, and last collected by veins back to the heart.

In addition to the dramatic variations within the body in different types of blood vessels, blood pressure in healthy people and patients shows a 24-hour circle with lower pressures in the evening, increasing rapidly in the morning, and maintaining at higher levels during the day (Sheng et al. 2013, Degaute et al. 1991). Blood pressure also shows seasonal cycles with higher levels during the winter and lower measures during the summer (Modesti et al. 2018).

The measured blood pressure used in research consists of systolic and diastolic pressure; and these two pressures are variables. Following the standard operation, blood pressures of a person are taken at a specific time of day on the left arm of a person. The measured blood pressures are thus the artery pressure on the left arm (corresponding to the elastic arteries), and they are generated by the blood on the wall of the artery at this location (Fig. 2.2) during the time when the pressures are measured.

From the discussion above, it can be seen clearly that blood pressure data used in research is simply a sample of the blood pressures measured in a special location of the body (i.e., left arm) taking at a special time of a day, on a special day of a week, and within a specific season of a year. These are the so-called data used to address a medical, health, or behavioral problem.

The blood pressure data described above presents a typical example for us to understand other variables used in research by carefully distinguishing a study character and measured variables.

2.2   Relationship Between Study Variables and Study Character

In the previous section, we can see that variables are used to investigate a character, although they are not equal. Since a study character is often complex in research studies, the relationship between a study character and the variables used to measure the character are more complex than we often think of. In this section, we will discuss three relationships that are critical for quantitative epidemiology: (1) Variables as a proxy of a study character; (2) many variables for one study character; and (3) one variable may reflect multiple characters.

2.2.1   Study Variables as a Proxy of the Study Character

Variables devised for a study character are used as *a proxy of the character* (left part of Fig. 2.3). As long as the type and number of variables are well devised, they will provide a good proxy of the study character to address a specific question. Using the

Fig. 2.3 Study variables
as approximate of study
character

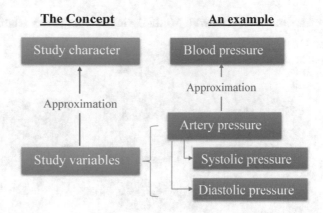

blood pressure in Sect. 2.1 as an example again, the concept "blood pressure" is the character. To study hypertension, two pressures on the artery, systolic and diastolic measured at the left arm are used as variables (right part of Fig. 2.3). These two variables are widely used in studying hypertension since they provide a best proxy of the artery blood pressure.

Since variables function as a proxy of the study character, unexpected results are likely in research studies in which a study variable used to measure a character does not provide a good proxy of the study character. This is one important point as to why it is essential (1) to distinguish study variables from the study character that these variables are used to measure and (2) to understand the relationship between the two.

2.2.2   Multi-variables for One Study Character

One character-multiple variables relationship: A study character often consists of multiple attributes. Technically, one variable can measure only one attribute; consequently, more than one variable can be used to measure one study character (Fig. 2.4a). This relationship can be illustrated using a number of examples. The character of physical development consists of several attributes such as height, weight, head circumference, and length of the four extremities; all of which are variables to study development. The character of Covid-19 infection consists of multiple attributes, and it can be investigated using a list of variables, including clinical symptoms of cough, headache and fever, antibody test for previous infection, and virial nucleotide test for current infection. Coronary heart disease as a character also possesses many attributes and it thus can be examined using clinical signs and symptoms, blood chemistry, ECG, chest X-ray, CT scan, and cardioangiography. Cigarette smoking as a character has multiple attributes and it can thus be measured using many variables such as ever smoked in life, age of smoking onset, days smoked in the past month, number of cigarettes smoked in a typical day, serum cotinine level (biomarker), and nicotine dependence.

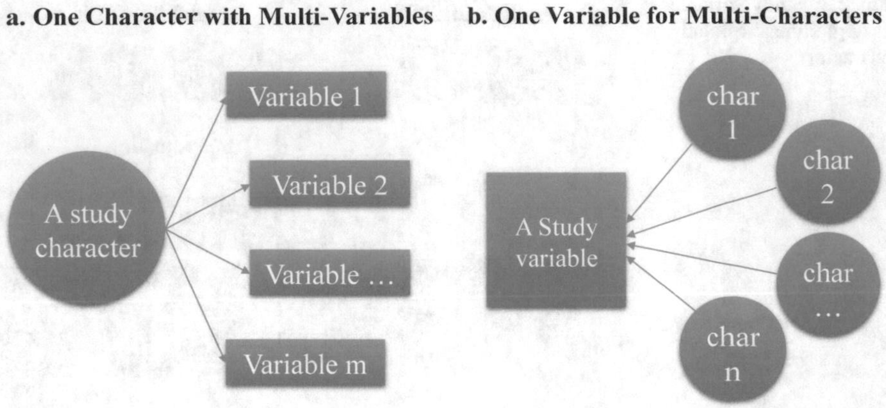

a. One Character with Multi-Variables　　**b. One Variable for Multi-Characters**

Fig. 2.4 Relationships between study character and study variable

As a reference, Table 2.1 lists several characters with multiple variables that are commonly used in epidemiology. From the discussion above and the example in Table 2.1, it can be seen that an *obvious advantage of one character-multiple*

Table 2.1 Examples of one study character with multi-variables

Study character	Study variable
Physically related	
Overweight and obese	Body image, height, weight, BMI, percent body fat (PBF) from body composition test, hydrostatic weighting, and DEXA scan
Coronary heart disease	Self-report, signs and symptoms, blood tests for biomarkers, chest X-ray, CT scan, and angiography
Covid-19	Self-report, contact history, signs and symptoms, antibody test, and viral test, clinical diagnosis, and asymptotic infection.
Mentally related	
Depression	The Center for Epidemiologic Studies Depression Scale (CES-D), Beck Depression Inventory (BDI), the Patient Health Questionnaire – 9 (PHQ-9),
Post-traumatic stress disorder (PTSD)	PTSD Symptom Scale (PSS), PTSD Checklist for DEM-5 (PCL-5), UCLA Child/Adolescent PTSD Reaction Index for DSM-5
Suicidality	Suicidal ideation, suicide attempt, self-injury, and other suicidal behaviors
Sociobehaviorally related	
Quality of life	The Quality of Life Scale (QOLS), McGill Quality of Life Questionnaire (MQOL), Measuring Health-Related Quality of Life (HRQOL)
Social capital	Connections with peers, neighbors, colleagues; connection with social organizations; participate in group activities; personal social capital scale
Cigarette smoking	Ever smoked cigarettes in life, days smoked in the past 30 days, number of cigarettes smoked during a typical day, urine cotinine test

variables is that it allows us to select variables most suitable for a research project, considering the reliability of the measures, validity, and cost to measure the variable.

2.2.3   One Variable for Multiple Characters

Another important phenomenon commonly seen in epidemiology is that one variable could be a proxy for multiple characters that are not explicitly defined (Fig. 2.4b). A typical example is education. In epidemiology, levels of education show a protective effect for almost all medical, health, and behavioral problems. In practice, education is measured with several alternative scales, including continuous measures (e.g., years of schooling) and categorical from simplest of binary (e.g., literacy vs. illiteracy) to multi-categorical (e.g., less than high school, high school, college or more). However, receiving education is a selective process in almost all countries across the world, including the impact from parental (genetic and parenting), informational (awareness of the opportunity for education), financial (affordable), and societal (education is available) factors. Information extracted from a variable to measure education reflects so many different characters. Caution is thus needed when a variable for education is used to investigate a medical, health, or behavioral problem.

Another example in the literature is being bilingual. A study reported that being capable of speaking a foreign language – bilingual – is protective factor for Alzheimer's disease (Chertkow et al. 2010). Speaking a foreign language can be a variable for many different characters, such as opportunities to learn another language (many people in European countries speak multiple languages since childhood), children of parents with higher education have more opportunities to learn a foreign language, and language intelligence may affect one's ability to master a foreign language, to name a few. It is thus very difficult if not impossible to conclude if the ability to speak another language is protective against Alzheimer's disease.

Other similar variables commonly used in epidemiology include handwashing, healthy diet, physical activities, computer use, and chronological age. Handwashing could be a response to a health education program, a personal habit, living in an environment equipped with handwashing facilities, and higher level of education, having a job in hospital. People who practice a healthy diet may have higher levels of education, more income, and live in a better off community that supports a healthy diet; levels of physical activity may be related to age, lifestyle, socioeconomic status and neighborhood conditions. Using a computer could be a reflection of education, occupation, socioeconomic status, sedentary lifestyle, etc. Chronological age measures the duration a person has lived and can be determined accurately (i.e., with date of birth from birth certificate); however, chronological age is also a very good approximate of biological and psychological age of a person.

The phenomenon of one variable – multiple characters presents a challenge to researchers in epidemiology, including descriptive, etiological, translational, and methodological studies. The one-variable and multi-character phenomenon is often the origin of bias due to confounding and the use of control variables in epidemiological research. This phenomenon also makes it challenging to interpret findings from quantitative analysis. Further research is highly needed to clarify issues in all research studies in general and in quantitative epidemiology in particular.

2.3   Data and Database

After study variables are determined, instruments/tools will be developed or used to measure the character of study subjects – animals, humans, or organizations – to generate data. When data becomes available, quantitative analysis can be conducted to address a research question regarding a study character that is abstractive. This section will focus on the concept of and skills to build a database after an introduction of the basic concept of data and measurement levels.

2.3.1   Data – Results from Measuring Variables

Research data are generated by measuring a collection of variables for a group of characters. For example, to study the relationship between being overweight (a character used as independent variable X) and hypertension (another character used as outcome Y), standing height, body weight, and derived body mass index (BMI) are often used to assess being overweight as the independent X; while three repeated measurements of systolic and diastolic blood pressure, and the mean of these three repeated measures are used to assess blood pressure as outcome Y (Fig. 2.5).

Fig. 2.5 Generate data through measurement

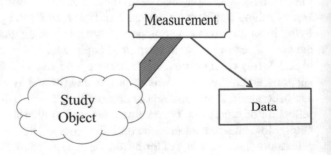

With BMI data, subjects can be classified into underweight (BMI<18.5), normal weight (18≤BMI<25), overweight (25≤BMI<30), or obese (BMI>30) based on the criteria recommended by CDC. With blood pressure data, subjects can be classified as normal (blood pressure <120/80 mmHg), hypertensive (blood pressure ≥ 90/140) or marginal hypertensive (blood pressures are between normal and hypertensive) based on the criteria recommended by the World Health Organization. These redefined variables are also used as data for quantitative analysis.

Likewise, to study if internet abuse – a character, can increase the risk of suicidality – another character among adolescents (the study population), data are often collected on such measures as the duration in hours online in a typical day during the weekdays and during weekends – two variables to quantify internet abuse as the influential factor X; and data are also collected regarding suicidal behaviors, such as suicidal ideation, attempt, and self-injury – outcome variables to quantify suicidality Y. With these data, more variables for both internet use and suicidal behaviors can be derived for quantitative analysis to examine the relationship between internet abuse and suicidality.

2.3.2   Levels of Measurement

In the previous section, we discussed that data are generated by measuring study variables to reflect a study character for quantitative analysis. A related issue is to understand the level of measurement. Six levels of measurement are established in quantitative analysis.

1. Count measure: In this simplest measure, data are obtained by simply counting the number of events, such as blood cells, hospital days, and number of COVID-19 cases.
2. Binary measure: This measure is used to divide study participants into two categories, such as gender (male vs. female), smoking status (smokers vs. non-smokers), laboratory test (positive vs. negative), clinical diagnosis (sick vs. not sick), and end status of life (alive vs. death).
3. Multi-categorical measure: More than two categories are used, such as racial/ethnic groups (White, Black, Hispanic, Asian, and other), country of origin (United States, Europe, Latin America, and Asia), and marital status (never married, married/live with partner, divorced/separate, other).
4. Ordinal measure: Similar to the binary and multi-category measures except that the categories are ranked. Typical examples include the Likert scale for attitudes from totally disagree to totally agree; frequency measures from none to daily; and satisfactory measures from not satisfied at all to completely satisfied.
5. Interval measures: Different from the category and ordinal measures, an interval measure classifies and ranks participants using a distance scale. Scores computed from a measurement instrument in mental and health behaviors are typical interval measures. Temperature is another example of an interval measure.

6. Ratio measure: This measure functions the same as interval measures. The difference between a ratio measure (e.g. weight) and an interval measure (e.g. body temperature measured with a thermometer or depression scores obtained from PHQ-9) is that an object with weight equal to zero means no weight at all, while a person with PHQ-9 score equal to zero does not mean that this person is absolutely depression free.

Statistically, data measured at levels 1–3 are categorical, data measured at levels 5–6 are continuous, and data measured at level 4 can be used as both continuous and categorical in quantitative analysis.

2.3.3   Organization of Data with Database – NHANES Data as an Example

To conduct quantitative analysis, data must be organized in a way that can be read, processed, and analyzed by a computer. A database is a collection of different types of original data. Dataset for a study can be generated with data from one or multiple projects. Epidemiologists often build their own database in teaching and research. Traditionally, quantitative epidemiology uses data collected by investigators themselves. Nowadays, in the era of data sciences and big data, access and use of secondary data has become a new trend (Chen and Chen 2020).

To gain understanding of the concept of a database and to develop skills for database construction, we use the 2017–18 NHANES data as an example. In the Practice Section of Chap. 1, we introduced the NHANES Project. Here, effort will be devoted to actually accessing the data. Tasks include downloading the original data to a computer, directly reading and converting the downloaded data, and preparing for further processing and analyses. The DEMO_J dataset from NHANES is used as a practical example, and SAS Program 2.1 shows the method for accessing the data.

```
********************************************************************************
* SAS PROGRAM 2.1: ACCESS TO 2017-18 NHANES DEMOGRAPHIC DATA IN 5 STEPS
* 1 DOWNLOAD DEMO J.XPT DATA FROM NHANES WEBSITE TO QUANTLAB\A_DATA\ORIGINAL
********************************************************************************;
* 2 SPECIFY LOCATION IN YOUR COMPUTER TO SAVE THE DATA ANALYZABLE USING SAS;
LIBNAME SASDATA "C:\QUANTLAB\A_DATA";
* 3 SPECIFY FILE NAME AND LOCATION OF THE DOWNLOADED DATA FILE DEMO_J.XPT;
LIBNAME XPTDATA XPORT "C:\QUANTLAB\A_DATA\ORIGINA\DEMO_J.XPT" ACCESS=READONLY;
* 4 READ THE XPORT SAS DATA INTO ANALYZABLE SAS DATA WITH SAME FILE NAME;
PROC COPY INLIB=XPTDATA OUTLIB=SASDATA; RUN;
* 5 CHECK VARIABLES IN DEMO_J;
PROC CONTENTS DATA = SASDATA.DEMO_J; RUN;
********************************************************************************;
```

The SAS Program consists of 5 steps in four parts: (1) Program notation, (2) specification of location to save the processed SAS data, (3) specification of location where the original data downloaded from NHANES (XPT type), (4) SAS Procedure **PROC COPY** to convert the exportable data **DEMOJ.XPT** into analyzable SAS data **DEMO_J**, and (5) SAS Procedure **PROC CONTENTS** to check the converted data.

Fig. 2.6 SAS Output showing the first 14 variables in DEMO_J

Alphabetic List of Variables and Attributes			
#	Variable	Type	Len	Label
29	AIALANGA	Num	8	Language of ACASI Interview
13	DMDBORN4	Num	8	Country of birth
14	DMDCITZN	Num	8	Citizenship status
17	DMDEDUC2	Num	8	Education level - Adults 20+
16	DMDEDUC3	Num	8	Education level - Children/Youth 6-19
31	DMDFMSIZ	Num	8	Total number of people in the Family
30	DMDHHSIZ	Num	8	Total number of people in the Household
32	DMDHHSZA	Num	8	# of children 5 years or younger in HH
33	DMDHHSZB	Num	8	# of children 6-17 years old in HH
34	DMDHHSZE	Num	8	# of adults 60 years or older in HH
36	DMDHRAGZ	Num	8	HH ref person's age in years
37	DMDHREDZ	Num	8	HH ref person's education level

In the SAS program above, **DEMOJ.XPT** is the original dataset provided by NHANES for data sharing. Such datasets cannot be analyzed directly but are used for sharing among researchers who use different statistical software packages such as SPSS, R, and SAS. Since the commercial software SAS will be used, the program is devised to convert **DEMOJ.XPT** into a SAS dataset.

By executing the SAS Program 2.1, SAS output shows N = 9254 observations in the dataset **DEMO_J** with P = 46 variables arranged alphabetically. Fig. 2.6 presents a snapshot of the first 12 variables in the dataset. This dataset can be processed and analyzed using the SAS software.

2.3.4 Select Variables to Form a Workable Dataset

There are a total of 46 variables in the dataset **DEMO_J**, but not all of them are needed for a study. The following SAS program shows how to select a subset of 9 variables from **DEMO_J**, and store them in a temporary dataset labeled as **TEMP**.

```
*********************************************************************************
*  SAS PROGRAM 2.2: SELECT 8 VARIABLES FROM DEMO_J AND STORE IN DATASET TEMP
*  USE THESE VARIABLES TO PRACTICE RECODING, RENAMING, AND RELABLING
*********************************************************************************;
* 1 READ DATA INTO A NEW DATASET CALLED TEMP;
DATA TEMP; SET SASDATA.DEMO_J;
* 2 SELECT NINE VARIABLES, PLUS SEQN TO BE USED LATER FOR DATA LINKAGE;
KEEP RIDAGEYR RIAGENDR RIDRETH3 DMDMARTL DMDYRSUS DMDEDUC2 DMDFMSIZ INDHHIN2 SEQN;
* 3 CHECK THE DATA FOR ALL 8 VARIABLES;
PROC CONTENTS DATA=TEMP; RUN;
*********************************************************************************;
```

The program first reads the data stored in the SAS dataset DEMO_J using the SAS keyword SET and put the results in the new dataset named as TEMP. The SAS keyword KEEP is used to select the variables needed from DEMO_J and stored them in TEMP. Executing this program generates the SAS output in Fig. 2.7 with the nine selected variables listed alphabetically for all 9254 subjects.

Fig. 2.7 Selected variables from DEMO_J, 2017–18 NHANES

Alphabetic List of Variables and Attributes			
#	Variable	Type	Len	Label
6	DMDEDUC2	Num	8	Education level - Adults 20+
8	DMDFMSIZ	Num	8	Total number of people in the Family
7	DMDMARTL	Num	8	Marital status
5	DMDYRSUS	Num	8	Length of time in US
9	INDHHIN2	Num	8	Annual household income
2	RIAGENDR	Num	8	Gender
3	RIDAGEYR	Num	8	Age in years at screening
4	RIDRETH3	Num	8	Race/Hispanic origin w/ NH Asian
1	SEQN	Num	8	Respondent sequence number

To check the actual data for these variables, you can use SAS **PROC PRINT**. For example, the following SAS program allows you to check data for the first 10 observations, as shown in Fig. 2.8.

```
* CHECK DETAILED DATA IN DATASET DEMO_J;
PROC PRINT DATA = TEMP (OBS=10); RUN;
```

Obs	SEQN	RIAGENDR	RIDAGEYR	RIDRETH3	DMDYRSUS	DMDEDUC2	DMDMARTL	DMDFMSIZ	INDHHIN2
1	93703	2	2	6	.	.	.	5	15
2	93704	1	2	3	.	.	.	4	15
3	93705	2	66	4	.	2	3	1	3
4	93706	1	18	6	.	.	.	5	.
5	93707	1	13	7	.	.	.	7	10
6	93708	2	66	6	7	1	1	2	6
7	93709	2	75	4	.	4	2	1	2
8	93710	2	0	3	.	.	.	3	15
9	93711	1	56	6	6	5	1	3	15
10	93712	1	18	1	5	.	.	4	4

Fig. 2.8 Dataset for 10 observations showing the NP structure of a database. Note: the dot "." indicates missing data

2.3.5   Database with N*P Structure

From the discussion and the examples of NHANES demographic data in Figs. 2.6, 2.7, and 2.8, the NP structure of a dataset for analysis can be summarized in Table 2.2. Understanding dataset structure is very important for quantitative epidemiology. In most of the quantitative analysis, software processes a dataset by individual variables or columns. To access individual subjects, special commands are needed. We will see them in the following section about variable recoding.

Table 2.2 Matrix database structure of N (observations) and P (variables)

Observation	Var(1)	Var(2)	Var(3)	...	Var(p-2)	Var(p-1)	Var (p)
Obs (1)	1,1	1,2	1,3	...	1, p-2	1,p-1	1,p
Obs (2)	2,1	2,2	2,3	...	2,p-2	2,p-1	2,p
Obs (3)	3,1	3,2	3,3	...	3,p-2	3,p-1	3,p
...	...	...	...	...	...	...	...
Obs (n-2)	n-2,1	n-2,2	n-2,3	...	n-2,p-2	n-2,p-1	n-2,p
Obs (n-1)	n-1,1	n-1,2	n-1,3	...	n-1,p-2	n-1,p-1	n-1,p
Obs (n)	n,1	n,2	n,3	...	n,p-2	n,p-1	n,p

2.4   Variable Recoding

In quantitative analysis, data can be both numerical (digits) and character (letters); but numerical data are preferred for analysis. Variable recoding can be used to convert non-numerical variables into numerical. In addition to non-numerical to numerical converting, variable recoding serves a number of functions in data processing. In this section, five recoding methods will be introduced: Recording by converting to numerical, recoding by rescaling, recoding by regrouping, recoding by recreating, and recoding measurement instruments. These methods are commonly used in quantitative analysis.

2.4.1   Recoding by Converting to Numerical

This method is simple and commonly used. For example, we can convert sex/gender of male (M) and female (F) into (M or male = 1 and F or female = 2); we can convert race of White, Black, Hispanic, Asian, and Other into: White = 1, Black = 2,

Hispanic = 3, Asian = 3, and Other = 5. The converted numerical numbers do not carry any numerical meaning and they are used simply as labels. For example, coding male = 1 and female = 2 does not mean being female is one unit larger than being male; and White = 1 does not mean being White is the smallest among all 5 racial groups.

2.4.2　Recoding by Rescaling

Two types of rescaling are often used: (1) Rescaling to the international standard and (2) harmonizing multiple variables into a narrow range.

Rescaling to international standard (i.e., kilogram for weight, centimeter for height, mol or nmol for concentration, Celsius for temperature). For example, in survey studies, feet and inches are often used to measure height and weight, and Fahrenheit is often used to measure temperature. In this case, recoding must be conducted. For height, 1 feet = 30.48 centimeters and 1 inch = 2.54 centimeters; for weight, 1 pound = 0.45359 kilograms; for temperature, $°C = (°F - 32)/1.8$.

Rescaling to harmonize multiple variables within a relatively narrow range. In multivariate analysis, different variables with different ranges are often used. For example, age for adolescents has a numerical range of 12–17, their family income can range from zero to millions of dollars. A 5-item scale on a 5-point Likert scale will have a mean scale score ranging from 1 to 25; while a same scale with 50 items will have a total score ranging from 1 to 250. In these cases, the variables can be rescaled. (1) *Harmonizing by division*: If the range is too large, dividing the variable by a constant – for example, dividing income by 1000. (2) *Harmonizing by regrouping:* For example, if the age range is very large, say from 20 to 100, the variable can be grouped into 10-year age groups for analysis. (3) *Harmonizing using mean score*: If the variables involve multiple scales, computing mean scores rather than total scores bring the best results.

2.4.3　Recoding by Regrouping

It is a common practice to collect very detailed data either in the lab or in the field to conduct research. For example, detailed data regarding demographic variables (e.g., age, race, education, marital status, and family members), very detailed laboratory test results (blood cell platelet counts, blood pressure, blood fats), very detailed medical and health insurance (list of all insurance companies), and detailed scores of many psychosocial testing scale scores. These variables are often recoded through regrouping for analysis. We already discussed by grouping age into 5- or 10-year age groups, but some other examples include: blood pressure in mmHg can be grouped into hypertensive (systolic >140 and diastolic >90) and normotensive; detailed education levels can be grouped into 1 (less than high school), 2 (high school, including those with and without a diploma), and 3 (college or higher); detailed income in dollars into 1(low), 2(medium), and 3 (high); detailed physical activities can be regrouped into 1(low), 2 (moderate), and 3 (high); detailed scale scores for depression can be regrouped into 1 (mild), 2 (moderate), and 3 (severe); detailed BMI measures can be regrouped into 1 (underweight), 2 (normal weight), 3 (over-weight), and 4 (obese).

2.4.4   Recoding by Recreating

While recoding through regrouping creates a variable for measuring the same character with different measurement widths, recoding by recreating generates a variable to measure a new character with several pieces of data. For example, in studies examining a health behavior, one question is used to assess the recency of a behavior, plus several other questions. Using cigarette smoking as an example, survey respondents were first asked if they had ever smoked cigarettes in their life, even a few puffs (yes/no)? For participants who responded positively to this question, they were further asked when was the last time they smoked with answer options (1 = last month, before last month but within the last 6 months, 2 = before 6 months but within the last 12 months, 3 = 12 months ago but within 2 years, and 4 = two years ago) – recency question. Based on data from the two questions, three new variables can be created by recoding:

1. Never-smokers: Persons who never smoked cigarettes in life, which include all participants who responded negatively to the first question regarding if they ever smoked in life.
2. Current smokers: Persons who smoked in the past 30 days, which include persons who ever smoked cigarettes in life (positive response to the first question) and last time smoking is within the past 30 days (answer option 1 to question 2).
3. Ex-smokers: Persons who ever smoked but not in the past year, which include persons who had ever smoked cigarettes, but last time smoking was 1 year ago.

Another typical example is to create a variable to measure substance abuse during pregnancy using data from multiple survey questions. In this type of study, survey data are often collected in different parts of the questionnaire about (1) gender (male or female), (2) if pregnant at the time of survey (yes/no), and (3) if used any of the substances during the past year, including alcohol, tobacco, marijuana, or opioids. With data from these three questions, a new binary variable to measure substance use during pregnancy (yes/no) can be created. Participants will be coded as having used a substance during pregnancy if they self-identified as female, being pregnant at the time of survey, and reported using one of the listed substances.

A third example is to create a new variable to measure the interaction between two variables. For example, the relationship between depression and poor quality of sleep could differ between smokers and nonsmokers, showing as an interaction. In this case, a new variable will be created to measure the interaction between smoking and depression and used to examine their effect on quality of sleep. This method is discussed in detail in Chap. 8 in this book.

2.4.5   Recoding Measurement Instruments

Instruments are tools for measuring subjective characters objectively, such as mental health status (i.e., QOL, anxiety, stress, depression, and suicidality), health related attitudes (sexual openness, perceived vulnerability), beliefs (self-efficacy for condom use, HIV stigma), and behaviors (resilience, social support, social capital). In this type of measurement, multiple items are used to measure one character named as the underling construct. Scores of individual items are summarized to generate scale scores for analysis.

Recoding a measurement instrument takes <u>four steps</u>. First, individual items must be checked for missing data and for distribution of the response of individual items. There will be more or less normal distribution of respondents along with the measurement scale. For example, if a 5-point Likert scale is used, fewer subjects will be scored with either 1 or 5 with most being 3, and lesser frequent for 2 and 3.

Second, it is essential to check revise-stated items and code them back. In most instruments, measurement items are stated in one direction with a few exceptions. For example, in the well-known 10-item CES-D scale, two items are stated reversely: "I felt hopeful about the future" "I was happy" with a 4-point measurement scale (0 = rarely or none of the time; 1 = some or a little of the time, 3 = occasionally or a moderate amount of time, and 4 = all of the time). In recoding, these two items must be reversely coded (5 – item score) such that higher scored indicating more frequent depressive symptoms.

Third, reliability analysis must be conducted (detailed later in this chapter). A published instrument usually has its reliability quantitatively established. The most commonly used indicator is Cronbach's alpha with the criteria of alpha = 0.7 for early-stage exploratory research, 0.8 for applied research, and 0.9 for research to make important decisions (Nunnally and Bernstein 1994). Cronbach's alpha provides a measure of the amount of information contained in the data. An alpha = 0.8 indicates that 80% of the data is information and the remaining 20% are errors.

Last, scale scores must be computed. Computing scale scores should only be done if (a) a reliability analysis is completed, (b) an alpha coefficient is estimated, and (c) the estimated alpha coefficient suggests adequate information in the data. There are two ways to compute scale scores:

1. *Total score*: This score is created by summing up all item scores.
2. *Mean score*: This score is created by computing total scores first, then dividing by total scale items.

2.5   Recoding and Analysis of Demographic Data as an Example

Demographic factors are widely used in epidemiological studies, particularly studies with survey data. Data on demographic factors present the best case to practice variable recoding. NHANES data contains a large array of demographic data. In this section, a SAS program will be provided as an example to practice variable recoding using the NHANES data. Following the recoding, practices are arranged to compute sample statistics. These skills can be used to create Table 1 in Practice.

2.5.1   Recode to Create a New Dataset

With the knowledge and skills described above, SAS Program 2.3 shows how to recode, re-create, and re-label new variables using the five variables RIDAGEYR, RIAGENDR, RIDRETH3, DMDMARTL, and DMDEDUC2 from the original data. In addition, consistent with NHANES technical documentation, only adults 20 years of age and older participated in survey data collection, thus we will limit our data to participants in this age range. With SAS Program 2.3 below, a new dataset named as **DATCH2** (stand for dataset created in chapter 2) will be created and saved in the data folder.

```
*********************************************************************************
* SAS PROGRAM 2.3: RECODE VARIABLES FROM DATASET TEMP, SECTION 2.3
* SELECT FIVE VARIABLES FROM THE ORIGINAL DATA STORED IN WORK DATASET TEMP
* RENAME/RECODE FOR CONVENIENCE OF USE
*********************************************************************************;
* 1 USE PROC FREQ TO CHECK ORIGINAL VALUES OF THE 5 VARIABLES IN TEMP DATASET
*     THESE VALUES ARE NEEDED TO SUPPORT VARIABLE RECODING;
PROC FREQ DATA = TEMP;
TABLES RIDAGEYR RIAGENDR RIDRETH3 DMDMARTL DMDEDUC2;
WHERE RIDAGEYR GE 20; RUN;
* 2 CREATE A NEW DATA NAMED AS DATCH2 AND PUT IT IN THE DEFINED DATA FOLDER
      READ DATA FROM TEMP THAT WAS CREATED FROM ORIGNAL DEMO_J;
DATA SASDATA.DATCH2; SET TEMP;
IF RIDAGEYR GE 20;                    * INCLUDE ADULTS 20 AND OLDER;
* 3 RENAME VARIABLE GENDER;
GENDER        = RIAGENDR;
* 4 RENAME VARIABLE AGE;
AGE           = RIDAGEYR;
* 5 RECODE AGE IN TO 10-YEAR AGE GROUPS BY RE-GROUPING;
IF 20 LE AGE LT 30 THEN AGE10G = 1; ELSE
IF 30 LE AGE LT 40 THEN AGE10G = 2; ELSE
IF 40 LE AGE LT 50 THEN AGE10G = 3; ELSE
IF 50 LE AGE LT 60 THEN AGE10G = 4; ELSE
IF 60 LE AGE LT 70 THEN AGE10G = 5;
ELSE AGEG10G = 6;
* 6 RENAME AND RECODE RACE FROM THE ORIGINAL 7 GROUPS TO 5;
IF RIDRETH3 EQ 3 THEN RACE5 = 1;          * WHITE;
IF RIDRETH3 EQ 4 THEN RACE5 = 2;          * BLACK;
IF RIDRETH3 IN (1 2) THEN RACE5 = 3;      * HISPANIC;
IF RIDRETH3 EQ 6 THEN RACE5 = 4;          * ASIAN;
IF RIDRETH3 EQ 7 THEN RACE5 = 5;          * OTHER;
* 7 RENAME AND RECODE EDUCATIONAL ATTAINMENT;
IF DMDEDUC2 IN (1 2) THEN EDUCATION = 1;   * LESS THAN HIGH;
IF DMDEDUC2 IN (3 4) THEN EDUCATION = 2;   * HIGH SCHOOL;
IF DMDEDUC2 EQ 5    THEN EDUCATION = 3;   * COLLEGE+;
* 8 COLLAPSE MARITAL STATUS INTO 3 LEVELS BECAUSE OF SMALL NUMBERS IN SOME GROUPS;
IF DMDMARTL EQ 5 THEN MARRIAGE = 1;
IF DMDMARTL IN (1 6) THEN MARRIAGE = 2;
IF DMDMARTL IN (2 3 4) THEN MARRIAGE = 3;
* 9 CREATE A NEW VARIABLE NEVER MARRIED;
IF MARRIAGE NE . THEN NV_MARRID = (MARRIAGE EQ 1); * LIMIT TO NO MISSING TO AVOID
ERROR;
*10 RELABEL THE 6 NEWLY RENAMED/CREATE VARIABLES;
LABEL  AGE        = "AGE IN YEAR",
       AGE10G     = "1=20~29, 2=30~39, 3=40~49 4=50~59 5=60~69 6=70~80",
       GENDER     = "GENDER 1=MALE 2=FEMALE",
       RACE5      = "1=WHITE 2=BLACK 3=HISP 4=ASIAN 5=OTHER",
       EDUCATION  = "1=LESS THAN HIGH 2=HIGH SCHOOL 3=COLLEGE+",
       MARRIAGE   = "1=NEVER MARRIED 2=MARRIED/STYWITH PARTNER 3=DIVORCE/WIDOWED",
       NV_MARRID  = "1=NEVER MARRIED, 0=OTHERWISE";
*11 KEEP 7 NEW VARIABLES, 3 UNCODED VARIABLES (FOR CHAPTER 3), PLUS SEQN;
KEEP AGE AGE10G GENDER RACE5 EDUCATION MARRIAGE NV_MARRID DMDYRSUS DMDFMSIZ INDHHIN2
SEQN; PROC CONTENTS; RUN;
*********************************************************************************;
```

By executing SAS Program 2.3 above, a permanent dataset `DATCH2` should be in the location (folder) that was defined with `LIBNAME SASDATA "C:\QUANLAB\A_DATA\"` in Sect. 2.3. The **PROC CONTENTS; RUN** is used to check recoded variables. The **PROC PRINT** `DATA = SASDATA.DATCH2(OBS=10)` show values for the first 10 observations. Make corrections when needed by going back to the beginning of this program.

2.5.2   SAS Program to Estimate Statistics for Continuous Variables

For continuous variables, range (minimum to maximum), mean, and standard deviation (SD) for the total sample and by gender are needed. SAS Program 2.4 shows how to compute them using the variable AGE as an example.

In SAS Program 2.4, a work dataset named A is created first to read `DATCH2` in the location defined in SAS Program 2.1. The **PROC MEANS** is thus used to compute statistics using dataset A. The SAS key word `VAR` specifies the variables used for analysis (multi-variables can be specified). The two program lines started by the SAS key word `WHERE` is unique. It allows us to compute the statistics for a specific gender and total sample. SAS Program 2.4 will compute the statistics for male since the computing for female is blocked. If you want to compute the results for females, just block the program for male by adding "*" at the beginning of the line and removing the "*" for female. To compute results for the total sample, block both. If done correctly, the mean age (SD) = 51.85 (17.93) for male, 51.17 (17.70) for female, and 51.50 (17.81) for the total sample.

```
********************************************************************************
* SAS PROGRAM 2.4. COMPUTING MEAN SD MIN MAX OVERALL ABD BY GENDER
********************************************************************************;
* 1 CREATE A WORK DATASET A BY READING THE NEWLY CREATED DATASET DATCH2;
DATA A; SET SASDATA.DATCH2; RUN;
* 2 CONDUCT ANALYSIS, OVERALL AND BY GENDER;
PROC MEANS DATA = A;
VAR AGE;
* 3 BLOCK BOTH USING * TO COMPUTE RESULT FOR THE TOTAL SAMPLE;
WHERE GENDER EQ 1;          * FOR MALE;
*WHERE GENDER EQ 2;         * FOR FEMALE;
RUN;
********************************************************************************;
```

2.5.3   SAS Program to Estimate Statistics for Categorical Variables

SAS Program 2.5 shows how to compute the frequency and percentage for categorical variables. The **PROC FREQ** command is designated to count frequencies and estimate various rates for categorical variables defined by TABLES. Since we need results by gender, all four variables are cross-tabled with the variable **GENDER**. Multiple TABLES can be specified under one **PROC FREQ** command.

```
********************************************************************************
* SAS PROGRAM 2.5. COMPUTING FREQ AND % FOR CATEGORICAL VARIABLES
********************************************************************************;
* CONTINUE AFTER PROC MEANS WITH DATA A;
PROC FREQ DATA = A;
* COMPUTE RESULTS BY AGE GROUP;
TABLES AGE10G * GENDER;
* COMPUTE RESULT FOR FIVE RACIAL GROUPS;
TABLES RACE5 * GENDER;
* COMPUTE RESULT BY LEVELS OF EDUCATION;
TABLES EDUCATION * GENDER;
* COMPUTE RESULT BY MARITAL STATUS;
TABLES MARRIAGE * GENDER;
RUN;
********************************************************************************;
```

SAS Program 2.4 and 2.5 will be used in Practice to create Table 1 after completion of all contents in this chapter.

2.6   Data Errors and Their Impact

Up to now, we know how to access and process data, and use the processed data to compute statistics. However, not much attention has been paid to data errors and their impact on analytical results. *Quality results can only be derived with quality data.* One important source that affects data quality is measurement errors. It is somewhat straightforward to understand measurement error in daily life. Measurement error is simply the difference between the value from our measurement and the true value we intent to measure. As showed in Fig. 2.9, given the true body height, any measure either smaller or larger than the true height is counted as errors in data.

However, this daily life understanding of measurement error is inadequate for quantitative epidemiology for several reasons as discussed in next section.

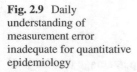
Fig. 2.9 Daily understanding of measurement error inadequate for quantitative epidemiology

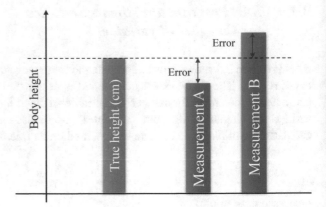

2.6.1 Concept of Errors in Data

To understand data quality for quantitative epidemiology, several concepts must be described. First, we have to admit that *the true value of a variable is philosophically an unknown*. Scientific studies are simply efforts to approach as close as possible to the true values but can never get the true value. Therefore, errors *are not avoidable; and the key is to understand and measure the error and work around the error to obtain valid results*.

As discussed in Chap. 1 on the paradigm for quantitative epidemiology and the descriptions of variables and data in previous sections of this chapter, research data are collected from multiple subjects that are sampled in a study population. First, errors can be introduced due to the definition of a study population and sampling. As described in Sects. 1.3, 1.4, and 1.5 in Chap. 1, differences between population and study population are conceptual, and can be handled conceptually. Sampling errors are an issue that also has been solved successfully in statistics and quantitative epidemiology. Sampling error is the foundation of hypothesis testing for statistical inference.

Second, errors can also be introduced by selecting different times to collect data. This is because almost all characters in medical, health, and behavior studies show variations at different times of a day, in different days of the week, and different seasons of the year. This type of error can be addressed through research design to obtain data representing different points in time. If data are collected at one specific point in time, potential errors can be adjusted based on documented changes in the character over time, although only a few studies in the literature have ever considered this type of data error or simply treated it as a limitation to a study.

Third, *random error* can contribute to data errors. Random error is also known as uncontrolled error. Taking body weight as an example, with the same scale to measure the weight of one person, two data collectors may not get exactly the same results after ruling out any possible mistakes. The same is true for almost all measures, including surveys and laboratory tests. Random errors are very common, and we will illustrate the impact of random errors on data quality in the following section.

Fourth, *systematic error* represents another source of data error. Different from random error, systematic error is often stemmed from some known cause that can be corrected. For example, if a scale to measure body weight is not correctly adjusted, weight data collected using the scale could be systematically higher or lower than the actual weight; when reporting age, people tend to use 5, 10, 16, 18... for milestone events in life or round up to an interval of 5, such as 15, 20, 25, ...; when answering questions about sensitive topics, such as income and drug use, people tend to under-report; and while answering socially desirable questions, people tend to over-report such as physical activity, attitudes against social stigma, and number of sex partners, etc. We must try our best to avoid systematic errors for quality research. In the next section, we will discuss the impact of systematic errors.

2.6.2   Influences of Random Error and Systematic Errors

To demonstrate the impact of random and systematic errors, we generated four sets of data each with 10 observations (n = 10, Table 2.3). Data (1) in Table 2.3 contains 10 values sampled from a population with mean μ = 3.5 and standard deviation σ = 1.0. Because of random sampling error, the sample mean $\overline{X} = 3.7$, variance

$$\left(\sum\left(x-\overline{X}\right)^2\right)=4.5, \text{ and standard deviation } (SD = \sqrt{\frac{\sum\left(x-\overline{x}\right)^2}{n-1}}) =0.7, \text{ both differ-}$$

ing from the population measure. The differences in the mean (3.7 vs. 3.5) and SD (0.7 vs. 1.0) between the sample and the population are simply due to sampling error. Student t-test is the method to test the difference in mean (you may do it yourself). If there are no other errors, Data (1) represents one set of data from all potential samples of a population.

However, random errors can occur in data collection, in addition to error due to random sampling. Data (2) in Table 2.3 consists of a set of data selected from the same population with μ = 3.5 and σ = 1.0. However, in data collection, random measurement errors are introduced. Assuming the error follows a normal distribution with mean = 0 and SD=1.5: $e \sim N(0, 1.5)$. Because of the random error, distribution of the data will be more diverse after SD was increase by 1.5. This makes the data like being collected from a sample with a population σ = 1.0 + 1.5 = 2.5. With the data, the computed sample mean $\overline{X} = 3.2$, not significantly different from the population mean μ = 3.5, but the SD = 2.1, which is significantly greater than 1.0, although smaller than σ = 2.5 (due to random sampling error). In other words, SD = 2.1 contains both sampling errors and mismeasurement errors due to random factors.

Data (3) in Table 2.3 contains a set of data with systematic errors that results in a reduction in the population mean by 0.5 units. As a result, such data looks like they were sampled from a population with μ = 3.0 (3.5 − 0.5). With this reduction, the sample mean $\overline{X} = 2.7$ is significantly smaller than the population mean μ = 3.0.

Last, Data (4) in Table 2.3 shows a set of data that contains both random and systematic errors. Because of the errors, the sample mean $\overline{X} = 2.6$ is under-estimated and the sample SD = 1.6 is over-estimated.

Table 2.3 Random and systematic errors affecting data quality differently

Observation (n)	Data (1) No error	Data (2) Random error	Data (3) Systematic error	Data (4) Rand. & syst. error
1	3.2	−0.9	3.8	−0.6
2	4.6	3.8	1.1	3.6
3	2.6	1.5	4.4	3.7
4	3.6	4.1	2.7	4.7
5	3.3	1.8	2.3	2.7
6	4.3	5.6	1.8	2.5
7	4.0	1.6	3.0	1.6
8	3.8	6.1	4.1	2.6
9	4.7	4.5	1.3	1.0
10	2.9	3.6	2.0	4.6
Mean	3.7	3.2	2.7	2.6
Variance	4.5	41.4	12.1	24.4
SD	0.7	2.1	1.2	1.6

Note: Data in the table are all simulated based on random distribution using r function rnorm(). The data in the first column are generated with mean=3.5 and SD=1 and used as reference. Data in the Random Error column is generated by an error factor with zero mean and 1.5 standard deviation. This type of error will increase the SD from 1.0 to 2.5 with no significant impact on the mean. In the Systematic error column, SD remained as 1.0 as in the data with no error, a systematic error reduced the true mean from 3.5 to 3.0. The last column contains simulated data with both random error (0, sigma=1.5) and systematic error (reduction in mean by 0.5).

2.6.3   Systematic Errors and Validity

Validity can be defined by bias, or the distance from a sample estimate to its population value. Data (3) in Table 2.3 show the existence of systematic errors (by purposefully subtracting 0.5 from the sample mean). This systematic error can make the sample mean deviate from the population mean (from 3.5 to 3.2; not 3.0 because of sampling error, although the systematic error was 0.5 units). In practice, different sizes of systematic errors are possible in all types of measurements as described in the Sect. 2.6.1 on the concept of errors in data.

Figure 2.10 further illustrates the relationship between system error and bias. For a variable with population mean $\mu = 1.5$ and $\sigma = 1.2$, the distribution is described by the red line. A study with data collected from the population has a distribution (blue line) with a sample mean $\overline{X} = 3.5$ and SD = 2.0. Based on the definition, bias due to systematic errors is thus the difference between the sample and population mean: $\mu - \overline{X} = 3.5 - 1.5 = 2.0$.

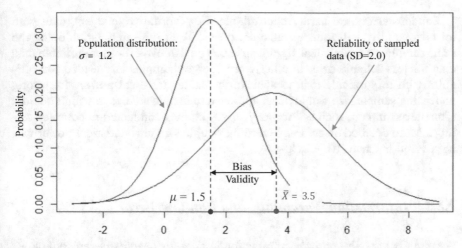

Fig. 2.10 Concepts of validity (bias) and reliability of sampled data

Systematic errors directly threaten the validity of research findings in quantitative epidemiology. Measures must be taken to avoid systematic errors in quantitative epidemiology.

2.6.4   Random Errors, Data Reliability, and Statistical Power

Replicability is the essence for scientific research; it determines the reliability of study results. From the example in Table 2.3, random errors can reduce reliability of collected data by amplifying the standard deviation or SD. Fig. 2.11 shows the relationship between SD and reliability for the same variable with a sample size n=2000 selected from the same population. Data points with smaller SD tend to locate in a small area of the data space, showing high reliability, while data points with larger SD tend to scatter everywhere in the data space, showing low reliability.

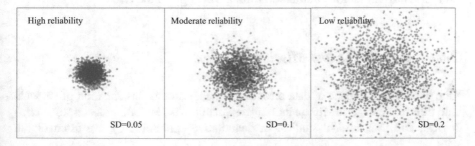

Fig. 2.11 Random errors reducing reliability of data by introducing extra variations that amplify the true standard deviation

Random errors are hardly controllable. In quantitative analysis, data with lower reliability will reduce statistical power. With the same variable and the same sample size, statistical significance can be achieved for more reliable data than for less reliable data. In other words, larger samples are needed for variables with less reliable data to achieve the same statistical power. Therefore, increasing sample size would be an approach to handle studies in which random errors are common, such as for many survey studies conducted in complex settings. More detailed discussion regarding sample size and statistical power will be covered in Chap. 10.

2.6.5   Information, Variability, and Random Error

Variation is the only source of information *in data for* quantitative epidemiology. We collect data because data contains information that can be extracted to address research questions. Although the concept of information is rather broad, quantitatively, variation in a variable is the only source of information; and constant variables provide little information. For example, if the body height is the same for all individuals in a study sample, such data provides little information for further analysis. If all students who completed the Quantitative Epidemiology course received a perfect score, such scores as data provide no information about the performance of the faculty who taught the class and the competence of students who completed the class.

Quantitatively, variance (and SD is standardized measure of variance) of a variable in the data provides a measure of the amount of information in the data for the variable. Consistent with the examples described in the previous paragraph, variables with constant values provide no information since its variance (and SD) = zero; and variables with larger variations (greater variance or bigger SD) provide a greater amount of information. However, *here comes a problem:* random errors do not provide information, but add variance to the data as shown in Table 2.3 and Fig. 2.10. Thus, in the reality, the information is often entangled with random errors in data regardless of the method for data collection, and the goal of quantitative analysis is to extract the information from the data given the error.

2.6.6   Data Error and Misclassification

One important influence of data error is its impact on the classification of subjects into different categories for quantitative epidemiology, including descriptive, etiological, and translational studies. In quantitative epidemiology, we often divide subjects into groups based on a variable. For example, we use measured blood pressure to dichotomize subjects into two groups of hypertensive (systolic pressure >140 and diastolic >90) and normal (otherwise); we used PHQ-9 scores to divide subjects into five levels of depression: minimal (0–4), mild (5–9), moderate (10–14), moderate severe (15–19), and severe (20+). But remember, this classification is made for individual participants, not the mean for a population; thus, any type of data error, including random errors, would lead to misclassification if it occurred right around a cutoff point.

Misclassification will lead to biased estimates of proportion, prevalence, and incidence used to describe the level, and distribution of medical, health, and behavioral problems in a population over time and across a geographic area. For example, errors in detecting the COVID-19 virus will lead to incorrect assessment of the pandemic with regard to level and time trend as well as differences between different populations living in different countries and regions.

Misclassification in the outcome variable presents a significant threat to etiological research (Szklo and Nieto 2004). Table 2.4 presents an example with hypothetical case control data. Data with no error (therefore no misclassification) are presented in the upper panel. There are 200 subjects in the sample. Of the 100 subjects with the study disease (cases), 20 were exposed to the risk factor with 20% proportion of exposure; of the 100 subjects with no disease (control), 10 were exposed with 10% proportion of exposure. The odds ratio (OR) = 2.00 (20/10); this result suggests that exposure to the risk factor is associated with a two-fold increase in disease risk.

For some reason, errors occurred in the exposed group with 4 cases out of 20 (20%) misclassified as controls, reducing the cases from 20 to 16 and increasing the controls from 10 to 14. Assuming no changes in the total (n=100), there would be 84 cases and 86 controls in the un-exposed group (mid-panel of Table 2.4). The computed OR reduced to 1.14 (16/14). This hypothetic data demonstrates the impact of misclassification in attenuating the true relationship seen between the exposure and outcome.

Table 2.4 Impact of misclassification on causal inference, hypothetic data

Misclassification	Exposure	No exposure	Total	Proportion exposure
No misclassification				
Cases (disease)	20	80	100	20%
Control (no disease)	10	90	100	10%
Odds ratio (OR)				OR = 2.0 (20/10)
4 Cases classified as control				
Cases (disease)	16	84	100	16%
Control (no disease)	14	86	100	14%
Odds ratio (OR)				OR = 1.14 (16/14)
2 Control classified as cases				
Cases (disease)	22	78	100	22%
Control (no disease)	8	92	100	8%
Odds ratio (OR)				OR = 2.75 (22/8)

Likewise, the bottom panel of Table 2.4 presents another hypothetic scenario. In this scenario, 2 controls are misclassified as cases in the exposed group; and the cases and controls would be 84 and 86 respectively to keep the total=100. With a misclassification as small as only 2 cases, the estimated OR = 2.75 (22/8), increasing by 37.35% (0.75/2.00).

In medicine and health, misclassification is also not avoidable even if there is no error in the data. This is because not only the overlap of the distribution of a variable (i.e., blood pressure) between a patient and a non-patient population, but a cutoff point must be used to separate patients from non-patients.

2.7 Data Quantitative Assessment – Assessment of Measurement Tools

It is very hard if not impossible to quantitatively assess all errors in a data set, and this would be a big topic in data sciences. From a quantitative epidemiology perspective, data quality is determined, to a great extent, by the tools used to collect data. In this section, we describe six basic concepts/methods that are used in research for data quality assessment: Sensitivity, specificity, reliability, accuracy, positive predictive value, and negative predictive value.

2.7.1 Understanding Sensitivity in General

Sensitivity is the smallest unit of an object a measurement tool can measure. In chemistry, the sensitivity of an instrument or a measurement method is defined by the minimum amount of chemicals that can be detected by the instrument/measurement method. Quantitatively, higher sensitivity measures provide more information for in-depth research.

This concept of sensitivity can also be used in quantitative epidemiology. For example, measuring income using $1 as a unit would be more sensitive than using $100 as a unit, and using $100 as a unit would be more sensitive than using $1000 as a unit; and using dollar counting would be more sensitive than using categories of low, middle, and high incomes.

Although increasing sensitivity will provide more information, higher sensitivity measures are more likely to be subject to measurement errors, reducing data quality. Using income again as an example, using the number of dollars other than $100 or $1000 will provide more information. However, as the sensitivity (information) increases, error in data also increases. Few people can remember exactly how much money they make in a year or month; however, most people do have an idea how many hundreds or thousands of dollars they make in a year.

2.7.2   Sensitivity, Specificity, and Accuracy in Epidemiology

In epidemiology, sensitivity and specificity are introduced together to assess the performance of a test. As shown in Table 2.5. To assess the sensitivity and specificity, a sample of subjects correctly confirmed with and without disease is recruited. These subjects are thus tested with a testing method and results are recorded as shown in the table. With data in the table, sensitivity, specificity and accuracy will be estimated respectively using following formula.

Sensitivity is the ratio of subjects with the disease and tested positive over the total number of subjects with the disease. Therefore, sensitivity measures the capability of the testing method to detect subjects with the disease among all subjects with the disease who are tested. Here we can see the difference between the sensitivity defined here and the concept of sensitivity in general described previously. Sensitivity in general is defined for continuous variables and the sensitivity defined here is based on categorical variables.

Table 2.5 Understanding the specificity and sensitivity of a test in research

Test result	True disease condition		Predictive values
	Disease	No disease	
Positive	A = True positive	B = False positive	PPV = A/(A + B)
Negative	C = False negative	D = True negative	NPV = D/C + D)
Sensitivity/specificity	Sensitivity = A/ (A + C)	Specificity = D/ (B + D)	Accuracy = (A + D)/ (A + B + C + D)

Note: *PPV*: Positive predictive value; *NPV*: Negative predictive value.

Different from sensitivity, specificity is the ratio of subjects with no disease and tested negative over the total number of subjects with no disease. Therefore, specificity measures the capability of a test to identify subjects who do not have the disease among all subjects that do not have the disease who are tested.

The relationship between sensitivity and specificity is discussed in detail in many books. The main point is the tradeoff between the two to minimize data errors since increases in sensitivity will result in declines in specificity, and vice versa.

Accuracy is a measure that is also very useful in epidemiology. It measures the ability of a test to correctly detect both true positive and true negative cases. The method to compute accuracy is also shown in Table 2.5.

In addition, two other indicators commonly used in epidemiology are positive predictive value (PPV) and negative predictive value (NPV). As shown in Table 2.5, PPV is a measure of the proportion of tested positive among all who are true positive. PPV thus provides a measure of accuracy of the test for positive results. Similarly, NPV is the proportion of tested negative among all those who are true negative; it provides a measure of accuracy of the test from the negative test result perspective.

2.7.3   Sensitivity and Specificity Analysis with Data

In this section, we will demonstrate the analysis using NHANES data on high blood pressure. In the 2017–18 NHANES, two sets of data can be used to measure high blood pressure. The first dataset is BPQ_J.XPT, which contains data for self-reported high blood pressure (yes, no; N = 6161). The second dataset is BPX_J. XPT, which contains measured blood pressures (N = 8704). Both systolic and diastolic blood pressure was repeatedly measured. High blood pressure can be defined by computing the mean blood pressure from 3 consecutive measures and the computed blood pressures are thus used to define high blood pressure using WHO standards if systolic blood pressure is greater or equal to 140mmHg or if diastolic blood pressure is greater or equal to 90 mmHg.

To conduct the analysis, first locate the two datasets from the NHANES website and save them into the folder **ORIGINAL** within the folder **A_DATA** under the folder **QUANTLAB**. Then use SAS Program 2.7 to convert the two datasets, combine them, and conduct the analysis.

```
****************************************************************************************
* SAS PROGRAM 2.7. PREPARE DATA AND CONDUCT ANALYSIS TO ASSESS A TEST
****************************************************************************************;
* SPECIFY PLACE TO SAVE THE PROCESSED SAS DATA;
LIBNAME SASDATA "C:\QUANTLAB\A_DATA";
* LOCATION OF THE ORGINAL DATASET BPQ_J, CONVERT AND SORT THE DATASET;
LIBNAME XPTDATA XPORT "C:\QUANTLAB\A_DATA\ORIGINA\CDQ_J.XPT" ACCESS=READONLY;
PROC COPY INLIB=XPTDATA OUTLIB=SASDATA; RUN;
PROC SORT DATA = SASDATA.CDQ_J; BY SEQN; RUN;
* LOCATION OF THE ORGINAL DATASET BPX_J,CONVERT AND SORT THE DATA;
LIBNAME XPTDATA XPORT "C:\QUANTLAB\A_DATA\ORIGINA\BPX_J.XPT" ACCESS=READONLY;
PROC COPY INLIB=XPTDATA OUTLIB=SASDATA; RUN;
PROC SORT DATA = SASDATA.BPX_J; BY SEQN; RUN;
* CREATE A NEW DATASET BY COMBINING THE TWO SORTED DATASETS;
DATA A; MERGE SASDATA.CDQ_J SASDATA.BPX_J; BY SEQN; RUN;
* CREATE VARIABLES NEEDED AND CODING;
DATA A; SET A;
IF BPXSY1 NE .;    *INCLUDE SUBJECTS WITH MEASURED BLOOD PRESSURE;
IF BPQ020 GT 2 THEN BPQ020=.; *CODE MISSING DATA;
HBP_Q = 2-BPQ020;  * REPORTED HIGH BLOOD PRESSURE RECODED WTIH 1=YES 0=NO;
* COMPUTE MEASURED BLOOD PRESSURE BASED ON THREE REPEATED MEASURES;
SYSTBP = (BPXSY1+BPXSY2+BPXSY3)/3;
DYSTBP = (BPXDI1+BPXDI2+BPXDI3)/3;
* DEFINE HIGH BLOOD PRESSUE WITH MEASURED DATA USING THE WHO STANDARD;
HBP_X = 0;
IF SYSTBP GE 130 OR DYSTBP GE 90 THEN HBP_X = 1; RUN;   * PURPOSEFULLY NOT USE >=140;
* STATISTICAL ANALYSIS;
PROC FREQ DATA = A;
TABLES HBP_Q * HBP_X/NOPERCENT NOROW; RUN;
****************************************************************************************;
```

Figure 2.12 displays the analytical results from SAS Program 2.7. The output is not in the standard format as discussed in Fig. 2.12. Of the total 997 subjects with high blood pressure determined on measured blood pressures, 635 (63.7%) were self-reported as having high blood pressure. Therefore, the sensitivity = 63.7%, not very impressive for self-reported high blood pressure.

Of the 4162 subjects with no high blood pressure based on the measured blood pressure, 3024 (72.7%) reported also having no high blood pressure. Thus, the

Fig. 2.12 Consistency
between self-reported and
measured blood pressure,
output from SAS
Program 2.7

Frequency Col Pct	Table of HBP_Q by HBP_X		
		HBP_X	
HBP_Q	0	1	Total
0	3024 72.66	362 36.31	3386
1	1138 27.34	635 63.69	1773
Total	4162	997	5159

specificity = 72.7% for self-reported high blood pressure. Relative to sensitivity, the estimated specificity is better.

Based on the results, the accuracy of self-reported high blood pressure = $(635 + 3024)/5159 = 70.9\%$. This result suggests that among 100 subjects with self-reported data on high blood pressure, more than 70 would be correct when the measured blood pressure was used as a reference.

2.7.4   Reliability of a Measurement Tool and Its Assessment

Reliability is referred to as measurement consistency in general. Reliability of data is determined by the method/test used to obtain the data. Reliability of data for objective measures is relatively easy to determine. For example, to assess the reliability of a scale in measuring bodyweight, you can use the scale to measure the same person multiple times at different settings; the scale, or data collected using the scale, will be reliable if differences between different measures are relatively small; otherwise, it will be unreliable. Blood pressure measurement is a typical example. The same measure is conducted three times, and the mean of the three is used as the final measure. The reliability of blood pressure measured using this method is high. Students can demonstrate this after learning the method in this section.

Survey data are used most often used in epidemiology. It is hard if not impossible to assess the reliability of a single survey question or data collected using the question because of several challenges. Data collected by asking one participant is inadequate; data collected by asking a participant the same questions multiple times are inappropriate because of memory; and data collected by asking the same question to multiple participants once are also inadequate since it is not possible to separate variance of the variable with random errors that are directly related to reliability (as described earlier in this section on system and random errors).

The advancement in psychometrics makes it possible to quantitatively assess the reliability of data, with one wave of data collected using the instrument. The well-known 9-item Patient Health Questionnaire (PHQ-9, Kroenke et al. 2001; Cameron et al. 2008) is a typical example. This scale uses nine wellp-composed questions to assess the frequency of depressive symptoms in the last 2 weeks (0 = not at all, 1 = several days, 2 = more than half of the days, 3 = nearly daily):

1. Little interest or pleasure doing things
2. Feeling down, depressed, or hopeless
3. Trouble falling or staying asleep, or sleeping too much
4. Feeling tired or having little energy
5. Poor appetite or overeating
6. Feeling bad about yourself or that you are a failure or have let yourself or family down
7. Trouble concentrating on things, such as reading the newspaper or watching television
8. Moving or speaking so slowly that other people could have noticed; or the oppo-site – being so fidgety or restless that you have been moving around a lot more than usual
9. Thoughts that you would be better off dead or of hurting yourself in some way

The data collected using the scale, the reliability of data or the reliability of the PHQ-9 can be assessed quantitatively.

In general, for an instrument with k items, its reliability can be estimated using the Cronbach alpha (Cronbach 1951) with the following formula:

$$\alpha = \frac{k}{1-k}\left(1 - \frac{\Sigma_{i=1}^{k}\sigma_i^2}{\sigma^2}\right), \tag{2.1}$$

where σ_i^2 represents the variance of individual items (or information carried by individual items in a scale), and σ^2 represents the total variance of the scale itself. The range of α varies from 0 to 1. A good instrument or data collected using the instrument is considered reliable if $\alpha \geq 0.8$ and excellent if $\alpha \geq 0.9$.

According to this formula, Cronbach α can be increased by (1) adding items to a measurement scale (increasing k), (2) reducing the variance of individual items (minimizing respondent error by constructing and pilot testing individual questions for a scale), and (3) increasing the variance of the total scale score (each item covers a specific area of the construct to be measured).

Technically, it has been accepted that Cronbach α provides a measure of the amount of information and error provided by a scale in addition to the role to assess reliability and internal consistency (Tavakol and Dennick 2011). This conclusion is very useful for quantitative epidemiology. For example, a measurement scale with Cronbach $\alpha = 0.8$ means the data contains 80% information and 20% error. As mentioned early, this method can be used to assess the reliability of blood pressure measurement using thee repeated measures, treating the 3 measures as 3 items.

2.7.5   Reliability Analysis with Real Data

The reliability test will be illustrated using PHQ-9 data in NHANES for depression. First, locate and download the DPQ_J.XPT (depression) from 2017–18 NHANES and saved it into the folder **ORIGINAL** within the folder **A_DATA** under the folder **QUANTLAB**. Then use SAS Program 2.8 to convert the data and conduct the analysis.

```
********************************************************************************
* SAS PROGRAM 2.8. COMPUTE CRONBACH ALPHA FOR PHQ-9 FROM 2017-18 NHANES DATA
********************************************************************************;
* PLACE TO SAVE THE PROCESSED SAS DATA;
LIBNAME SASDATA "C:\QUANTLAB\A_DATA";
* LOCATION OF THE ORGINAL DATA;
LIBNAME XPTDATA XPORT "C:\QUANTLAB\A_DATA\ORIGINA\DPQ_J.XPT" ACCESS=READONLY;
PROC COPY INLIB=XPTDATA OUTLIB=SASDATA; RUN;
* CHECK THE CONVERTED DATA;
PROC CONTENTS DATA =   SASDATA.DPQ_J; RUN;
** CONDUCT ANALYSIS TO ESTIMATE CRONBACH ALPHA;
PROC CORR ALPHA DATA = SASDATA.DPQ_J;
VAR DPQ010 DPQ020 DPQ030 DPQ040 DPQ050 DPQ060 DPQ070 DPQ080 DPQ090;
RUN;
********************************************************************************;
```

2.7.6   Main Results and Interpretation

Figure 2.13 presents the main findings from SAS Program 2.8. First, the table "Cronbach Coefficient Alpha" contains the result we need. Two coefficients are presented, raw and standardize. Raw coefficient is for instruments with all items measured using the same rating scale as in the PHQ-9; and standard coefficient is for instruments with individual items measured with different rating scales. Since all PHQ-9 items are measured using the same 3-level rating scale, the estimated Cronbach alpha = 0.84, suggesting good reliability.

The second part of the outcome in Fig. 2.13 provides data to see if the instrument can be improved further by dropping "bad" items that may not contribute to the measurement. Using results in the first row for DPQ010 as an example. The result says that this item has an item-to-total correlation of 0.5552. If this item is removed (deleted), the raw Cronbach alpha will be 0.829. Obviously, this alpha is smaller than 0.845, the coefficient with no item removed. This result suggests that DPQ010 cannot be removed from the scale.

When this method is used to check the remaining 8 items, removal of any of these items will lead to a reduction in the estimated raw Cronbach alpha coefficient. This result suggests that all 9 items are needed or the PHQ instrument is adequate for assessing depressive symptoms.

Cronbach Coefficient Alpha	
Variables	Alpha
Raw	0.844845
Standardized	0.851364

Cronbach Coefficient Alpha with Deleted Variable				
	Raw Variables		Standardized Variables	
Deleted Variable	Correlation with Total	Alpha	Correlation with Total	Alpha	Label
DPQ010	0.555165	0.829312	0.547195	0.838164	Have little interest in doing things
DPQ020	0.680741	0.815840	0.688453	0.823554	Feeling down, depressed, or hopeless
DPQ030	0.570932	0.830242	0.556152	0.837257	Trouble sleeping or sleeping too much
DPQ040	0.614095	0.824035	0.595047	0.833288	Feeling tired or having little energy
DPQ050	0.560928	0.828654	0.553280	0.837548	Poor appetite or overeating
DPQ060	0.617507	0.823517	0.642589	0.828369	Feeling bad about yourself
DPQ070	0.572093	0.827660	0.577976	0.835036	Trouble concentrating on things
DPQ080	0.525571	0.832890	0.539231	0.838969	Moving or speaking slowly or too fast
DPQ090	0.423325	0.843653	0.438225	0.848997	Thought you would be better off dead

Fig. 2.13 Reliability assessment of HPQ-9, output from SAS Program 2.6

2.8 Practice

2.8.1 Data Processing and Statistical Analysis

1. Spend time to practice how to access and acquire original data using SAS Program 2.1 as an example, gain familiarity with data folder systems and get to know where is what for data processing.
2. Practice on how to select specific variables from a long list of variables in the original data using SAS Program 2.2.
3. Spend time to study and practice variable recoding and data processing using SAS program 2.3. By the time when you complete this practice, you should be able to build the dataset **DATCH2** with all the variables as described in the chapter.
4. Practice SAS Program 2.6 to assess a measurement tool, including the method to create the cross-table and use the results in the table to compute sensitivity, specificity, accuracy, PPV, and NPV. Repeat the same analysis first, then redefine hypertension using systolic blood pressure >=140, keep diastolic blood pressure >=90 as in the SAS program.

5. Practice SAS Program 2.7 to assess the reliability of an instrument. Try to repeat all steps in the programs first, and then repeat the same analysis for the data by gender and racial groups. Reliability often varies by demographic factors. Use the same method to assess the reliability of blood pressure (systolic and diastolic blood pressure separately) based on the three measurements (as three items).
6. Practice SAS Program 2.4 for continuous variables and 2.5 for categorical variables to replicate results in Template Table 1 below by limiting the subjects within the age range of 20–69 years old with 5-year age intervals.

A Template of Table 1. Characteristics of the study sample

Variable	Male	Female	Total
Sample size, n (%)	2174 (48.07)	2349 (51.93)	3419 (100.00)
Age in year			
20–29, n (%)	407 (18.72)	421 (17.92)	828 (18.31)
30–39, n (%)	393 (18.08)	466 (19.84)	858 (18.99)
40–49, n (%)	382 (17.57)	431 (19.83)	813 (17.97)
50–59, n (%)	431 (19.83)	488 (20.77)	919 (20.32)
60–69, n (%)	561 (25.80)	543 (23.12)	1104 (24.41)
Mean (SD)	45.93 (14.72)	45.58 (14.72)	45.75 (14.53)
Race, n (%)			
White	651 (29.94)	679 (28.91)	1330 (29.41)
Black	527 (24.24)	589 (25.07)	1116 (24.67)
Hispanic	527 (24.24)	591 (25.16)	1118 (24.72)
Asian	342 (15.73)	381 (16.22)	723 (15.98)
Other	127 (5.84)	109 (4.64)	236 (5.22)
Educational attainment[a], n (%)			
Less than high school	447 (20.59)	413 (17.61)	860 (19.04)
High school	1217 (56.06)	1331 (56.76)	2548 (56.42)
College or more	507 (23.35)	601 (25.63)	1108 (24.53)
Marital status[a], n (%)			
Never married	506 (23.30)	461 (19.65)	967 (21.40)
Married/live with parents	1356 (62.43)	1348 (57.46)	2704 (59.85)
Divorced/windowed	310 (14.27)	537 (22.89)	847 (18.75)

Note: [a]Numbers not adding up due to missing. Actual sample, not weighted. As a template, only five demographic and socioeconomic factors are included. In a typical public health and epidemiological studies, 8–10 variables are often used while in clinic-based studies, more variables are included

2.8.2 Work on Your Study Project

1. Use all the methods practiced in this chapter to create a dataset for your own project. You can do this by simply adding more variables to **DATCH2**; you can also do this by accessing new data from NHANES. After done, save all your data to the **A_DATA** folder.

2. Create a temporary Table 1 for your own study project with the newly created dataset. Please use SAS Programs 2.4 and 2.5 and Template Table 1 from your own practice to make Table 1 for your study. Be advised, the table is simply a first draft, and it can be revised later as your study progresses.
3. Use the actual data to further improve your study project, including the definition of the study population, study variables, study hypothesis, analytical methods, and expected findings. Please complete this step of work with reference to the Template described in Chap. 1.
4. Revise your project title and add substantive information, such as sample size and demographic composition to your abstract.

2.8.3 Study Questions

1. Use your own examples to discuss the difference and connections between study characters, variables, data, and information in quantitative epidemiology.
2. In this chapter, we have learned that constant variables provide little information, and only variations (i.e., SD) in a variable contain information. In practice, two studies A and B both collected data for the same variable; the SD of the variable in Study A is larger than that in Study B. Can we conclude that data from Study A is more informative than the data from Study B? Why or why not?
3. Name the methods commonly used in data processing.
4. Understand potential sources of data error that can be introduced from different steps in research, starting from study population, sampling, variable selection, measurement, data processing, and recoding.
5. What are random errors and systematic errors; how do each of the two errors affect reliability and validity of data used in quantitative epidemiology?
6. How does the sensitivity used in laboratory tests (i.e., based on the continuous measure) differ from the sensitivity used (i.e., based on the binary measure) in quantitative epidemiology?
7. What are the main impacts of data errors for quantitative epidemiology?

References

Cameron, I.M., Crawford, J.R., Lawton, K., Reid, I.C.: Psychometric comparison of PHQ-9 and HADS for measuring depression severity in primary care. Br. J. Gen. Pract. **58**(546), 32–36 (2008)

Chen, X., Chen, D.: Statistical methods for global health and epidemiology. Springer (2020)

Chertkow, H., Whitehead, V., Phillips, N., Wolfson, C., Atherton, J., Bergman, H.: Multilingualism (but not always bilingualism) delays the onset of Alzheimer disease: Evidence from a bilingual community. Alzheimer Dis. Assoc. Disord. **24**(2), 118–125 (2010)

Cronbach, L.J.: Coefficient alpha and the internal structure of tests. Pyschometrika. **16**(3), 397–334 (1951)

Degaute, J., van de Borne, P., Linkowisk, P., Cauter, E.V.: Quantitative analysis of the 2-hour blood pressure and heart rate patterns in young men. Hypertension. **18**(2), 199–210 (1991)

Kroenke, K., Spitzer, R.L., Williams, J.B.: The PHQ-9: Validity of a brief depression severity measure. J. Gen. Intern. Med. **16**(9), 606–613 (2001)

Modesti, P.A., Rapi, S., Rogolino, A., Tosi, B., Galanti, G.: Seasonal blood pressure variation: Implications for cardiovascular risk stratification. Hypertens. Res. **41**, 475–482 (2018)

Nunnally, J.C., Bernstein, I.H.: Psychometric theory, 3rd edn. McGraw-Hill, New York (1994)

Sheng, Y., Wang, K., Xu, L., et al.: A cyclic function mode for 24-h ambulatory blood pressure monitoring in Chinese patients with mild to moderate hypertension. Acta Pharmacol. Sin. **34**(8), 1043–1051 (2013)

Szklo, M., Nieto, F.J.: Epidemiology beyond the basics. Jones and Bartlett Publishers (2004)

Tavakol, M., Dennick, R.: Making sense of Cronbach's alpha. Int. J. Med. Educ. **2**, 53–55 (2011)

Chapter 3
Quantitative Descriptive Epidemiology

Current status informs future directions.

Descriptive study is often used at the beginning of a project to examine a medical, health, or behavioral problem in public health and medicine. Although, it is common practice to describe a problem using words; quantitative epidemiology focuses on the application of descriptive statistical methods and visualization techniques for description. Information provided using a quantitative method is thus less subjective, and more concise and accurate than words. The commonly used descriptive statistics include sum, mean, standard deviation (SD), proportion, quantile, interquarter range (IQR), rate, ratio, and 95% confidence intervals; and the commonly used visualization techniques include histograms, pie charts, bar charts, line charts, scatter plots, and mapping. With these quantitative methods and techniques, numbers and figures are generated to describe the distribution of a medical, health, or behavioral problem in a population to assess who are at high risk by geographic area to locate the hot spots, and over time to assess temporal trends.

3.1 Introduction

Descriptive epidemiology is so familiar with us that few have even considered it in research. Using vital statistics to track historical trends of an infectious disease, a chronic disease, overweight and obesity for populations in a country belongs to descriptive epidemiology. In all textbooks, the study of disease distribution is often presented first to introduce epidemiology. In most papers published in peer-reviewed journals, Table 3.1 for sample characteristics (used as Table 1 in a published paper) can also be considered as descriptive epidemiology. With advancement in methods and data, descriptive epidemiology is used more and more often in research and result presentation in recent days.

Table 3.1 Life Expectancy at birth for the US population, overall and by gender and race

Year	Total	Male	Female	White	Black
1900–02	49.24	47.88	50.70	49.64	33.80
1909–11	51.49	49.86	53.24	51.90	35.87
1919–21	56.40	55.50	57.40	57.42	47.03
1929–31	59.20	57.71	60.90	60.86	48.53
1939–41	63.62	61.60	65.89	64.92	53.85
1949–51	68.07	65.47	70.96	69.02	60.73
1959–61	69.89	66.80	73.24	70.73	63.91
1969–71	70.75	67.04	74.64	71.62	64.11
1979–81	73.88	70.11	77.62	74.53	68.52
1989–91	75.37	71.83	78.81	76.13	69.19
1999–01	76.86	74.13	79.47	77.43	71.81
2009–11	78.60	76.13	80.98	78.88	74.99

Data source: Arias et al. 2020. U.S. Decennial life tables for 2009–2011, United States Life Tables. *National* Vital Statistics *Reports*, vol 69 no 8. Hyattsville, MD: National Center for Health Statistics

Historically, epidemiology was established by studying the distribution of infected disease cases. The most common example is the identification of the cause of cholera in London by plotting individual patients on the street map (Snow 1857). Linking the distribution of an infectious disease with potential exposure is used as a classic approach for etiological study of infectious diseases even today. For example, geographic distribution is a major technique used in examining the origin and spread of many infectious diseases, such as the COVID-19 pandemic which was first detected in Wuhan, China in 2019 and subsequently observed in many other countries across the globe.

The classic case-control studies of smoking and lung cancer by Doll and Hill (1950) can be considered as a population distribution study. This is because the study reached the conclusion essentially by comparing the proportion of smokers between lung cancer patients (cases) and non-cancer patients (controls). By comparing the proportion (distribution) of smokers among the cases and controls, the researchers were able to determine if smoking was associated with the risk of lung cancer, and if yes, how much the risk was.

In introducing epidemiology, a common misconception is to include the distribution of determinants, risks, or influential factors as part of the research focus. A systematic understanding of the distribution of determinants or risk factors is central to environmental health; the focus of epidemiology is on the distribution of diseases, unhealthy lifestyles, and health-related behaviors. We examine determinants or factors related to these problems in etiological studies and target the modifiable factors through interventions to prevent disease and promote health.

3.1.1 Univariate Descriptive Analysis

Prior to quantitative study of a problem in a population across geographic area over time, knowledge is needed regarding the distribution of variables used to describe a problem. Understanding the distribution of a specific health outcome is considered as *univariate descriptive analysis*.

If a continuous variable is used to measure a health outcome, we would like to know if the distribution is normal because many analytical methods require normally distributed data. Typical examples include examination of development using body height and weight, investigation of hypertension using systolic and diastolic blood pressure, and evaluation of response to a treatment for people living with HIV using viral load. If the distribution deviates from normal, measures should be considered to convert the distribution to normal. For example, viral load of HIV is often not normally distributed, but can be converted into normal by taking algorithm transformation.

Categorical variables are used most often to measure health status. Typical examples include severity of a disease (asymptotic, light, moderate, and severe), clinical stage of cancer (Stage I, Stage II, etc.), levels of addiction (none, light, moderate and heavy), and health attitudes and beliefs, etc. In these cases, descriptive analysis is conducted first to check if the number of participants in each group is adequately large. If not, re-grouping operations must be conducted to ensure robustness of the statistics for distribution, including the rate, ratio, or proportion for individual groups.

In some cases, if a continuous variable is not normally distributed, converting it into a categorical variable provides a remedy. When converting a continuous variable into categorical, objective cutoff points must be used, such as percentiles. It is worth noting that, in theory, converting a continuous variable into categorical will result in a loss of information; however, it will reduce the impact of error in data.

Methods to conduct univariate descriptive analysis will be covered later in Sect. 3.2.

3.1.2 Bivariate Descriptive Analysis

Bivariate descriptive analysis is the method we routinely use to gain insight into the distribution of medical, health, and behavioral problems with regard to the 3 W's (i.e., whom, when, and where). When a variable is assessed against another variable, it is termed as bivariate descriptive analysis. When analyzing the prevalence of hypertension by racial groups, information is obtained on the distribution of the disease across the population; when plotting smoking rates by year since the 1950s when the tobacco control program started in the US, information is generated on the distribution of smoking behavior changes over time; while mapping the incidence of COVID-19 by state in a country or by country in the world, information is obtained on geographic distribution of the disease.

If a health outcome is described along with a categorical variable, univariate descriptive analysis is used to determine if the number of participants is adequate for individual categories (groups). Too few subjects in a group will reduce the robustness of the analytical results for the group. Let us take five racial groups of White, Black, Hispanic, Asian, and Native Americans as an example. Before in-depth analysis, information must be obtained on the number of participants per group. In many studies, results are not provided for minority groups (such as Asian/ Native American) not because of negligence but rather due to an inadequate number of participants.

In addition to categorical variables (e.g., gender, race, marital status), health outcomes can be described against a continuous variable, such as income and days of smoking. In this case the continuous income in dollar is often converted into (i) lower, (ii) medial, and (iii) high; and the days of smoking are often converted into (i) nonsmokers (zero days of smoking), (ii) light smokers (some days of smoking), and (iii) heavy smokers (smoke almost every day).

Results from bivariate descriptive analysis provide the most information about the distribution of variables in epidemiology. We will introduce various methods to conduct the analysis, including analysis of population distribution in Sect. 3.4, temporal distribution in Sect. 3.5, and geographic distribution in Sect. 3.6.

It is worth noting that both univariate and bivariate distributions are useful to describe study samples. However, results from bivariate analysis provide further information and are useful for hypothesis generation and in-depth studies. More detailed discussion will be covered in Chap. 5 on exploratory bivariate analysis.

3.2 Data Preparation for Descriptive Analysis

Data from various sources can be used for descriptive analysis. Typical examples include data from the National Center for Health Statistics, the Census Bureau, and the National Survey on Drug Use and Health. For training purposes, we will use the 2017–18 NHANES data to demonstrate different types of descriptive analysis.

3.2.1 SAS Program for Data Processing

SAS Program 2.1 to 2.3 in Chap. 2 demonstrated how to create a dataset using the **DEMO_J.XPT** from 2017–18 NHANES. In the dataset **DATCH2** created for Chap. 2, six demographic variables were renamed, and recoded for analysis, including **AGE** AGE10G **GENDER** RACE5 EDUCATION MARRIAGE NV_MARRID. There were three variables included but not processed. These three variables were

DMDYRSUS (years in the US), DMDFMSIZ (family size), and INDHHIN2 (household income). We will create DATCH3 by reading DATCH2 and process these variables. This is achieved using SAS Program 3.1 below.

```
************************************************************************
* SAS PROGRAM 3.1 DESCRIPTIVE ANALYSIS USING 2017-18 NHANES DATA
************************************************************************;
LIBNAME SASDATA "C:\QUANTLAB\A_DATA";
** CREATE DATCH3 BY SELECTING SUBJECTS AND RECODE VARIABLES;
DATA SASDATA.DATCH3; SET LIB.DATCH2;    * READ OLD DATA DATCH2 INTO NEW DATCH3;
* EXCLUDE SUBJECTS WITH MISSING DATA ON AGE;
IF AGE NE .;
* RECODE ADDITIONAL VARIABLE FOR USE IN ANALYSIS;
YRSINUS      = DMDYRSUS;        * RENAME AS YEARS IN THE USA;
IF DMDYRSUS IN (77, 99) THEN YRSINUS = .; * RECODE MISSING;
*RENAME VARIABLE FAMILY SIZE;
FAMISIZE = DMDFMSIZ;
*RENAME HOUSEHOLD INCOME;
HHINCOME = INDHHIN2;
IF INDHHIN2 IN (77, 99) THEN HHINCOME = .;    * RECODE MISSING;
* RELABEL NEW VARIABLES;
LABEL  YRSINUS     = "YEARS IN USA, CATEGORY 1: <1, 9: 50+"
       FAMISIZE    = "FAMILY SIZE: NUMBER OF PERSIONS IN FAMILY",
       HHINCOME    = "ANNUAL HOUSEHOLD INCOME: 1 FOR <5000 TO 15 FOR 100K+";
* KEEP ONLY THE NEW VARIABLES NEEDED FOR ANALYSIS;
KEEP AGE AGE10G GENDER RACE5 YRSINUS EDUCATION MARRIAGE FAMISIZE HHINCOME SEQN;
RUN;    PROC CONTENTS; RUN;
************************************************************************;
```

3.2.2 Check the Data Before Analysis

As a routine, we must check the newly created data to see if all variables are correctly created, appropriately labeled, and examine the status of missing data. To check variables in the dataset, the program codes **PROC CONTENTS** can be used immediately after the dataset is created. Figure 3.1 will be the expected results if correctly done.

#	Variable	Type	Len	Label
				Alphabetic List of Variables and Attributes
3	AGE	Num	8	AGE IN YEAR,
4	AGE10G	Num	8	1=20~29, 2=30~39, 3=40~49 4=50~59 5=60~69 6=70~80,
6	EDUCATION	Num	8	1=LESS THAN HIGH 2=HIGH SCHOOL 3=COLLEGE+,
9	FAMISIZE	Num	8	FAMILY SIZE,
2	GENDER	Num	8	GENDER 1=MALE 2=FEMALE,
10	HHINCOME	Num	8	ANNUAL HOUSEHOLD INCOME: 1: <5000, 15 100K+
7	MARRIAGE	Num	8	1=NEVER MARRIED 2=MARRIED/STYWITH PARTNER 3=DIVORCE/WIDOWED,
5	RACE5	Num	8	1=WHITE 2=BLACK 3=HISP 4=ASIAN 5=OTHER,
1	SEQN	Num	8	Respondent sequence number
8	YRSINUS	Num	8	YEARS IN USA, CATEGORY 1: <1, 9: 50+

Fig. 3.1 The 9 variables in the newly created dataset **DATCH3** plus **SEQN**

3.3   Univariate Distribution

As described in the previous section, the purpose of univariate descriptive analysis is to provide information on the distribution of a study variable itself. Different methods will be used for continuous and categorical variables. In this section, we will demonstrate the methods for univariate descriptive analysis using real data created using SAS Program 3.1 in the previous section.

3.3.1   Univariate Descriptive Analysis with Continuous Variables

The distribution of a continuous variable can be assessed using various statistical methods. We demonstrate the use of **PROC UNIVARIATE** from SAS. This method generates almost all the information needed to know the distribution of a continuous variable. SAS Program 3.2 demonstrates the use of this method in describing the distribution of two continuous variables, family size and age, included in the dataset **DATCH3** just created in Sect. 3.2.

```
******************************************************************************
* SAS PROGRAM 3.2 UNIVARIATE ANALYSIS FOR CONTINUOUS VARIABLES
******************************************************************************;
** DATA PREPARATION: READ DATA FROM THE NEWLY CREATED DATASET DATCH3;
LIBNAME SASDATA "C:\QUANTLAB\A_DATA\";
DATA A; SET SASDATA.DATCH3;RUN;
** 1 SIMPLE UNIVARIATE ANALYSIS WITH ONE VARIABLE;
PROC UNIVARIATE DATA = A;
VAR FAMISIZE;
RUN;
** 2 ANALYSIS WITH HISTOGRAM TO CHARACTERIZE DISTRIBUTION
PROC UNIVARIATE DATA = A;
VAR AGE;
HISTOGRAM /ENDPOINTS = (20 TO 85 BY 5);
RUN;
** 3 ANALYSIS WITH PERCENTILE SPECIFIED;
PROC UNIVARIATE DATA = A NOPRINT;
VAR AGE;
* SPECIFY THE PERCENTILE;
OUTPUT OUT=UNI_PCNT  PCTLPTS=2.5 5 25 50 75 95 97.5 PCTLPRE=P;
RUN;
* SHOW THE ESTIMATED PERCENTILE CUTOFF POINTS;
PROC PRINT DATA = UNI_PCNT NOOBS; RUN;
******************************************************************************;
```

Run the first analysis of SAS Program 3.2 above, and it will produce five blocks of results: (i) Moments, including sample size N, mean, variance, standard deviation, skewness, and kurtosis; (ii) Basic Statistical Measures, including mean, median, and mode; (iii) Test for Location: $\mu = 0$, (iv) Quantiles, including 0% or minimum, 1%, 5%, 10%, 25% (quantile 1, Q1), 50% (Median), 75% (quantile 3, Q3), 90%, 95%, 99%, and 100% or maximum; and (v) Extreme Observations. Of the five, (i), (ii), and (iv) are used most often in practice. Figure 3.2 displays the first

Moments					Basic Statistical Measures			
N	5569	Sum Weights	5569		Location		Variability	
Mean	2.97198779	Sum Observations	16551	Mean	2.971988	Std Deviation	1.66769
Std Deviation	1.66768809	Variance	2.78118357	Median	3.000000	Variance	2.78118
Skewness	0.6881598	Kurtosis	-0.4001642	Mode	2.000000	Range	6.00000
Uncorrected SS	64675	Corrected SS	15485.6301			Interquartile Range	2.00000
Coeff Variation	56.1135579	Std Error Mean	0.02234736				

Fig. 3.2 Moment and basic statistical measures of family size, output of univariate analysis SAS Program 3.2

two blocks of results from the univariate distribution analysis; and the result for block iv was not displayed.

Results from the univariate analysis indicate that, in the US, the average family size is 2.97 persons per family (SD=1.67). The variable is about normally distributed since the mean is very close to the median 3.00. The inter-quarter range = 2, suggesting that 75% of families in the US have 4–6 people in them.

Age is used in the second univariate analysis in SAS Program 3.2 with a histogram added to visually see the distribution in addition to the five block of statistics. Results from the analysis indicate the mean age of subjects in the 2017–18 NHANES was 51.05 (SD=17.81), median age was 53, and IQR was 30.

We often think that age is a continuous variable and could be normally distributed. The histogram in Fig. 3.3 shows that the age distribution of the subjects in the 2017–18 NHANES data are not normally distributed but have more of an even distribution. This characteristic cannot be revealed numerically without a histogram.

In descriptive epidemiology, is it sometimes also useful to estimate specific percentile points, such as 2.5% percentile for two-sided statistical tests, and tertial, quartile, and quintile to convert a continuous variable into categorical. This can be achieved using the last univariate analysis in SAS Program 3.2. By running this analysis, a simple table will be generated as $P2\_5 = 21$, $P5 = 23$, $P25 = 36$, $P50 = 53$, $P75 = 66$, $P95 = 80$, and $P97\_5 = 80$. This result shows that 2.5% of the sample has an age up to 21, 5% with an age up to 23, and 25% with an age up to 36, etc.

With this information, the continuous variable, age, can be converted into categorical (say a 4-level) variable using age 26, 53 and 66 as the cutoff ages. This objective converting ensures a similar number of subjects per level. It is used very often in studies to convert non-normal continuous variables into categorical for statistical analysis.

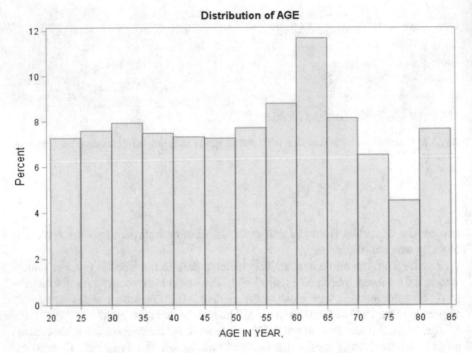

Fig. 3.3 Age distribution, result from second univariate analysis of SAS Program 3.2

3.3.2 Categorical Variables

It is much easier to conduct univariate descriptive analysis for categorical variables than for continuous variables with statistical software. SAS Program 3.3 shows such analysis with several example variables. It contains three different analytical methods. Analysis 1 in the program shows the use of **PROC FREQ** to analyze more than one variable in one program statement; Analysis 2 shows the same analysis with a plot to visualize the distribution, and Analysis 3 shows a pie chart analysis.

```
*********************************************************************************
* SAS PROGRAM 3.3 ANALYZE CATEGORICAL DEMOGRAPHIC VARIABLES (REPLACE HEALTH STATUS)
*********************************************************************************;
** READ DATCH3 DATA, THIS CAN BE OMITTED IF CONTINUED FROM SAS PROGRAM 3.2;
LIBNAME SASDATA "C:\QUANTLAB\A_DATA\";
DATA A; SET SASDATA.DATCH3; RUN;
** 1 SIMPLE ANALYSIS USING PROC FREQ;
PROC FREQ DATA = A;
TABLES GENDER RACE5 EDUCATION MARRIAGE;
RUN;
** 2 PROC FREQ ANALYSIS PLUS A BAR CHART;
PROC FREQ DATA = A;
TABLES RACE5/PLOTS=FREPLOT; RUN;
** 3. PIE CHART ANALYSIS;
PROC GCHART DATA = A;
* DEFINE PIE CHART;
PIE EDUCATION; RUN;
*********************************************************************************;
```

As an example, Fig. 3.4 shows part of the results from Analysis 1 in SAS Program 3.3: Distribution by male-female gender and racial groups. The remaining results are left for students to review and interpret. Based on the results, of the 5569 adult subjects in the NHANES sample, 2702 (48.52%) were male and 2867 (51.48%) were female. With regard to race, the number of subjects varied dramatically across racial groups with White individuals accounting for 34.75% and Asians for 14.56%.

Fig. 3.4 Partial results from SAS Program 3.3 Analysis 1

1=MALE 2=FEMALE,				
GENDER	Frequency	Percent	Cumulative Frequency	Cumulative Percent
1	2702	48.52	2702	48.52
2	2867	51.48	5569	100.00

1=WHITE 2=BLAKC 3=HISP 4=ASIAN 5=OTHER,				
RACE5	Frequency	Percent	Cumulative Frequency	Cumulative Percent
1	1935	34.75	1935	34.75
2	1298	23.31	3233	58.05
3	1252	22.48	4485	80.54
4	811	14.56	5296	95.10
5	273	4.90	5569	100.00

Despite these large variations, 811 subjects in the total sample were Asian, the smallest group of the first four. Therefore, sample sizes for the four racial groups are reasonably large and are adequate to obtain robust statistical estimates and for significant tests to draw statistical conclusions.

The racial distribution is visualized by running Analysis 2 in SAS Program 3.3 as seen in Fig. 3.5. The figure provides a measure better for comprehension of the

Fig. 3.5 Bar plots showing the distribution of racial groups from SAS Program 3.3 Analysis 2

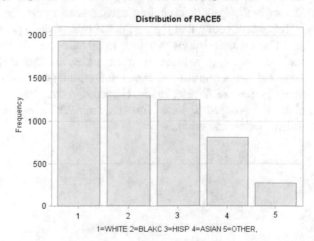

number of subjects by group. The same method showed in Analysis 2 can be used to analyze other variables.

Analysis 3 and results for a pie chart in SAS Program 3.3 are not presented; they are reserved for students to practice.

3.4 Population Distribution

Population distribution is used most often in epidemiology. The goal is to describe the distribution of a variable of interest, say incidence of influenza, mortality of heart disease, prevalence of marijuana use, over one population character, such as gender, age, race/ethnicity, income, etc. It is called bivariate distribution because two variables are involved, one measuring a medical, health, or behavioral problem and another measuring a population character.

3.4.1 Determine the Variables

Variables to measure a medical, health, or behavioral problem are obvious. This variable is determined during the process when a research project is established with a testable hypothesis. For example, to study factors related to high blood pressure, measured systolic and diastolic blood pressure or a diagnosis of hypertension would be the variable; to examine mental health status, scores from a scale to assess depressive symptoms would be the variable; to study opioids, self-reported use or results from a biopsy would be the variable.

Variables used to measure population characters are more than the character of a study population since one character can be measured using more than one variable (see Chap. 2). In epidemiology, demographic factors and socioeconomic status are often used to characterize a study population. In Sect. 3.2, a set of population measures are introduced, including age, gender, race, education, years living in the United States (for first-generation immigrants), marital status, family size, and income.

It is worth noting that the traditional male-female gender is based on biological sex. This measure is now extended to include a number of sexual minority groups, such as lesbian, gay, bisexual, transgender, and queer (LGBTQ). There are also more detailed definitions in racial and ethnic groups. In the US, commonly used racial groups are: White, Black, Hispanic, Asian, Native, and other. Race and ethnicity are grouped to have Non-Hispanic White, Non-Hispanic Black, Hispanic, Asian, Native, and other.

3.4.2 Add Data for Bivariate Descriptive Analysis

To conduct a study about population distribution, we need two pieces of data: data that classifies a population into subgroups and data for a health outcome variable to be described. Results of descriptive studies are often presented using tables and bar charts. Here we demonstrate the distribution of reported hypertension for adults in the US by age, gender, and racial groups, using a table using SAS Program 3.4. Variables for description: hypertension (yes/no) and age when having had hypertension the first time.

```
*******************************************************************************
* SAS PROGRAM 3.4: ADD BPQ_J TO DATCH3_1 TO CREATE DATCH3 FOR BIVARIATE ANALYSIS
*******************************************************************************;
** 1 PROCESS BPQ_J THAT WAS DOWNLOADED AND SAVED IN CHAPTER 2;
*  CONVERT BPQ_J INTO SAS DATASET;
LIBNAME XPTDATA XPORT "C:\QUANTLAB\A_DATA\ORIGINA\BPQ_J.XPT" ACCESS=READONLY;
PROC COPY INLIB=XPTDATA OUTLIB= SASDATA; RUN;
DATA TEMP1; SET LIB.BPQ_J;
*  BPD035-AGEONSET, BPQ020-HYPERTENSION, BPQ050A-ANTIHYPERTENSIVE MEDICATION, SEQN;
KEEP BPD035 BPQ020 BPQ050A SEQN;
*  CHECK THE DATA FOR THE 4 VARIABLES;
PROC CONTENTS DATA=TEMP1; RUN;
** 2 READ IN DATCH3 TO TEMP2;
DATA TEMP2; SET LIB.DATCH3; RUN;
** 3 ADD TEMP1 AND TEMP2 TO CREATE TEMP;
*  SORT THE TWO DATASETS TO BE COMBIED;
PROC SORT DATA = TEMP1; BY SEQN; RUN;
PROC SORT DATA = TEMP2; BY SEQN; RUN;
*  DATASET COMBINATION BY ID SEQN;
DATA TEMP; MERGE TEMP1 TEMP2; BY SEQN;
* CHECK THE DATA FOR THE 5 VARIABLES FOR DISTRIBUTION STUDY;
PROC CONTENTS DATA = TEMP; RUN;

** 4 CREATE PERMANENT DATASET USING THE SAME DATASET NAME;
DATA SASDATA.DATCH3; SET TEMP;
* RECODE AGE INTO A 5-YEAR AGE GROUPS AS 20-24 25-29 30-34...75-79
  THIS METHOD IS MUCH MORE EFFICIENT THAN THOSE IN SAS PROGRAM 2.2;
AGEG5 = INT(AGE/5)*5;
* RECODE AGE INTO A 10-YEAR AGE GROUPS DIFF FROM AGE10G IN CHAPTER 2;
AGEG10 = INT(AGE/10)*10;
* RENAME VARIABLE GENDER;
IF 12 <= BPD035 <= 80 THEN AGEHYPR = BPD035;
* CODE IF HAVING HAD HYPERTENSION;
IF BPQ020 IN (1 2) THEN HBP = (BPQ020 = 1);
* CODE ON ANTIHYPERTENSIVE MEDICATION;
IF BPQ050A IN (1 2) THEN HBPMED = (BPQ050A = 1);
* LABEL ALL VARIABLES;
LABEL AGEG5   = "AGE GROUP: 20: 20-24, 25: 25-29 ... 75: 75-79",
      AGEG10  = "AGE GROUP: 20: 20-29, 30: 30-39 ... 70: 70-79",
      AGEHYPR = "AGE OF HYPERTENTION ONSET",
      HBP     = "HIGH BLOOD PRESSURE 1=YES 0 = NO";
KEEP AGE AGEG5 AGE10G AGEG10 GENDER RACE5 AGEHYPR HBP HBPMED SEQN;
* CHECK THE DATA AND VALUES FOR THE 5 VARIABLES;
PROC CONTENTS; RUN;
PROC FREQ; RUN;
*******************************************************************************
```

Note to SAS Program 3.4: Three variables from SAS Program 3.1 (YRSINUS FAMISIZE HHINCOME) were not included on purpose. They are left for students to add for your own practice and research if you need.

By executing the simple SAS program **PROC PRINT** DATA=SASDATA.CHAP3(OBS=10); **RUN;** you should see the results in Fig. 3.6. It shows the first 10 observations in the new dataset just created. The dataset will be used to study distributions of hypertension among the US population by age, gender, and race.

Obs	SEQN	GENDER	AGE	AGE10G	RACE5	MARRIAGE	YRSINUS	FAMISIZE	HHINCOME	AGEG5	AGEG10	AGEHYPR	HBP	HBPMED
1	93705	2	66	5	2	3		1	3	65	60	50	1	1
2	93708	2	66	5	4	2	7	2	6	65	60	50	1	1
3	93709	2	75		2	3		1	2	75	70	71	1	1
4	93711	1	56	4	4	2	6	3	15	55	50		0	
5	93713	1	67	5	1	3		1	6	65	60		0	
6	93714	2	54	4	2	2		3	7	50	50		0	
7	93715	1	71		5	2		5	8	70	70		0	
8	93716	1	61	5	4	2	7	3	15	60	60		0	
9	93717	1	22	1	1	1		1		20	20		0	
10	93718	1	45	3	2	1		7	10	45	40	39	1	1

Fig. 3.6 First 10 Observations of the Newly Created Dataset, SAS Program 3.4

3.4.3 Racial Distribution of Hypertension Among US Adults

Pie charts are a method commonly used to analyze the distribution of a medical, health, or behavioral event by subgroups of a population. SAS Program 3.5 demonstrates the use of a pie chart with the number of subjects who have ever been told by their doctors they had hypertension (**HBP**). In the program, a new dataset A is created by reading data directly from the permanent dataset **DATCH3** saved in the defined location. SAS Procedure **PROC GCHART** was used to draw a pie chart. Several titles are defined to describe the chart. The GROUP = GENDER was used to draw the chart by gender and the option ACROSS=2 was used to have the two pie charts on one page; otherwise, the two charts will be presented on two separate pages.

```
***************************************************************************************
SAS PROGRAM 3.5 RACIAL DISTRIBUTION OF HYPERTENSION AMONG US ADULTS
***************************************************************************************
* 1 READ DATA AND SELECT SUBJECTS WITH HYPERTENSION;
LIBNAME SASDATA " C:\QUANLAB\A_DATA\";
* SELECT HYPERTENSIVE SUBJECTS FOR COMPUTING PROPORTIONS BY SEX AND RACE;
DATA A; SET SASDATA.DATCH3;
IF HBP EQ 1;
* CREATE SEX AND RACE WITH LETTER FOR PLOTTING, ALLOW FOR 5-LETTERS;
IF GENDER EQ 1 THEN Sex = "M";
IF GENDER EQ 2 THEN Sex = "F";
IF RACE5  EQ 1 THEN RACE = "White"; ELSE
IF RACE5  EQ 2 THEN RACE = "Black"; ELSE
IF RACE5  EQ 3 THEN RACE = "Hisp."; ELSE
IF RACE5  EQ 4 THEN RACE = "Asian"; ELSE
RACE = "Other";
* DROP OTHER VARIABLES AND KEEP SEX, RACE, AND HBP FOR FIGURE;
KEEP SEX RACE HBP;
* CHECK DATA;
PROC CONTENTS; RUN;
PROC FREQ DATA = A; RUN;

* 2 DRAW PIE CHART WITH PROC GCHART;
PROC GCHART DATA = A;
* DEFINE PIE CHART;
PIE RACE/GROUP = SEX NOHEADING CLOCKWISE PERCENT=INSIDE VALUE =NONE ACROSS=2
         MIDPOINTS="White" "Black" "Hisp." "Asian" "Other" LEGEND;
* ACROSS=2: PLOT M AND F IN ONE PAGE, MIDPOINTS DETERMINE THE ORDER OF SLICES;
RUN;
***************************************************************************************
```

Figure 3.7 is produced using SAS Program 3.5. From the figure, the following information can be derived. First, the racial distribution of hypertensive patients in the US
differs by gender. For example, among Whites, more males (36.35%) were hypertensive
than females (29.90%); however, a reverse gender pattern was revealed for Blacks with
a higher proportion of females than males who were hypertensive (33.67% vs. 27.62%).

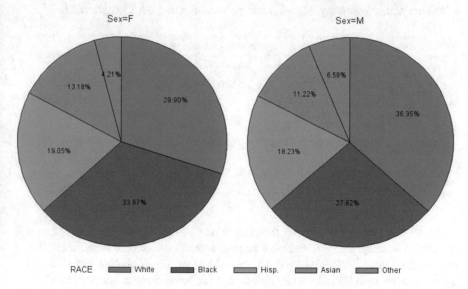

Fig. 3.7 Racial distribution of hypertension among US adults 20 years of age and older, the
2017–18 NHANES data

Second, there were substantial racial differences in the proportion of subjects
who were hypertensive in the study sample. The proportion was much higher for
Whites, Blacks, and Hispanics than Asians and other. However, these results must be
interpreted with caution. We already counted the sample size by race in the Template
Table 1 in in Practice from Chap. 2, and the total number of Whites, Blacks, and
Hispanics was much greater than that of Asians and others. Be advised, this proportion distribution is not a measure of the risk for hypertension. More hypertensive
patients are likely for a larger population given the same level of risk exposure.

3.4.4   Distribution of the Hypertension by Age

Bar charts and line charts are two methods to describe age distributions in addition
to tabulation. To demonstrate the use of this method, SAS Program 3.6 is provided.
In this program, a new dataset A is created by reading all subjects from the permanent dataset DATCH3 saved in the defined location SASDATA regardless of their
hypertension status. We need data for participants with and without high blood pressure to estimate the prevalence rate. One strength of the prevalence rate is that it is
not affected by sample size, or the number of participants across comparison groups.

Instead of **PROC GCHART** for pie chart, another plot procedure **PROC SGPLOT** from SAS is used. The command VBAR AGEG5 is used to ask for a vertical bar chart by the defined 5-year age group; the command RESPONSE = HBP STAT=PERCENT is used to ask the program to generate a bar chart with % of HBP (high blood pressure or hypertension). Other lines of command are self-explanatory. Figure 3.8 is generated using SAS program 3.6.

```
********************************************************************************
SAS PROGRAM 3.6 DISTRIBUTION ANALYSIS HYPERTENSION AND MEDICATION BY AGE
********************************************************************************;
* 1 READ IN DATA FROM THE NEWLY CREATED PERMANENT DATA FOR ANALYSIS;
DATA A; SET SASDATA.DATCH3; RUN;
* 2 PLOT DISTRIBUTIONS BY AGE USING PROC SGPLOT;
PROC SGPLOT DATA = A;
VBAR AGEG5 /RESPONSE = HBP STAT=PERCENT;
XAXIS LABEL ='5-YEAR AGE GROUPS';
YAXIS LABEL ='PREVALENCE OF HYPERTENTION';
RUN;
* 3 TABLE ON % OF MEDICATION BY 5 RACIAL GROUPS;
PROC FREQ DATA = A;
TABLES RACE5* HBPMED;
WHERE HBP EQ 1;      * LIMIT TO SUBJECTS WITH HYPERTENSION;
RUN;
********************************************************************************;
```

Results in Fig. 3.8 show that the prevalence of hypertension increased as age increased from 20 to 24 to reach the peak at age 60–64, before it declined. Based on these results, US adults aged 50 and older are the high-risk population for hypertension, which is also a key risk factor for heart disease and stroke. The US

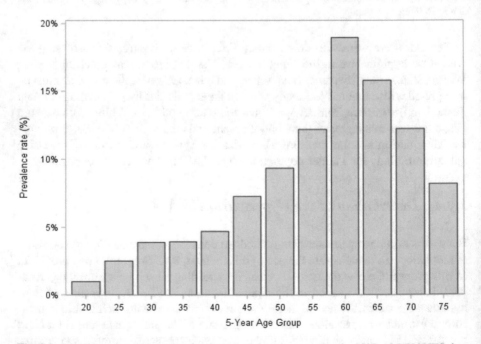

Fig. 3.8 Prevalence rate of hypertension for US adults by age group, the 2017–18 NHANES data

Department of Health and Human Services, and CDC should prioritize this high-risk group in decision-making and resource allocation for chronic disease control and prevention; translational studies should focus on prevention intervention programs to reduce risk of hypertension starting before age 55; and hospital administrators and clinicians must be prepared to treat the large number of hypertensive patients in the high-risk age range.

It is worth noting that SAS Program 3.6 can be revised to plot the same data by gender and race. This can be done by adding a useful SAS command `WHERE` before `RUN`. For example, by adding `WHERE GENDER = 1`, results for males can be plotted; and by adding `WHERE RACE5 = 1`, results for Whites can be plotted. By replacing `AGEG5` with `AGEG10`, the data by 10-year age groups can be plotted.

Furthermore, SAS Program 3.6 can be used to draw line charts as well by replacing `VBAR AGEG5 /RESPONSE = HBP STAT=PERCENT` with `VLINE AGEG5 /RESPONSE = HBP STAT=PERCENT MARKERS`. Here, the key word `VLINE` is used to ask the program to draw a line chart vertically across age groups with `RESPONSE = HBP` for the Y-axis using %. The key word `MARKERS` asks the program to put a dot for each data point. We leave all of these alternatives for students to practice themselves.

Results from Part 3 in the SAS Program indicate that HBP patients who were on medication were 81.66% for Whites, 85.55% for Blacks, 83.12% for Hispanics, 87.8% for Asians, and 80.46% for other.

The same methods can be used to describe different types of distributions for other variables in the dataset and for variables of your choice.

3.5   Temporal (Time) Distribution

As the term suggests, temporal or time distribution describes the trend of a medical, health, or behavioral outcome measure over time. Since two variables, one variable of interest (i.e., a medical, health, or behavioral problem) and another variable of time are needed, temporal distribution is also bivariate. Depending on the purpose and data, the unit of time measurement can be very short, such as a minute, hour, day, week, and month or be very long, such as a year, every 5 years, and decades. To examine historical and stable trends, longer time units can be used, such as a year, 5-years, and 10-years; to examine current and rapidly changing events, shorter time units are more relevant, such as minutes, hours, and days.

Temporal or time distribution is relatively simpler than population distribution since time is one-dimensional, while populations are multi-dimensional. Two methods commonly used in describing time trends are: tabulation and line graphs. Tabulating a set of medical, health, or behavioral problems by year is often the first step toward time trend analysis. With tabulated data, line graphs can be generated to provide a visual presentation. We will introduce the two methods using life expectancy of the US population.

3.5.1 Historical Trends in Life Expectancy at Birth for US Population

Overall health status of a population and historical trends of the status provide the first and most fundamental knowledge for all people in the medical and health professions. Such information is particularly important for planners and decision makers at the state, national, and global levels to grasp the overall condition, to make public health diagnoses, and to form plans and policies and to make decisions. Many indicators are used to describe health status at the population level. Typical examples include total deaths and deaths by leading causes (such as cancer, heart diseases, diabetes, and suicide), infant and child mortality, maternal mortality, crude mortality rate, age-standardized mortality rate, and life expectancy at birth.

Among various indicators, life expectancy is used most often in both academia and the mass media to describe the current status and historical trends of the health of a population. Life expectancy is computed by exposing a standard population of 100,000 at birth to the observed age-specific mortality rates from birth to the highest ages of a population. Life expectancy estimated using this method is thus not biased by age composition of a study population, and is ideal for describing long-term trends, which compares health status over time for a population in the same state or country. As such, life expectation is also ideal for comparison of health status across population subgroups within a country and health status across multiple countries in the globe.

3.5.2 Data Sources

Table 3.1 from Sect. 3.1 at the beginning of this chapter summarizes the life expectancy at birth for the US population overall, by sex, and by White-Black race from 1900–02 to 2009–2011 (Arias et al. 2020). Results in the table show a substantial increase in life expectancy for the US population since 1900–02. Overall, the US population in the 2010s lived approximately 30 years longer compared to 100 years prior (29.36 = 78.60–49.24). Further, the improvement was much more for Blacks (41.19 = 74.99–33.80) than for Whites (29.24 = 78.88–49.64), and more for females (80.98–50.70 = 30.28) than for males (76.13–47.88 = 28.25). Despite the great achievement in population health, there are large differences in life expectancy up to 2000–2011.

3.5.3 Visualization with a SAS Program

Despite detailed information in Table 3.1, it is not easy to gain a comprehensive understanding of the time trends and gender/racial differences with so many numbers as shown in a table. SAS Program 3.7 demonstrates the method to generate a line chart for a quick and more wholesome understanding of the health status of the US population during this long period of time.

The program consists of three parts. Part 1 is the so-called "data step" with the command **DATA** A to create a new dataset; the command INPUT YEAR $ TOTAL MALE FEMALE WHITE BLACK instructs the program to read the data in the specified order ($ following YEAR indicates this is a character not a numerical variable); and DATALINES prepares to add original data from Table 3.1 (marked in yellow).

Part 2 is used to check if the dataset A is created correctly. Other SAS functions can also be used to check data, such as **PROC FREQ** DATA = A; **RUN; PROC PRINT** DATA = A (OBS=10); **RUN;**

Part 3 is for plotting by calling SAS Procedure **PROC SGPLOT**. Several functions are illustrated, including labeling th e axis, suppressing the axis label, and adding text to figure (see Fig. 3.9).

```
*************************************************************************
SAS PROGRAM 3.7 TRENDS OF LIFE EXPECTANCY OF US POPULATION
*************************************************************************;
* 1 INPUT DATA;
DATA A; INPUT YEAR $ TOTAL MALE FEMALE WHITE BLACK;
DATALINES;
1900-02     49.24  47.88  50.70  49.64  33.80
1909-11     51.49  49.86  53.24  51.90  35.87
1919-21     56.40  55.50  57.40  57.42  47.03
1929-31     59.20  57.71  60.90  60.86  48.53
1939-41     63.62  61.60  65.89  64.92  53.85
1949-51     68.07  65.47  70.96  69.02  60.73
1959-61     69.89  66.80  73.24  70.73  63.91
1969-71     70.75  67.04  74.64  71.62  64.11
1979-81     73.88  70.11  77.62  74.53  68.52
1989-91     75.37  71.83  78.81  76.13  69.19
1999-01     76.86  74.13  79.47  77.43  71.81
2009-11     78.60  76.13  80.98  78.88  74.99
;
RUN;
* 2 CHECK DATA;    PROC CONTENTS; RUN;
* 3 DRAW LINE CHART WITH PROC SGPLOT;
PROC SGPLOT DATA = A;
SERIES X = YEAR Y = TOTAL/MARKERS;*HIGHLIGHT TOTAL WITH A MARKER;
SERIES X = YEAR Y = MALE;
SERIES X = YEAR Y = FEMALE;
SERIES X = YEAR Y = WHITE;
SERIES X = YEAR Y = BLACK;
YAXIS LABEL   = 'Life expectancy (years old)';
XAXIS DISPLAY = (NOLABEL);        * REMOVE X-AXIS LABEL;
INSET 'Temporal distribution study'/ POSITION = BOTTOMRIGHT BORDER;
RUN;
*************************************************************************
```

Compared to data in Table 3.1, Fig. 3.9 delivers a much clearer picture about the achievements in health status of the US population overall and by gender and race over a 110-year period. The improvement in health status over this long period is not homogenous but varied with more rapid improvement before the 1950s, slowed down from 1950 to 1970, followed with a sudden increase during 1970–80.

Although females lived longer than males over this long period, the gender difference also varied much over time with an increasing difference up to 1979–81 before it started to narrow. The life expectancy of Whites is close to the

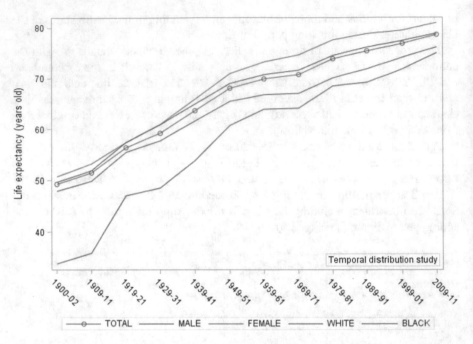

Fig. 3.9 Trends in life expectancy (years) of US population, 1900–2011

national average while the life expectancy for Blacks, although started as 15.44 years lower than White, increased rapidly to catch up the national average of males with several rapid increasing periods, particularly between 1909–11 and 1919–21.

The same tabulation method in Table 3.1 and SAS Program 3.7 can be used to describe long term trends for many other medical, health, and behavioral problems, such as declines in infectious diseases since the 1900s, the decline in tobacco use since the 1950s, increases in overweight and obesity, and cardiovascular diseases since the 1980s, and increases in suicide since the 1990s in the US.

3.5.4   Short-Term Trends with High Time Resolutions

By changing the time measure from years to days, weeks, and months, the same method described in the previous section can also be used to describe daily, weekly, and monthly trends for urgent medical and health issues, such as daily or weekly incidences, hospitalizations, and deaths from a novel infection such as the SARS-CoV-2 virus; and seasonal variations in respiratory diseases such as pneumonia and influenza.

Short-term trends with high time resolutions are frequently used for surveillance and monitoring in epidemiology. Plotting daily cases over time represents the best examples of this type of descriptive analysis. Description of short-term trends are often conducted using spreadsheets, such as MS Excel. This method is simple and has been widely used in epidemiology. Fig. 3.10 presents daily cases of COVID-19 in China over the first 3 months from December 8th, 2019 to February 21st, 2020 (China CDC 2020). The figure is re-generated using data derived from a published study (China CDC 2020). Several features in the figure are innovative.

First, two related statistics are presented in one figure: the green bars represent the daily confirmed cases based on either the clinical symptoms, viral test results, or both and data for the blue bars are derived by asking individual patients the first time they noticed they had COVID-19 symptoms (onset).

Second, a piece of information hidden in the figure is the latent period – the time from onset to clinical visit. By inspection, we can see the mode of cases (highest frequency) for onset was on January 26 and the mode for confirmed cases was on February 4th. It will take roughly an average of 9 days for a patient to visit a doctor after experiencing their first symptoms.

Lastly, a sub-figure is used to show the early trend of the epidemic when the daily cases were rather few. Information regarding the early trend for a novel infectious disease is very important, and such information will be masked when more cases are detected later on in an epidemic. This complementary method is used often in practice.

Information derived from such short-term time distribution is also essential for surveillance, planning intervention strategies, and evaluating intervention programs.

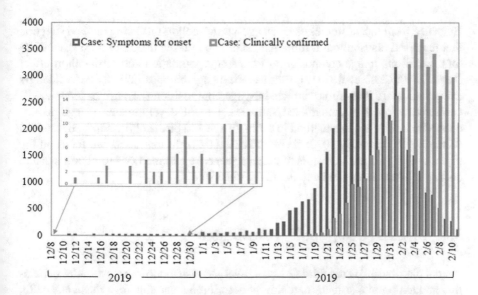

Fig. 3.10 Example of time plot of daily COVID-19 cases in China during the first 3 months. Note: Recreated based on published studies by China CDC (2020)

3.5.5 7-Day Moving Average

7-Day moving average is one method that has been commonly used in surveillance of emerging epidemics. As described early, the daily cases of a new epidemic cannot be determined accurately because of many practical and technical limitations. Therefore, the reported cases by day often fluctuated dramatically. Figure 3.10 is an example, particularly during the early period of the epidemic. More dramatic fluctuations are reported in many studies, particularly studies as seen in daily news report and online. One way to solve the problem is to compute 7-day moving average to better reflect the underlying time trends.

The method is simple. Instead of reporting the number of cases on a daily basis, an average of cases in 7 days is computed and used for the day, including the reporting day, 3 days before, and 3 days after. The formula is slightly modified to compute the moving average for the first 3 days. For day 1, data for 4 days (day 1 plus 3 days after) are available, the moving average will thus be computed by summing up the cases of the first 4 days, divided by 4; For day 2, data for first 5 days are available (1 day before, 3 days after), the moving average will thus be computed by summing up the cases during the first 5 days, then divided by 5; likewise, the moving average for day 3 will be computed by summing up the daily cases for the first 6 days, divided by 6.

The same method is used to compute the moving average for the last 3 days.

3.5.6 Caveats

Evidence from recent studies using an age-period-cohort modeling method suggests that temporal distribution or time trends could be biased due to two important factors: variations in age composition of the study population and birth cohort effect (Chen 2020; Chen et al. 2018). Bias caused by age composition can be avoided by using indicators that are not affected by age composition (i.e., life expectancy) or corrected using age-standardized statistics. Recent developments in age-period-cohort modeling led to a method to estimate age and birth cohort-adjusted statistics (Chen 2020; Din et al. 2020; Yu et al. 2019, 2020). In this book, we focus on the direct use of various indicators to describe time trends; methods to obtain age and cohort-adjusted rates can be found in the cited studies.

3.6 Spatial (Geographic) Distribution

Spatial distribution is the third group of bivariate distribution analyses after population and temporal distribution. It aims at describing a variable on a medical, health, and behavioral outcome over another array - geographical location. Since geographic location can be presented on a plane with two dimensions, geographic mapping presents one of the most widely used techniques for distribution studies. Although spatial distribution can be three-dimensional by adding altitude, in this book we describe the distribution over a two-dimensional space. Therefore, the term geographic distribution and spatial distribution are used interchangeably.

Mapping of a health-related outcome provides the most efficient approach to gain a quick and visual comprehensive understanding of a problem. Before software is available for mapping with a computer, maps used to describe geographic distribution of a health-related outcome are often created manually. Today, rapid advancements in data and software for geographic mapping make it highly efficient to visualize data with a map. Many software packages can produce impressive epidemiological maps, including free open-source software R. In this book, we demonstrate the use of **PROC GMAP** from SAS, a software we have used for a long time in research. We will use COVID-19 data by states in the US to demonstrate how to draw maps with data.

3.6.1 Data Preparation

Two pieces of data are needed to visualize a medical, health, or a behavioral event: map data and the data to be mapped. Map data are the data used to draw the map for the target area. Map data often come with the software for mapping. For example, **PROC GMAP** from SAS provides data for many countries in the world. The GMAP is the tool used to access the data.

Data to be mapped are measures of medical and health problems. These data must be arranged to match the map data. For example, if a disease will be mapped by countries in the world, the data must be organized by countries that exactly match with the map data; and if a disease in the US is mapped by state, the disease data must be organized by states.

3.6.2 SAS Program for Geographic Mapping of COVID-19

To demonstrate the use of **PROC GMAP** in describing geographic distribution of an event, the US COVID-19 cases, up to July 31, 2020 are used. Four indicators are mapped: total count, p rate, g rate, and pg rate. Of the four indicators, g rate and pg rate are derived based on the newly developed measures for epidemiology (Chen et al. 2020), and the computing methods are included in SAS Program 3.8). With the data, SAS Program 3.8 demonstrate the method for geographic mapping, starting with data processing.

```
**********************************************************************************
SAS PROGRAM 3.8 GEOGRAPHIC DISTRIBUTION USING PROC GMAP, US DATA
TOTAL COVID-19 CASES BY STATE UP TO JULY 31, 2020; 2019 POPULATION IN 1000
GEOGRAPHIC AREA IN SQUARE KM FOR INDIVIDUAL STATES
**********************************************************************************;
** CREATE A DATASET TO HOLD THE ORIGINAL DATA;
*  READ IN DATA: STATE NAME, COVID CASES, POPULATON AREA;
DATA A; INPUT ST $ COVID POP AREA;
* CREATE STANDARD ID FOR MAPPING USING THE INPUTED STATE NAME;
STATE = STFIPS(ST);
* COMPUTER P RATE;
PRATE=COVID/POP;
* COMPUTER G RATE;
GRATE=(COVID/AREA)*1000;
* COMPUTER PG RATE;
PGRATE = (COVID /(POP * AREA))* 10000;

** ORGINAL DATA FOR SAS PROGRAM TO READ;
DATALINES;
AL      87867           4903            135767
AK      2990            732             1723337
AZ      174010          7279            295234
AR      42511           3018            137732
CA      493588          39512           423967
CO      46809           5759            269601
CT      49810           3565            14357
DE      14877           974             6446
DC      12126           706             177
FL      465030          21478           170312
GA      186352          10617           153910
HI      1989            1416            28313
ID      20721           1787            216443
IL      180118          12672           149995
IN      66154           6732            94326
IA      44582           3155            145746
KS      27812           2913            213100
KY      30151           4468            104656
LA      116280          4649            135659
ME      3937            1344            91633
MD      89365           6046            32131
MA      117612          6949            27336
MI      90574           9987            250487
MN      55188           5640            225163
MS      59881           2976            125438
MO      50323           6137            180540
MT      3965            1069            380831
NE      26211           1934            200330
NV      48312           3080            286380
NH      6583            1340            24214
NJ      181660          8882            22591
NM      20600           2097            314917
NY      416633          19454           141297
NC      122148          10488           139391
ND      6602            762             183108
OH      91159           11689           116098
OK      39105           3957            181037
OR      18493           4218            254799
PA      112936          12802           119280
RI      19022           1059            4001
SC      89016           5149            82933
SD      8764            885             199729
```

```
TN      105959      6833        109153
TX      420946      28996       695662
UT      40797       3206        219882
VT      1414        624         24906
VA      90801       8536        110787
WA      55803       7615        184661
WV      6642        1792        62756
WI      56934       5822        169635
WY      2726        579         253335
;
RUN;

** DRAW MAP FOR TOTAL COVID CASES BY STATE USING DATA A;
PROC GMAP MAP=MAPS.US DATA = A ALL;
* TELL SAS PROGRAM STATE IS THE UNIT FOR MAPPING;
ID STATE;
* TELL THE PROGRAM TO DRAW CHORO MAP WITH COVID DATA;
CHORO COVID;        * MAP ON COVID COUNT*;
RUN; QUIT;

*************************************************************
REPLACE COVID WITH PRATE, GRATE, AND PGRATE FOR THE
REMAINING 3 INDICATORS
*************************************************************;
```

3.6.3   Mapping Results and Interpretation

Figure 3.11 presents the mapping results using SAS Program 3.8. With official US data, of the four maps, Fig. 3.11a presents the total count of COVID-19 cases up to July 30, 2020. States with more cases are a darker blue while states with fewer cases are a lighter blue. Information in this map indicates states with more cases (darker blue) need to arrange more resources for COVID-19 treatment than states with less cases (lighter blue).

Figure 3.11b presents p rates of COVID-19 for all US states. A p rate is the ratio of total COVID-19 cases over a 100,000 population. It removed the impact of population size that differs across states, and thus p rate provides a measure of COVID-19 risk across status. As a piece of information for public health diagnosis: After the population size id is considered, the states colored with a darker blue are more problematic than those colored with a lighter blue.

As a new indicator in epidemiology, Fig. 3.11c presents g rates of COVID-19 by states in the US. G rate for a state is the ratio of total COVID-19 cases over the total area of a state, and it provides a measure of *case density*. People living in high density of COVID-19 cases are more likely to be infected than people living in low density of COVID-19 cases. Like p rates that adjust for population size, g rates consider the difference of geographic area across states to assess risk of infection from COVID-19. As a piece of information for public health diagnosis: After geographic size is considered, states colored with darker blue are riskier for COVID-19 spreading than states colored with lighter blue.

As a natural extension of the previous two indicators, Fig. 3.11d presents pg rates that provides a measure of COVID-19 spread considering both population and geographic area. It is thus the least biased measure of the risk of COVID-19 spread. Based on Fig. 3.11d, US states are grouped in to two high-risk regions divided by a

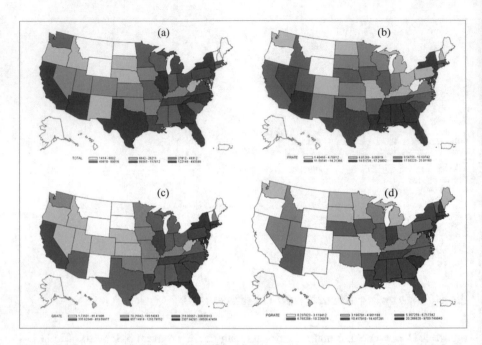

Fig. 3.11 Geographic distribution of COVID-19 cases in the US with four different indicators: Total count (**a**), population-based P rate (**b**), geographic area-based G rate (**c**) and both population and geographic area-based PG rate (**d**). These four measures form a 4D indicator system for descriptive epidemiology.

band of 5 low-risk states in the middle (Montana, Wyoming, Colorado, New Mexico, and Texas) and three low risk states on the west (Alaska, Oregon, and California). Information provided by PG rate is best among all four measures for public health diagnosis about the risk of COVID-19 spread in the US. Overall, the 4D indicator system provides the most comprehensive information to describe the characteristics of an medical, health and behavior problems in a popoulation.

3.6.4 Applications of the Geographic Mapping Method

The SAS **PROC GMAP** introduced above can be used to map many other medical, health, and behavioral problems in the US. In addition to incidence, deaths and mortality rates can be mapped for various types of diseases and health risk behaviors. **PROC GMAP** in SAS Program 3.8 can be revised to map county data for individual states and model country data across the globe (Yu 2020).

3.7   Utilities of Descriptive Epidemiology

It is relatively easier to conduct descriptive analyses, but many of us are not fully aware of the significance of information derived from descriptive epidemiology. Based on the information covered in this chapter, descriptive epidemiology can be used to reveal underlying time trends, detect high-risk populations, and identify hot geographic spots with increased disease risks. We will discuss three significant utilities of such information in epidemiology: (i) support public health diagnosis to prioritize, plan, and make decisions; (ii) inform etiological research; and (iii) evaluate public health policies and regulations.

3.7.1   Make Public Health Diagnosis, Support Prioritizing, Planning, and Decision-Making

Descriptive analysis is used to provide information on a medical, health, or behavioral problem over time, across population subgroups and different geographic areas. Data on population distribution is essential to make a *public health diagnosis* with a detected at-risk population for precision intervention; data on spatial or geographic distribution is a direct measure of hotspots to prioritize strategies and optimize allocation of limited resources for prevention and treatment; and data on time trends or temporal distribution of the past can also inform current work and plans for future.

A typical example is the report of daily cases of the COVID-19 pandemic. Descriptive data of the epidemic can be used to assess the condition of a neighborhood, community, city, county, state, country, and even the whole world. With such data, public health leaders and epidemiologists can make public health diagnoses about the problem. In addition to assessing an overall health condition, public health diagnosis can be made by subgroups of age, gender, and race/ethnicity. For example, the total number of cases can be used to assess the need for hospital beds and health professionals to treat the infection; countries and places with more cases and quicker increases in cases are hotspots that need extra attention; subgroups with disproportionately higher rates of infection consist of the high-risk populations to be prioritized for prevention; changes in the daily cases in the past inform whether the pandemic is getting worse or better in order to take proactive actions to curb the pandemic.

3.7.2   Inform Etiological Research

As discussed at the beginning of this chapter, descriptive study is often the first step to identify influential factors of a disease or health behavior problem. This is particularly true for studying infectious diseases, particularly diseases caused by new pathogens. When knowledge is limited, the very first step is to assess the distribution of the diseases in a population by age, race, and family history, distribution across different geographic regions and changes over time. Information derived from such descriptive studies will give clues for in-depth research. Modern infectious disease epidemiology was and has been inspired by the distribution study of cholera in London, including today's studies of the COVID-19 pandemic caused by the novel SARS-Cov-2 virus.

Descriptive studies are also important for etiological studies of chronic diseases. For example, it has been widely accepted that high testosterone is a risk factor for prostate cancer, based the Nobel Prize winning research conducted in the 1960s (Huggins and Hodges 1941), and is supported by the persistent effect of testosterone deprivation therapy. However, a study of the age distribution indicates that the risk of prostate cancer diagnosis peaks at around 65–75 years of age when testosterone levels become very low. Inspired by this descriptive information, a new theory of age-related testosterone decline has been proposed and supported with empirical data (Xu et al. 2015). Based on this new line of theory and data, it is not the higher levels of, but quicker declines in testosterone than normal aging that puts men at risk for prostate cancer (Wang et al. 2017).

3.7.3   Assist in Public Health Policy Evaluation

Descriptive methods can be used to evaluate massive disease control and prevention measures at the population level. Different from randomized controlled trials, no comparison group is used for public health policies and regulations to control and/or prevent a disease or promote health at the population level. In this case, descriptive epidemiology presents as an option. For example, to assess the effect of national tobacco control in the US, the Surgeon General has used the trends in the annual tobacco sales and prevalence rates of cigarette smoking as the primary measure in their report to the nation (DHHS 2014). The CDC used changes in the prevalence of alcohol in adolescents and young adults to demonstrate if the establishment and enforcement of legal drinking age of 21 reduced the number of underage drinking among US youth (Carpenter and Dobkin 2011). Although there might be no control group, a declining trend consistently associated with a public health policy and/or regulation evinces the effect of the intervention.

3.8   Practice

3.8.1   Data Processing and Statistical Analysis

1. Practice data processing and coding using SAS Program 3.1 to see if you can get the right data and code them as you want. Practice adding new variables to an existing dataset using SAS Program 3.4.
2. Practice the univariate analysis for both continuous and categorical variables using SAS Program 3.2. Find the categorical health outcome variable and conduct univariate distribution analysis.
3. Practice bivariate distribution analysis using SAS Program 3.3 covered in the text and analyze other variables of your own choice.
4. Practice distribution analysis by population, time, and geographic region using SAS Programs 3.4–3.8.
5. Practice distribution analysis using other software, such as MS excel and free software R.
6. Find data from published studies or governmental resources (i.e., CDC, World Bank, WHO) to practice population, time, and geographic distribution analysis using SAS and other software, such as MS excel and R.

3.8.2   Work on Your Own Study Project

1. Add variables needed for your own project to the dataset **DATCH3** and check data quality.
2. Code/recode/rename variables to increase the efficiency for data analysis; and conduct distribution analysis for your project and update your results.
3. Update Table 3.1 (Table 1 of your study) to include the variables you add; you may also remove variables you selected first or revise them from the analysis you conducted now using information from the analysis. Be advised, Table 3.1 often consists of two parts, part 1: demographic variables and part 2: outcome variables. Often more than one variable can be presented for one type of outcome. All variables are listed in three columns: male, female, and total.
4. This is also the time for you to change the research topic you previously selected if needed, based on your knowledge about the data and the descriptive analysis results.

3.8.3   Study Questions

1. Descriptive epidemiology uses both qualitative (using words) and quantitative methods. Please briefly discuss the strengths and weakness of these two approaches.
2. Select a disease (i.e., COVID-19, tuberculosis, breast cancer) of a country or state or city and try to give a public health diagnosis using the relevant data and univariate/bivariate descriptive analysis.
3. How can information from descriptive analysis be used to make a public health diagnosis, plans and decisions?
4. One task of epidemiology is to examine the distribution of a medical, health, or behavioral issue in a population across geographic area and time. Why is the distribution of determinants and risk factors not the focus of epidemiology?
5. What are the four indicators used in geographic mapping? Which of the four indicators provides the best information about overall disease risk considering both population size and geographic area?
6. Discuss the significance of knowledge gained from quantitative descriptive epidemiology in terms of your research and career development.

References

Arias, E., Minino, A., Curtin, S., Tejada-Vera, B.: U.S. decennial life tables for 2009-2011, United States life tables. In: National Vital Statistics Reports, vol. 69. National Center for Health Statistics, Hyattsville (2020)

Carpenter, C., Dobkin, C.: The minimum legal drinking age and public health. J. Econ. Perspect. **25**(2), 133–156 (2011)

Chen, X., Sun, Y., Yu, B., Gao, G., Wang, P.: Historical trends in suicide risk for the residents of mainland China: APC modeling of the archived national suicide mortality rates during 1987-2012. Soc. Psychiatry Psychiatr. Epidemiol. **54**(1), 99–110 (2018)

Chen, X., Yu, B., Chen, D.: A 4D system of count, p rate, g rate and pg rate for epidemiology and global health. In: Chen, X., Chen, D. (eds.) Statistical Methods for Global Health and Epidemiology, pp. 201–218. Springer (2020)

Chen, X.: Historical trends in mortality risk over 100-year period in China with recent data: an innovative application of age-period-cohort modeling. In: Chen, X., Chen, D. (eds.) Statistical Methods for Global Health and Epidemiology, pp. 219–242. Springer (2020)

China CDC Novel Coronavirus Pneumonia Emergency Response Epidemiology Team.: Vital Surveillance: The epidemiological characteristics of an outbreak of 2019 novel coronavirus disease (COVID-19) – China, 2020/China CDC Weekly. No. 8, pp. 1–10 2020

Din, Y., Chen, X., Zhang, Q., Liu, Q.: Historical trends in breast cancer among women in China from age-period-cohort modeling of the 1990-2015 breast cancer mortality data. BMC Public Health. **20**, 1280 (2020). https://doi.org/10.1186/s12889-020-09375-0

Doll, R., Hill, A.B.: Smoking and carcinoma of the lung; preliminary report. Br. Med. J. **2**(4682), 739–748 (1950)

Huggins, C., Hodges, C.V.: Studies on prostate cancer I. The effect of castration, of estrogen and of androgen injection on serum phosphates in metastatic carcinoma of the prostate. J. Urol. **167**(2, part 2), 948–951 (1941)

Snow, J.: On the origin of the recent outbreak of cholera at west ham. Br. Med. J. **1**(45), 934–935 (1857)

U.S. Department of Health and Human Services (DHHS): The Health Consequences of Smoking—50 Years of Progress: A Report of the Surgeon General. DHHS, Centers for Disease Control and Prevention, National Center for Chronic Disease Prevention and Health Promotion, Office on Smoking and Health, Atlanta (2014)

Wang, K., Chen, X., Bird, V.Y., Herke, T.A., Manini, T.M., Prosperi, M.: Association between age-related reductions in testosterone and risk of prostate cancer – an analysis of patients' data with prostate diseases. Int. J. Cancer. **141**, 1783–1793 (2017)

Xu, X., Chen, X., Hu, H., Dailey, A.B., Taylor, B.D.: Current opinion on the role of testosterone in the development of prostate cancer: a dynamic model. BMC Cancer. **15**, 806 (2015). https://doi.org/10.1186/s12885-015-1833-5

Yu, B., Chen, X.: Age and birth cohort-adjusted rates of suicide mortality among US male and female youths aged 10-19 years from 1999 to 2017. JAMA Netw. Open. **2**(9), e1911383 (2019). https://doi.org/10.1001/jamanetworkopen.2019.11383

Yu, B., Chen, X.: Age patterns of suicide with different methods for US whites: APC modelling analysis of the 1999-2017 national data. Epidemiol. Psychiatr. Sci. **29**, e180 (2020)

Yu, B.: Geographic mapping for global health research. In: Chen, X., Chen, D. (eds.) Statistical Methods for Global Health and Epidemiology, pp. 179–200. Springer (2020)

Chapter 4
Causal Exploration with Bivariate Analysis

Well begun is half done.

Etiological studies account for a major part of medical, health, and behavioral research. A solid investigation of the etiology of a problem often starts with bivariate analysis to explore if a proposed X ~ Y relationship is supported by data. If yes, further research will be planned to confirm the relationship by considering covariates and confounders.

Etiology, or aetiology, is derived from the ancient Greek words, *aitiología*, and refers to the study of causation, origination, or simple reason for something. Modern etiological research for medicine and public health started with infectious diseases and is characterized by well-developed research design, quality data collection and processing, and advanced quantitative analysis.

In this chapter, we start with an introduction to causal relationships, followed by discussions on causes and influential factors, outcome variables, variable selection, and bivariate analyses. In addition to theoretical discussion, various methods for bivariate analysis will be introduced using real data. Skills to interpret the analytical results will also be covered.

4.1 Importance of Bivariate Analysis of an X ~ Y Relationship

Etiological or causal inference research starts with a hypothetical X ~ Y relationship. It is rather hard if not impossible to ascertain if a hypothetical relationship is worth a full-scale investigation given the complexity of a closely connected real world, insufficient knowledge basis, and limitations of our research capability.

© The Author(s), under exclusive license to Springer Nature Switzerland AG 2021
X. Chen, *Quantitative Epidemiology*, Emerging Topics in Statistics and
Biostatistics, https://doi.org/10.1007/978-3-030-83852-2_4

4.1.1 Hypothetic Relations

Forming a hypothetic X ~ Y relation is a key step for quantitative epidemiological research studies. However, few researchers have ever thought what a hypothetic X ~ Y relation is. For example, in cancer research, tobacco smoking as X is often hypothesized to be associated with lung cancer as Y. Although this conceptualization could be formed through strict theoretical derivation, supported by data in the literature or from preliminary studies, but we do not know how and to what extent does this hypothetic X ~ Y relation reflect the smoking-lung cancer relationship in the real world?

No matter how an X ~ Y relation is formed and used in research, we have to admit that any hypothetic relation is simply a small part of the complex network relationship in the real world. As Fig. 4.1 shows, when we plan to use an influential factor X and an outcome Y to test a X ~ Y relation in a study, this X ~ Y relation is simply what we framed and believe that is one of many such relations within a domain in the broad universe.

Although there is a lack of confusion regarding the domain for epidemiology, since health, diseases, and behaviors are our targets of research; it is rather complex with regard to an X ~ Y relation we hypothesized for further research. When zooming into a focus area of interest within the domain, the relation soon becomes complex.

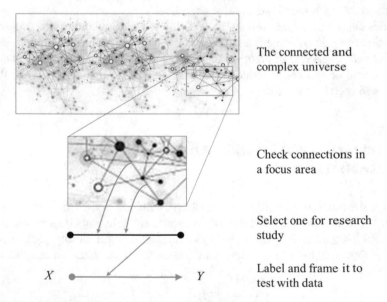

The connected and complex universe

Check connections in a focus area

Select one for research study

Label and frame it to test with data

Fig. 4.1 An epidemiological study targeting only one or two related causal paths from a focus area in the complex, multilevel and mega causal network within the universe

4.1.2   Key Points to Framing an X ~ Y Relation

When framing an X ~ Y relation, the first key step is to determine which is X and which is Y. With adequate knowledge, this may not be an issue. For example, it is well-known that exposure to stress is a X for heart disease Y; and it is also known that suffering from heart disease can also be X, increasing risk for stress Y. However, it will be very challenging to determine which is X and which is Y when knowledge is lacking; while research would no longer be needed if we have all the knowledge about the X and Y.

The second key step is to assess the distance between X and Y or closeness of a selected X ~ Y relation. Let us use the same stress and heart disease relationship above as an example. There might be many steps from exposure to stress to heart disease, including damages to endoepithelial cells in the walls of arteries, changes in the immune system and related infection, increases in blood pressure, accumulation of damages, and damage repairements. The longer the distance between X and Y, the more challenging it is to assess an X ~ Y relation.

The third key step is the measurement of X (with reference to Chap. 2). For tobacco exposure, both self-reported data on smoking behavior and biomarkers of nicotine exposure can be used. Self-reported data can measure years of smoking, frequency and amount of smoking, and even changes in smoking behavior. Biomarkers (i.e., nicotine metabolites cotinine and hydroxycotinine) provide objective measures. However, biomarkers reflect only recent exposure; and such measures are also subject to large variations in individuals with differences in toxicant metabolism capacity.

Likewise, the fourth key step is measurement of Y. For any disease or unhealthy risk behavior, a spectrum of measures can be used, including occurrence, progression, response to treatment, and prognosis. An X related to the occurrence of Y may not be associated with its progression. This phenomenon is rather common in chronic and non-infectious diseases. For example, exposure to carcinogens is an X of cancer occurrence, but the progress and prognosis of many cancers are not due to the same X but many other factors.

4.2   Causes, Risk, Protective, and Promotional Factors Versus Influential Factors

In epidemiology, cause, risk factor, protective factor, promotional factor, and influential factor are five of the most commonly used terms. Contemporary understanding of the term cause of a disease stemmed from infectious disease research. In examining infectious diseases, the goal is to identify the pathogenic organism(s) that causes a disease. Koch's Postulates for causal inference are considered as the milestone achievement in causal relationship research. However, this causal framework is inadequate to address non-infectious diseases. For example, tobacco use is associated with lung cancer in almost all reported studies, but not all lung cancer patients are smokers. New terms such as influential factors, including risk factors, protective factors, and promotional factors are proposed to facilitate research and communication.

4.2.1   Causes in Infectious Diseases and Koch's Postulates

The concept *cause of a disease* was established during the 18th and 19th centuries when infectious diseases were dominant. The high mortality of infectious diseases, such cholera and plague, encouraged scientists, particularly pathologists and biologists, to search for microorganisms as the cause of these diseases. A milestone achievement was the establishment of four guiding principles by Dr. Robert H. Koch, known as Koch's Postulates. To demonstrate if a microorganism is the cause of a disease, it must satisfy the following four conditions:

1. A large number of the microorganisms must be present in the person who suffers from the disease but not found in a person without the disease (first approval – direct evidence);
2. The microorganism must be isolated from a diseased person and grow in pure culture (second approval – confirm the evidence);
3. The cultured microorganism should cause the same disease after introduced into a host (often an animal) without the disease (third approval – repeatability);
4. The microorganism can be isolated from the incubated experimental host and it must be identical to the original microorganism (last approval – further confirm the evidence).

Koch's Postulates have been widely used in infectious disease research and continue to be used today. Figure 4.2 presents eight typical pathogenic bacteria and viruses identified as the biological causes of the corresponding diseases, including cholera, typhoid fever, pneumonia, HIV, Ebola, Polio, hepatitis C, and COVID-19.

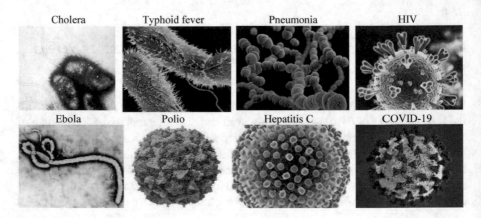

Fig. 4.2 Bacteria and viruses for eight common infectious diseases. (Source: CDC website)

4.2.2   Necessary and Sufficient Causes

Koch's postulates are challenged even in studying causal relationships for infectious diseases. Take COVID-19 as an example. Following Koch's postulates, the virus SARS-Cov-2 that causes COVID-19 can be isolated; the isolated virus can be successfully cultured; and the isolated virus can cause COVID-19 in animal models. However, a large proportion of carriers who have the pathogen in their body do not show any symptoms (Nishiura et al. 2020). This evidence indicates that infection of a pathogen is *insufficient* to cause a disease.

The challenge stimulates re-conceptualization of the causal logic to distinguish the essential cause from sufficient cause. As Fig. 4.3 shows, Koch's causal relationship (top panel) is expanded to include other factors that may interact with a pathogen to cause a disease (bottom panel). Conceptually, *essential cause is the cause without which the consequence cannot occur; but it will not definitely ensure the consequence.*

Applying the concept to an infectious disease, the pathogen for a disease is the essential cause since the disease will never occur if no pathogen invades the person. No streptococcus pneumoniae, no pneumonia; no HIV virus, no HIV/AIDS; and no SARS-Cov-2, no COVID-19. However, with the infection of a pathogen, a person may not develop the disease. Other factors must be present to complete the infection process so that it becomes a disease. These other factors are collectively named as sufficient cause.

A sufficient cause is thus conceptually the factor collection that is needed to generate the consequence given the essential cause. Using COVID-19 again as an example, the novel virus SARS-Cov-2 is a necessary cause since an individual will never suffer from the disease if not infected by the virus. However, whether infection with SARS-Cov-2 will lead to the disease depends on many other factors – the sufficient causes. Sufficient causes are often multiple, including factors related to a pathogen itself; intrapersonal factors (e.g., demographic, nutrition, pre-existing conditions) and exposure to the pathogen (i.e., frequency and duration).

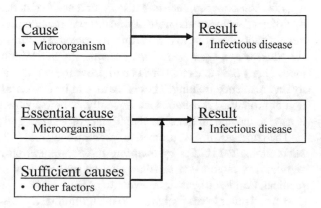

Fig. 4.3 Cause (top), essential cause, and sufficient causes (bottom) of an infectious disease

4.2.3 Risk Factors

Tremendous success in controlling and preventing infectious diseases promoted the well-known epidemiologic transition in the last century (Omran 2005). Koch's postulates are further challenged when used as guidance to investigate (1) non-infectious diseases, such as high blood pressure, heart diseases, stroke, and cancer; (2) mental health problems such as anxiety, stress, depression, and suicide; and (3) behavior-related issues, such as eating disorders, being overweight, sedentary lifestyles, alcohol and tobacco use, and use of illicit drugs.

In comparison to infectious diseases, no single essential cause can be determined for a non-infectious disease or a health-related behavior. For example, smoking is a strong risk factor for many diseases such as cardiovascular diseases and cancer; but many smokers do not suffer from these diseases. Receiving education shows consistent protective effects against almost all diseases and health risk behaviors; but the same diseases and health risk behaviors can be found among people with a college or graduate degree and among professors who educate the educated. Exercise has been proven to be protective for almost all diseases, too; but individuals who specialized in exercise as professions are not immune from both chronic and infectious diseases.

Since it is difficult to determine the essential cause of a non-infectious disease and a health-related behavior, a more general concept is used – risk factor. Conceptually, a *risk factor is any factor that is associated with increased likelihood (risk) of a negative health consequence*. Applying the concept in epidemiology, a risk factor is any factor that is associated with increased risk of a disease, a health status, or a health-related risk behavior. Applying this principle to infectious diseases, the pathogen SARS-Cov-2 is also a risk factor for COVIND-19.

4.2.4 Influential Factors for Risks, Protections, and Promotions

Since the concept of risk is conceived to describe factors that increase chances for a negative consequence, such as a disease or a health risk behavior, more general terms have been developed and used. Typical terms include protective factors and promotional factors. Relative to risk factors, a *protective factor* is the *factor that can reduce the chances of a negative health consequence*. In addition to protection, attention is increasingly paid to factors that can improve the health status, such as physical activity and resilience training. These factors can be termed as factors *for* health promotion or promotional factors. Consequently, a more abstractive term *influential factor* is used to include all three, including risk, protective, and promotional factors.

The concepts of risk, protective, promotional, and influential factors have facilitated etiological studies by *avoiding the determination of essential and* sufficient causes. Any factors can be influential as long as they may alter the chance for a medical, health, or behavioral event to occur.

Several other terms equivalent to the influential factors include *independent variable*, *explanatory variable* or *factor*, *predictor* or *predictor* variable. These terms provide information of the role of an influential factor in a mathematical equation, since an influential factor X is often put on the right side of an equation to calculate Y that is placed on the left of the equation. It looks like the X is used to predict Y or as an explanation of the changes in Y.

4.3 Selection of an Influential Factor X

In epidemiology, a challenge for many new investigators is to select an influential factor X to address a proposed X ~ Y relation through exploratory bivariate analysis. In Chap. 2 Sect. 2.2, details were provided on the concept of one character measured by multi-variables. In this section, we will provide guidance to help select an X to test a hypothetical X ~ Y relationship.

4.3.1 3D Matrix Framework for Variable Selection

Several lines of studies both in theory and empirical testing have generated a useful knowledge basis that can be used by epidemiologists to locate and select influential factors for research. Typical examples include causal concepts of genome-wide association research (Hu et al. 2018) and epigenetic-wide association research (Paul and Beck 2014) to select genetic variables; concepts of the human exposome in environmental-wide association research (Patel 2018) to select factors related to physical environment; and socioecological models for health behavioral research for social and behavioral factors (Golden and Earp 2012).

Based on the conceptual frameworks in published studies, a three-dimensional matrix framework is introduced to assist in variable selection. This matrix classifies all influential factors into three domains of (i) biophysical, (ii) psycho-mental, and (iii) socio-behavioral, all being assessed at three levels of (i) intrapersonal, (ii) contextual, and (iii) interactional, across the continuous timeline from past to current (Fig. 4.4).

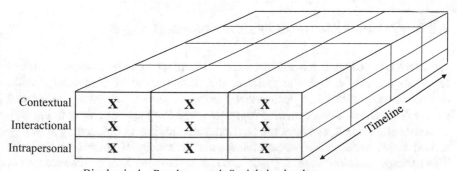

Fig. 4.4 3D Matrix Framework to select influential factors for exploratory analysis

4.3.2   Considering Factors by Domains and Measurement Levels

The 3D Matrix Framework provides guidance to think of intrapersonal factors. For example, when studying DNA and genetic factors, we can consider genes that primarily affect biology and/or physiology, or predominantly link to the psychology, emotion, and/or cognition of social interaction and behaviors. Likewise, when examining contextual factors, we may consider all factors from each of the three domains, including contextual factors that mainly affect the biophysical aspects, such as chemical pollutants, or psycho-mental and/or socio-behavioral aspects, such as social media and information, peer influences, neighborhood safety, social cohesion, and social capital (Chen et al. 2009, 2015).

In addition, the timeline provides another dimension to think of the same factors measured at different points in time, particularly the use of factors measured in the past to predict outcomes assessed in the current for more effective causal inference analysis. With this measurement approach, the reverse impact of the outcome on influential factors is minimized.

It is worth noting that practice is the best approach to develop skills for variable selection and the 3D Matrix Framework is simply a guide for beginners.

4.4   Determination of Outcome Y and Framing an X ~ Y Relation

After an influential factor X, the next step is to determine the outcome variable Y. With knowledge of X's, consequences from exposure to the selected X are outcomes Y. In medical, health, or behavioral research, outcome Y can be assessed at different stages from onset, to development, progression, and prognosis. The impact of exposure to the same X may differ for Y measured at different stages.

4.4.1   Outcome Measures by Developmental Stage

As described in Chap. 2, a health outcome as a character can be assessed from different angles. As an outcome variable, the development of a medical, health, or behavioral problem can be described using a general four-stage conceptual framework – Onset, Development, Progression, and Prognosis as shown in Fig. 4.5.

Although different measures can be used, categorizing an outcome by developmental stages increases the purposefulness and efficiency of quantiative analysis. This conceptualization makes it possible to assess the same X on different stages of a health outcome, better informing our understanding of the problem. This is

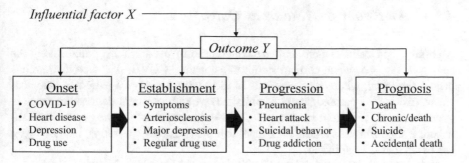

Fig. 4.5 Outcomes by developmental stage of a medical, health, or behavioral problem

because the same infleuntial factor X can have a different effect on the same health problem at different stages.

With outcomes measured by developmental stages, results from such analysis will provide data that is also useful to inform intervention programming. For example, knowledge on factors related to onset will be useful for prevention while knowledge on factors related to progression will be useful for patient treatment to prevent progression.

4.4.2   Onset as Outcome Y

As the name suggests, onset is the mark when a problem first occurs to or first detected in a person. Onset as outcome Y has been used often as an outcome measure in epidemiology. Taking COVID-19 as an example of an infectious disease, as discussed in Chap. 3, the first time when symptoms appear can be used to mark the clinical onset of the disease; and a transition from sero-negative to sero-positive can be considered as the mark of biological onset.

For non-infectious diseases, such as heart diseases and cancer, the onset Y is often determined when the disease is first diagnosed. For example, the age when first diagnosed with hypertension or a heart attack is often used in research to examine onset. In cancer research, in addition to clinical diagnosis, the onset can be determined using the carcinoma in situ (CIS) – detection of a small group of abnormal cells growing in a confined location with no spread to nearby tissue.

The onset Y of mental health problems such as depression, suicidal behavior, and substance use is often measured using self-reported data on age when a person first experienced the negative emotion, the behavior, or engaged in using the substance. Typical examples include age when first started to smoke cigarettes or engaged in binge drinking for the first time in life, age when using illicit drugs for the first time in life, and age when having experienced depressive symptoms for the first time in life.

4.4.3 An Established Status as Outcome Y

An established status of a problem is most commonly used as Y in epidemiology. As shown in Fig. 4.5, when clinical symptoms appear, "COVID-19" as a disease has been established; when atherosclerosis in the heart arteries of a patient is detected, "heart disease" is pathologically established; when a person's depression score is greater or equal to 9 from Beck's scale, "severe depression" for the person is established; if a person uses a drug on a regular basis (i.e., daily, weekly), his/her "drug use behavior" is established.

Relative to onset, an established health outcome Y is relatively stable. Such variables are thus good for etiological studies. With a stable Y, reliable and robust results can be obtained to assess a hypothetic X ~ Y relationship. If the outcome Y is volatile, it is not easy for different studies conducted at different conditions to obtain consistent result. It is critical to know this ahead of time.

4.4.4 Progression and Prognosis as Outcome Y

The remaining two types of outcomes in Fig. 4.5 are progression and prognosis related Ys. These two types of outcome measures are used often in clinical based studies and, no detailed discussion will be provided in this text.

4.4.5 X ~ Y Relations for Infectious and Non-Infectious Diseases

A key to successful bivariate analysis is to test theory-based hypotheses. The conceptual frameworks described in this and the previous two sections are useful to form theory-based X ~ Y relationships. Another issue that needs to be emphasized in etiological research is the distinction between infectious and non-infectious diseases.

With all infectious diseases, the onset, development, treatment, and prognosis are all correlated to *one specific microorganism - pathogen*. For example, the human immunodeficiency virus (HIV) is treated as the cause for onset, progression, AIDS, and death. The more virus, the quicker the onset of infection, the faster progression to AIDS, and the higher the likelihood of death. Therefore, the goal of treatment is to suppress the virus and the goal of prevention is to avoid contact with the virus.

However, this principle cannot be applied in studying many non-infectious and chronic diseases. Figure 4.6 presents the causal linkages between an infectious disease pneumonia (upper part) and chronic disease prostate cancer (lower part). Antibiotics against *S. pneumoniae* can treat the disease, suggesting that *pneumoniae*

Fig. 4.6 Difference in causal relationship between infectious and non-infectious diseases with pneumococcal pneumonia and prostate cancer as examples

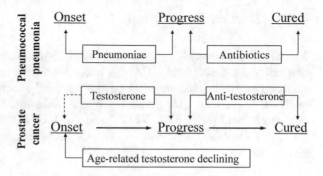

is the cause. In prostate cancer, removal of testosterone can treat the disease (Higgins and Hodges 1941); however, not the level of (dashed line) but the rapid decline in testosterone with age is associated with increased risk of onset of prostate cancer (Wang et al. 2017).

The same principle is applicable to many chronic and non-infectious diseases to conceive an X ~ Y relationship for research, including cancers in many other organs in addition to prostate, cardiovascular diseases, osteoporosis, and Alzheimer's disease, to name a few. In these cases, a different X for a different stage of a medical or health problem should be considered.

4.5 Data Preparation for Bivariate Analysis

After X and Y are determined using the method described in Sect. 4.4, it is now the time to introduce quantitative methods for bivariate analysis with empirical data to explore or test the hypothetic X~Y relation. In the analysis, an X ~ Y relation of tobacco smoking and hypertension is proposed as an example.

4.5.1 Data Sources for Variables

Data for X (smoking measures) and Y (blood pressure measures) are derived from the 2017–2018 NHANES. Building upon dataset **DATCH3** used in Chap. 3, additional data are added, including measured systolic and diastolic pressures (3 repeated measurements). With regard to tobacco smoking, self-reported data for cigarette smoking as well as biomarkers of tobacco exposure are included.

4.5.2 Dataset Preparation

Much has been covered on data processing in Chaps. 2 and 3, including reading and
converting **XPT** data from NHANES into a SAS dataset, selecting, recoding, and
relabeling variables, merging data using SEQN, and selecting subsets of subjects for
analysis. To facilitate data processing, please make sure to download the following
data from NHANES: BPX_J.XPT and SMQ_J.XPT save them in the folder
C:\QUANTLAB\A_DATA\ORIGINAL\. SAS Program 4.1 shows one way to
process the data.

```
**************************************************************************************
* SAS PROGRAM 4.1. DATA PREPARATION FOR BIVARIATE EXPLORATORY ANALYSIS
* A NEW DATASET DATCH4 WILL BE CREATED BY MERGING FOUR TEMP DATASETS INDEXED BY SEQN
**************************************************************************************
** 1 READ DATASET DATCH3 INTO TEMP1 AND CHECK DATA, HBP=REPORTED HIGH BLOOD PRESSURE;
LIBNAME SASDATA "C:\QUANTLAB\A_DATA\";
DATA TEMP1; SET SASDATA.DATCH3;
KEEP AGE GENDER RACE5 EDUCATION MARRIAGE YRSINUS HBP HBPMED SEQN; PROC CONTENTS; RUN;
** 2 CONVERT AND SAVE MEASURED BLOOD PRESSURES FROM BPX_J INTO TEMP2;
LIBNAME XPTDATA XPORT "C:\QUANTLAB\A_DATA\ORIGINAL\BPX_J.XPT" ACCESS=READONLY;
PROC COPY INLIB=XPTDATA OUTLIB=SASDATA; RUN;
DATA TEMP2; SET LIB.BPX_J;
KEEP BPXDI1-BPXDI3 BPXSY1-BPXSY3 SEQN;
PROC CONTENTS; RUN;
** 3 CONVERT AND SAVE SMOKING DATA FROM SMQ_J.XPT INTO TEMP3;
LIBNAME XPTDATA XPORT "C:\QUANTLAB\A_DATA\ORIGINAL\SMQ_J.XPT" ACCESS=READONLY;
PROC COPY INLIB=XPTDATA OUTLIB=SASDATA; RUN;
DATA TEMP3; SET LIB.SMQ_J;
* RENAME, RECODE, AND SELECT VARIABLES FOR USE;
EVERSMK  = SMQ020;
ONSETAGE = SMD030;
SMKNOW   = SMQ040;
SMKDAYS  = SMD641;
SMKNUMS  = SMD650;
LABEL    EVERSMK   = 'EVER SMOKED 100 CIGARETTES IN LIFE 1=Y 2=N',
         ONSETAGE  = 'AGE STARTED SMOKING REGULARLY 0-76 0=NEVER SMOKED REGULARLY',
         SMKNOW    = 'IF SMOKING NOW, 1=EVERY DAY, 2=SOMEDAY 3=NO',
         SMKDAYS   = 'DAYS SMOKED IN THE PAST 30 DAYS 0-30',
         SMKNUMS   = 'AVERAGE # CIGARETTES SMOKED PER DAY 1-60';
KEEP EVERSMK ONSETAGE SMKNOW SMKDAYS SMKNUMS SEQN; PROC CONTENTS; RUN;
** 4 CONVERT SAVE BIOMARKER DATA FOR SMOKING FROM COT_J.XPT INTO TEMP4;
LIBNAME XPTDATA XPORT "C:\QUANTLAB\A_DATA\ORIGINAL\COT_J.XPT" ACCESS=READONLY;
PROC COPY INLIB=XPTDATA OUTLIB=SASDATA; RUN;
DATA TEMP4; SET LIB.COT_J;
COTININE = LBXCOT;
H_COTININE = LBXHCT;
LABEL COTININE = 'COTININE LEVEL IN SERUM >0.015=SMOKING',
      H_COTININE= 'HYDROXYCOTININE IN SERUM >0.015=SMOKING';
KEEP  COTININE H_COTININE SEQN;
PROC CONTENTS; RUN;
** 5. SORT AND COMBINE THE 4 TEMP DATASETS INTO ONE AND SAVE AS DATCH4;
PROC SORT DATA = TEMP1; BY SEQN; RUN;
PROC SORT DATA = TEMP2; BY SEQN; RUN;
PROC SORT DATA = TEMP3; BY SEQN; RUN;
PROC CORT DATA = TEMP4; BY SEQN; RUN;
DATA TEMP; MERGE TEMP1 TEMP2 TEMP3 TEMP4; BY SEQN; RUN;
PROC CONTENTS DATA = TEMP; RUN;    * CHECK BEFORE MAKING THE DATASET PERMANENT;
DATA SASDATA.DATCH4; SET TEMP; PROC CONTENTS; RUN; * CREAT PERMANENT DATCH4;
**************************************************************************************
```

4.5.3 Variables in the New Dataset DATCH4

Figure 4.7 presents the SAS output from the last line of SAS Program 4.1 above, if programmed correctly.

#	Variable	Type	Len	Label
2	AGE	Num	8	AGE IN YEAR,
7	BPXDI1	Num	8	Diastolic: Blood pres (1st rdg) mm Hg
9	BPXDI2	Num	8	Diastolic: Blood pres (2nd rdg) mm Hg
11	BPXDI3	Num	8	Diastolic: Blood pres (3rd rdg) mm Hg
6	BPXSY1	Num	8	Systolic: Blood pres (1st rdg) mm Hg
8	BPXSY2	Num	8	Systolic: Blood pres (2nd rdg) mm Hg
10	BPXSY3	Num	8	Systolic: Blood pres (3rd rdg) mm Hg
17	COTININE	Num	8	COTININE LEVEL IN SERUM >0.015=SMOKING,
3	GENDER	Num	8	1=MALE 2=FEMALE,
5	HBP	Num	8	HIGH BLOOD PRESSURE 1=YES 0 = NO
18	H_COTININE	Num	8	HYDROXYCOTININE IN SERUM >0.015=SMOKING
12	LIFESMK	Num	8	EVER SMOKED 100 CIGARETTES IN ENTIRE LIFE 1=Y 2=N,
13	ONSETAGE	Num	8	AGE STARTED SMOKING REGULALRY 0-76 0=NEVER SMOKED REGULARLY,
4	RACE5	Num	8	1=WHITE 2=BLAKC 3=HISP 4=ASIAN 5=OTHER,
1	SEQN	Num	8	Respondent sequence number
15	SMKDAYS	Num	8	DAYS SMOKED IN THE PAST 30 DAYS 0-30,
14	SMKNOW	Num	8	IF SMOKING NOW, 1=EVERY DAY 2=SOMEDAY 3=NO,
16	SMKNUMS	Num	8	AVERAGE # CIGARETTES SMOKED PER DAY 1-60

Fig. 4.7 Variables in the newly created dataset DATCH4 using SAS Program 4.1

4.6 Exploring Categorical Variables

As an illustration, in this section bivariate analysis will be introduced using a categorical X for smoking measures and binary Y for reported high blood pressure.

4.6.1 Binary Measure of Y – High Blood Pressure

The outcome variable Y is measured using reported high blood pressure (HBP). This variable is based on the response (yes/no) of NHANES' participants to the question: "Have you ever been told by a doctor or other health professional that you had hypertension, also called high blood pressure?" It is a common practice to use self-reported diseases in epidemiology, which is fast, cost-effective, and valid. Findings from the survey data provides important evidence for more in-depth research.

4.6.2 Categorical Measures of X – Cigarette Smoking

Five variables will be used to measure cigarette smoking, including four behavioral measures and one biomarker measure.

1. Lifetime smoking (LIFESMK, binary), this variable is based on the data from the question: "Have you smoked at least 100 cigarettes in your entire life (yes/no)?"
2. Smoking now (SMKNOW, 3-level), this variable is based on the data from the question: "Do you now smoke cigarettes (not at all, some days, everyday)?"
3. Smoking now (SMKNOWBI, binary), created based on the 3-level variable SMKNOW by combining answer options "some days" and "everyday" into one group as smokers.
4. Smoking now (SMKDAYBI), created based on the number of smoking days in the past 30 days (SMKDAYS, 0–30) with data from the question: "On how many of the past 30 days did you smoke a cigarette?" Subjects who smoked at least on one day in the past 30 days were coded as smokers.
5. Smoking now (BIOSMKBI), created using cotinine (ng/ml) in serum. Subjects with cotinine level > 0.015 was coded as smokers.

4.6.3 SAS Program for Data Processing

SAS Program 4.2 presents an example on how to process and recode data to prepare for bivariate analysis and to test the hypothesis that smoking X is related to hypertension Y with X being measured in different ways.

The first part of the program shows how to process data for analysis by reading the newly created dataset DATCH4 into work dataset **A**; excluding subjects with missing data; coding system missingness; code missing due to skips in data collection into meaningful results (i.e., code missing days and average number of cigarettes of smoking as 0 for subjects who did not smoke in their lifetime); creating binary measures; labeling new variables and re-relabeling revised variables.

```
*********************************************************************************
* SAS PROGRAM 4.2 CHECK MISSING DATA AND PREPARE FOR RECODING
*********************************************************************************;
** 1 DATA PROCESSING;
LIBNAME SASDATA "C:\QUANTLAB\A_DATA\";
* READ DATCH4 INTO A WORK DATASET A;
DATA SASDATA.DATCH4; SET LIB.DATCH4;
* INCLUDE 5856 SUBJECTS WITH SMOKING DATA FROM 9027 TOTAL;
IF LIFESMK NE .;
* INCLUDE 5143 SUBJECTS WITH NO MISSING DATA ON HBP;
IF HBP      NE .;
* CODE SYSTEM MISSING AFTER CHECKING WITH PROC FREQ USING SAS PROGRAMS IN CHAPTER 2;
ARRAY MS LIFESMK SMKNOW SMKDAYS SMKNUMS ONSETAGE COTININE H_COTININE;
DO OVER MS; IF MS IN (0 99 777 999) THEN MS = .; END;
* REVERSE CODE SMKNOW FROM 3 TO 0 AS NO, 2 TO 1 AS SOME DAYS, 1 TO 2 AS EVERY DAY;
SMKNOW = 3-SMKNOW;
* RECODE LIFESMK FROM 2 TO 0 FOR NO AND KEEP 1 AS 1 FOR YES;
LIFESMK = 2-LIFESMK;
* RECODE MISSING OF SMOKING NOW AS NOT SMOKING BASED ON LIFETIME SMOKING;
IF LIFESMK EQ 0 AND SMKNOW = . THEN SMKNOW=0;
* RECODE MISSINGOF SMOKING DAYS AS ZERO;
IF LIFESMK EQ 0 AND SMKDAYS = . THEN SMKDAYS = 0;
* RECODE MISSINGOF NUMBER OF CIGARETTES SMOKED PER DAY AS ZERO;
IF LIFESMK EQ 0 AND SMKNUMS = . THEN SMKNUMS = 0;
* CREATE BINARY MEASURE FROM OTHER MEASURES;
IF SMKNOW NE .   THEN SMKNOWBI = (SMKNOW GE 1);
IF SMKDAYS  NE . THEN SMKDAYBI = (SMKDAYS GE 1);
IF COTININE NE . THEN BIOSMKBI = (COTININE GT 0.015);
LABEL LIFESMK  = 'EVER SMOKED 100 CIGARETTES IN LIFETIME 0=NO 1=YES',
      SMKNOW   = '0=NOT AT ALL 1=SOME DAYS 2= EVERYDAY',
      SMKNOWBI = 'IF SMOKING NOW DEFINED USING SMKNOW'
      SMKDAYBI = 'IF SMOKING NOW DEFINED USING DAYS SMOKED IN THE PAST 30 DAYS'
      BIOSMKBI = 'IF SMOKING NOW DEFINED USING BIOMARKER COTININE';
PROC CONTENTS; RUN;
** 2. CHECK IF MISSING ARE CORRECTLY CODED FOR THE VARIABLES TO BE ANALYZED;
PROC FREQ DATA = SASDATA.DATCH4;
TABLES HBP LIFESMK SMKNOW SMKDAYS SMKNUMS ONSETAGE SMKNOWBI SMKDAYBI BIOSMKBI;
RUN;
*********************************************************************************;
```

After completion of the data process, part 2 of SAS Program 4.2 is used to check if the processed data are exactly what we need and to make corrections for any mistakes. SAS Procedure **PROC FREQ** is often used for checking this.

4.6.4   Analytical Method and SAS Program

As depicted in Table 4.1 when both the exposure to influential factor X and outcome Y are categorical, the goal of analysis is to test if the proportions of exposure to X between subjects with [D/(B + D)] and without [C/(A + C)] the disease (outcome Y) are similar or different. If the two proportions are significantly different, exposure to X might be associated with Y.

The model described in Table 4.1 can be extended to include X with more than two levels.

Chi-square statistics are most commonly used to assess the association between two categorical variables. Chi-square tests can be conducted manually. With data processed using SAS Program 4.2 above, SAS Program 4.3 provides an efficient

Table 4.1 Categorical X and Categorical Y

Exposure (X)	Outcome (Y)		
	No disease	Disease	Total
No	A	B	A + D
Yes	C	D	B + C
Total	A + C	B + D	A + B + C + D

approach for such analysis to explore the relationship between different categorical measures of cigarette smoking and self-reported high blood pressure.

```
*******************************************************************************
* SAS PROGRAM 4.3 BIVARIATE ANALYSIS OF DIFFERENT CATEGORICAL MEASURES OF SMOKING;
*******************************************************************************;
* 1 ANALYSIS FOR TOTAL SAMPLE, NOPERCENT AND NOCOL TO SUPPRESS RESULTS NOT NEEDED;
DATA A; SET SASDATA.DATCH4; RUN;
PROC FREQ DATA = A;
TABLES LIFESMK * HBP /CHISQ NOPERCENT NOROW;
TABLES SMKNOWBI* HBP /CHISQ NOPERCENT NOROW;
TABLES SMKDAYBI* HBP /CHISQ NOPERCENT NOROW;
TABLES BIOSMKBI* HBP /CHISQ NOPERCENT NOROW;
TABLES SMKNOW  * HBP /CHISQ NOPERCENT NOROW;
 RUN;
* 2 EXAMPLES OF ANALYSES BY GENDER, CAN BE USED TO TEST BY AGE, RACE...;
PROC FREQ DATA = A;
TABLES BIOSMKBI* HBP /CHISQ NOPERCENT NOROW;
TABLES SMKNOW  * HBP /CHISQ NOPERCENT NOROW;
WHERE GENDER EQ 1;  *(1=MALE, CHANGE 1 TO 2 FOR FEMALE);
RUN;
* 3 THE SAME METHOD IN PART 2 TO ANALYZE BY RACE, AGE GROUP, AND OTHER VARIABLES;
*******************************************************************************;
```

SAS Program 4.3 is nothing new, and we have used it in previous chapters. For better review of the analytical results, two options are added to suppress unnecessary output from SAS, including NOPERCENT to suppress percentages of individual cell counts, and NOROW to suppress row percentages, respectively.

4.6.5 Outcome and Interpretation

Executing Part 1 of SAS Program 4.3 will produce a set of chi-square test results. Figure 4.8 shows a typical SAS output from the SAS program code TABLES LIFESMK * HBP /CHISQ NOPERCENT NOCOL. .

The first part of the output is a cross-table, corresponding to Table 4.1, with A = 2046, B = 959, C = 1227 and D = 902; total = A + B + C + D = 5134 (sample size). Two proportions by columns are already computed with D/(B + D) =48.47%, the proportion of smokers among subjects with HBP; and C/(A + C) = 37.49% the proportion of smokers among subjects without HBP. There were more smokers among subjects with HBP than those without (48.47% vs. 37.49%).

The second part is the statistics to test if the observed 10.98% more smokers (48.47–37.49%) among hypertensive subjects than among non-hypertensive

Fig. 4.8 A Typical SAS
Output by Executing SAS
Program 4.3

Table of LIFESMK by HBP			
LIFESMK(EVER SMOKED 100 CIGARETTES IN LIFETIME 0=NO 1=YES,)	HBP(HIGH BLOOD PRESSURE 1=YES 0 = NO)		
	0	1	Total
0	2046 62.51	959 51.53	3005
1	1227 37.49	902 48.47	2129
Total	3273	1861	5134

Statistics for Table of LIFESMK by HBP

Statistic	DF	Value	Prob
Chi-Square	1	58.9297	<.0001
Likelihood Ratio Chi-Square	1	58.6746	<.0001
Continuity Adj. Chi-Square	1	58.4782	<.0001
Mantel-Haenszel Chi-Square	1	58.9183	<.0001
Phi Coefficient		0.1071	
Contingency Coefficient		0.1065	
Cramer's V		0.1071	

subjects is real or simply due to sampling error. Among all 7 pieces of the results listed in this part of the output, only two are needed for the exploratory analysis: Chi-square value and Prob (probability).

From the results, the computed chi-square value = 58.93 and Prob<.0001. This result indicates that the probability to obtain the same difference of 10.98% between the two comparison groups due to sampling error is less than 1/1000. In another words, the difference is highly more likely to be real than be due to sampling error. Such results give us confidence to conclude that findings from the bivariate exploratory analysis suggest smoking cigarettes is positively associated with high blood pressure. Multivariate analysis should be conducted to verify the results by controlling for covariates and confounders.

Table 4.2 summarizes all results from executing Part 1 of SAS Program 4.3. Several pieces of information can be obtained from these results. Based on the chi-square value and difference in the proportion of smoking, among the five smoking behavior measures, self-reported lifetime smoking would be the best, followed by smoking determined using biomarkers, and reported days of smoking in the past 30 days. The rest are inadequate.

It seems to make sense that lifetime smoking performs better than other measures because it covers information regarding long-term exposure to tobacco, not

Table 4.2 Results from SAS Program 4.2 Part 1: Categorical measures of cigarette smoking

Smoking Behavior Measure	HBP, n (%)		Total	Missing	Chi-square (p-value)
	Yes	No			
Life time smoking (self-report)					
Yes	902 (42.4)	1227 (57.6)	2129	0	58.93(<.001)
No	959 (31.9)	2046 (68.1)	3005		
Current smoking (self-report)					
Yes	351 (18.9)	630 (19.3)	981	0	0.12 (0.734)
No	1510 (81.1)	2643 (80.7)	4153		
Current smoking (smoked in past 30 days)					
Yes	348 (26.6)	620 (23.3)	968	1161	5.45 (0.020)
No	959 (73.4)	2046 (76.7)	3005		
Current smoking (cotinine>0.015)					
Yes	1049 (62.7)	1943 (66.6)	2992	542	7.21 (0.007)
No	625 (37.3)	975 (33.4)	1600		
Current smoking					
Not at all	1510 (80.8)	2643 (80.8)	4153	0	0.41 (0.813)
Some day	70 (4.1)	135 (3.8)	205		
Every day	281 (15.1)	495 (15.1)	776		

Note: Biomarker-determined current smoking (cotinine >0.015 ng/ml)

like others that focus only on the recent exposure to tobacco. The binary measure of current smoking derived from the biomarker cotinine performs only next to self-reported lifetime smoking with $p < 0.01$. Although this biomarker only reflects recent exposure to tobacco, smoking rates determined by this measure are much higher than the self-reported rates of recent smoking, suggesting that there may be substantial underreporting.

If tobacco exposure is associated with hypertension, a dose-response relationship should exist. However, the 3-level measure of reported smoking behavior (not at all, some days, and every day) was not associated with high blood pressure with a Chi-square = 0.41 and p> > 0.05. This is very likely due to underreporting.

Evidence from the bivariate analysis suggests that among all five measures, three could be used for further analysis: lifetime smoking, whether smoked in the past 30 days, and biomarker cotinine-determined current smoking. Of the three, self-reported lifetime smoking contains no missing data while the other two contain a large number of subjects with missing data, which may affect statistical power in studies with small samples.

4.7 Exploring Continuous Measures of X

Several continuous measures for cigarette smoking in the NHANES data make it possible to also explore the use of different measures of cigarette smoking behavior to examine the smoking – hypertension relationship. These measures include days smoked in the past 30 days, average number of cigarettes smoked per day in a typical day in the past 30 days, years of smoking (from age of smoking onset to the age at the survey date), and biomarkers of tobacco exposure (i.e., serum cotinine and hydroxycotinine, ng/ml).

4.7.1 Data Preparation and Distribution of X

Data preparation includes a quality check of existing variables, creation of a new variable, years of smoking, and a data quality check after recoding. SAS Program 4.4 below is an example for data processing.

```
*************************************************************************************
* SAS PROGRAM 4.4 CHECK DATA AND PREPARE FOR ANALYSIS OF CONTINUOUS VARIABLES
*************************************************************************************;
** 1 READ DATCH4 INTO DATASET A (SECTIONS 1-3 ARE THE SAME AS IN SAS PROGRAM 4.2);
LIBNAME SASDATA "C:\QUANTLAB\A_DATA\";
DATA SASDATA.DATCH4; SET SASDATA.DATCH4;
** 2 INCLUDE SUBJECTS WITH NO MISSING ON KEY VARIABLES
* INCLUDE 5856 SUBJECTS WITH SMOKING DATA FROM 9027 TOTAL;
IF LIFESMK NE .;
* INCLUDE 5143 SUBJECTS WITH NO MISSING DATA ON HBP;
IF HBP     NE .;
** 3 CODE SYSTEM MISSING AFTER CHECKING WITH PROC FREQ, SAS PROGRAMS IN CHAPTER 2;
ARRAY MS LIFESMK SMKNOW SMKDAYS SMKNUMS ONSETAGE COTININE;
DO OVER MS; IF MS IN (0 99 777 999) THEN MS = .; END;
* RECODE MISSING OF SMOKING NOW AS NOT SMOKING BASED ON LIFETIME SMOKING;
IF LIFESMK EQ 2 AND SMKDAYS = . THEN SMKDAYS = 0;
* RECODE MISSINGOF NUMBER OF CIGARETTES SMOKED PER DAY AS ZERO;
IF LIFESMK EQ 2 AND SMKNUMS = . THEN SMKNUMS = 0;
** 4 CREATE A NEW VARIABLE SMKYRS FOR YEARS OF SMOKING;
SMKYRS = AGE - ONSETAGE;
RUN;
** 5 ANALYSIS TO CHECK DISTRIBUTION OF 4 CONTINUOUS VARIABLES AS EXAMPLE;
DATA B; SET SASDATA.DATCH4; RUN;
PROC UNIVARIATE DATA=SASDATA.DATCH4;
VAR SMKDAYS SMKNUMS SMKYRS COTININE H_COTININE;
HISTOGRAM SMKDAYS /MIDPOINTS=(0 TO 30 BY 5);
HISTOGRAM SMKNUMS /MIDPOINTS=(0 TO 60 BY 5);
HISTOGRAM SMKYRS  /MIDPOINTS=(0 TO 70 BY 10);
HISTOGRAM COTININE/MIDPOINTS=(0 TO 800 BY 100);
RUN;
*************************************************************************************;
```

Figure 4.9 depicts distributions of the four smoking measures. Three measures (COTININE, SMKNUMS, SMKDAYS) are not normal but skewed with a large number of zeros; only the variable SMKYRS (years of smoking) is approaching a normal distribution.

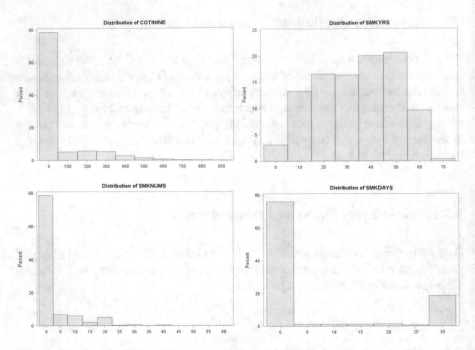

Fig. 4.9 Distribution of four continuous smoking measures in the dataset

4.7.2 Bivariate Analysis and Result Interpretation

SAS Program 4.5 shows the application of a Student t-test for bivariate analysis of the five continuous measures of cigarette smoking. The purpose is to assess if these measures significantly differ between subjects with and without high blood pressure; and if yes, which one has the biggest difference.

```
*********************************************************************************
* SAS PROGRAM 4.5 EXPLORATORY ANALYSIS USING STUDENT T-TEST
*********************************************************************************;
** COMPARE THESE MEASURES BETWEEN SUBJECTS WITH AND WIHTOUT HBP;
PROC TTEST DATA = B;
CLASS HBP;
VAR SMKDAYS SMKNUMS SMKYRS COTININE H_COTININE;
RUN;
*********************************************************************************
```

Figure 4.10 presents a typical example for the continuous measure years of smoking (SMKYRS). The distribution of this measure for the two groups deviated from normal as previously observed in Fig. 4.9. The two distributions also differed significantly from each other through the equal variances test (F = 1.21, $p < 0.05$). With an unequal variance in SMKYRS, Satterthwaite test, rather than Student t-test,

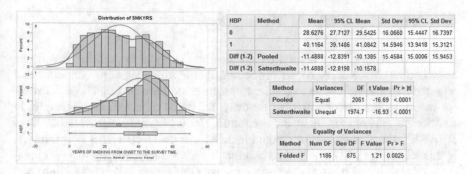

Fig. 4.10 Typical outputs from SAS Program 4.5 for bivariate analysis

was used with t = 2.25, and p = 0.0245, <0.05. This result suggests that hypertensive subjects, on average, smoked for 11.5 years more than normotensive subjects (40.1 vs. 28.6) at the $p < 0.05$ level.

Results from all analyses using SAS Program 4.5 are summarized in Table 4.3. Among the three measures of cigarette smoking from survey data, one derived measure (SMKYRS) and one reported measure (SMKNUMS) performed better than days smoked in the past 30 days (SMKDAYS). Among the two laboratory measures, H_COTININE performed better than COTININE. Since these measures each provide evidence of exposure to tobacco from different aspects, they can all be used in multivariate analyses.

Table 4.3 Mean differences in 5 continuous measures of smoking between hypertensive and normotensive subjects, US Adults 20–69, from the 2017–2018 National Health and Nutrition Examination Survey (NHANES)

Influential factor	Sample N	HBP (SD)	Normal (SD)	Difference (SD)	t (p-value)*
Days smoked	3973	6.93 (12.2)	6.01 (11.6)	0.92 (11.8)	2.25(0.0245)
# cigarettes smoked per day	3970	3.17 (7.02)	2.49(5.92)	0.68 (6.30)	3.01 (0.001)
Years of smoking	2063	40.11(14.59)	28.63 (16.07)	11.49 (15.46)	16.93(0.000)[a]
Cotinine, **ng/ml**	4555	62.47 (136.9)	55.71 (124.7)	6.76 (129.2)	1.66 (0.096)
Hydroxycotinine	4591	26.99(68.52)	20.78 (51.76)	6.20 (58.43)	3.21 (0.0005)

Note: *HBP* High blood pressure. *: Equal variance test was significant for all five influential factors; therefore, Satterthwaite test for unequal variances is used instead of Student t-test

One more piece of information revealed from the bivariate analysis is that the standard deviation (SD) is larger than the mean for four of the five measures, suggesting more errors in data for these variables.

4.8 Exploring Different Measures of Y

In Sects. 4.6 and 4.7, we demonstrated bivariate analysis to explore categorical and continuous measures of an influential factor using cigarette smoking and reported hypertension as an example. In practice, as described in Chap. 2, different measures can also be used to describe the same outcome. For example, in addition to self-reports, data on measured blood pressure are available from NHANES. We already have such data included for analysis in SAS Program 4.1. In this section we will show how to conduct bivariate analysis with different measures of high blood pressure, including binary (self-report and examination) and continuous (measured blood pressure readings, individual measures, and mean of 3 repeated measures).

4.8.1 Variables for Analysis

To show bivariate analysis in exploring potential measures for an outcome variable, two different measures of high blood pressure will be used.

A total of 10 variables will be used to measure the blood pressure as the outcome Y, including two binary and 8 continuous measures. The two binary measures include one that is based on the self-report as being used in the previous two sections; and another which is defined based on the measured diastolic and systolic blood pressure following the standard by the World Health Organization (WHO) (diastolic pressure greater/equal 90 mmHg and systolic pressure greater/equal to 140 mmHg).

The eight continuous measures include 3 repeated measures of both systolic and diastolic measures and the mean of the three repeated measures for systolic and diastolic pressure. The mean systolic and diastolic pressures are the standard used in medicine and public health to determine high blood pressure. Each of these eight measures provides important information regarding hypertension.

Five Xs for smoking as the influential factor are selected based on the analytical results reported in Sects. 4.6 and 4.7, including three reported measures and two laboratory-tested measures. The three reported measures are years of smoking (SMKYRS), days of smoking in the past 30 days (SMKDAYS), and mean number of cigarettes smoked in a typical day (SMKNUMS), and the two laboratory-tested measures include serum cotinine (COTININE, ng/ml) and hydroxycotinine (H_COTININE, ng/ml).

4.8.2   Data Processing

Data processing for the selected variables is shown in SAS Program 4.6. Parts 1 through 5 of the data processing in SAS Program 4.6 can be copied from SAS Program 4.4 since they are the same. Additional program codes are provided to re-code missing data (part 5), and re-code and label newly defined variables measuring blood pressure.

It is worth noting that all the variables processed using this SAS Program are included in dataset **DATCH4**. Smoking measures and reported high blood pressure (HBP) were processed through SAS Program 4.4. By processing measured blood pressures, we will have all the variables needed for the bivariate analysis.

```
****************************************************************************************
* SAS PROGRAM 4.6 DATA PROCESSING AND ANALYSIS OF DIFFERENT MEASURES OF AN OUTCOME
****************************************************************************************;
** READ DATCH4 TO PROCESS MEASURED BLOOD PRESSURE
LIBNAME SASDATA "C:\QUANTLAB\A_DATA\";
DATA SASDATA.DATCH4; SET SASDATA.DATCH4;
* 1 INCLUDE SUBJECTS WITH NO MISSING ON KEY VARIABLES
* INCLUDE 5856 SUBJECTS WITH SMOKING DATA FROM 9027 TOTAL;
IF LIFESMK NE .;
* INCLUDE 5143 SUBJECTS WITH NO MISSING DATA ON HBP;
IF HBP      NE .;
* 2 CODE SYSTEM MISSING AFTER CHECKING WITH PROC FREQ;
ARRAY MS LIFESMK SMKNOW SMKDAYS SMKNUMS ONSETAGE COTININE H_COTININE;
DO OVER MS; IF MS IN (0 99 777 999) THEN MS = .; END;
IF COTININE EQ 1620 THEN COTININE = .; * CODE AN OUTLIER;
IF H_COTININE EQ 1520 THEN H_COTININE = .; * CODE AN OUTLIER;
* 3 RECODE MISSING OF SMOKING NOW AS NOT SMOKING BASED ON LIFETIME SMOKING;
IF LIFESMK EQ 2 AND SMKDAYS = . THEN SMKDAYS = 0;
* 4 RECODE MISSINGOF NUMBER OF CIGARETTES SMOKED PER DAY AS ZERO;
IF LIFESMK EQ 2 AND SMKNUMS = . THEN SMKNUMS = 0;
* 5 CREATE NEW VARIABLE SMKYRS FOR YEARS OF SMOKING;
SMKYRS = AGE - ONSETAGE;
* 6 CODE ZERO DIASTOLIC PRESSURE AS MISSING;
ARRAY BPX BPXDI1-BPXDI3; DO OVER BPX; IF BPX EQ 0 THEN BPX = .; END;
** COMPUTING BLOOD PRESSURE AND DEFINE MEASURED HIGH BLOOD PRESSURE;
** COMPUTING BLOOD PRESSURE AND DEFINE HIGH BLOOD PRESSURE;
* 1 COMPUTE AVERAGE BLOOD PRESSURE;
DIASBP = (BPXDI1+BPXDI1+BPXDI1)/3;
SYSTBP = (BPXSY1+BPXSY2+BPXSY3)/3;
* 2 DEFINE HIGH BLOOD PRESSURE USING WHO CRITERIA;
HBPX = (DIASBP GE 90 | SYSTBP GE 130);
** LABEL NEWLY CREATED VARIABLES;
LABEL  SMKYRS = 'YEARS OF SMOKING FROM ONSET TO THE SURVEY TIME',
       DIASBP = 'MEASURED DIASTOLIC BLOOD PRESSURE, MEAN)',
       SYSTBP = 'MEASURED SYSTOLIC BLOOD PRESSURE, MEAN',
       HBPX   = 'HIGH BLOOD PRESSURE BASED EXAMINATION';
RUN;
****************************************************************************************
```

4.8.3   Using Plot to Show Liner Correlation

SAS Program 4.7 shows the bivariate analyses to associate the two computed mean systolic and diastolic blood pressure Ys with the five influential factor Xs. As an in-depth consideration, the variable HBP_MED (defined in Chap. 3, y/n with y = under antihypertensive medication) is used here. For hypertensive subjects, their measured blood pressures will no longer be valid in detecting factors associated with hypertension.

```
*********************************************************************************
* SAS PROGRAM 4.7 BIVARIATE ANALYSIS OF CONTINUOUS OUTCOME MEASURES
*********************************************************************************;
DATA C; SET SASDATA.DATCH4; RUN;
** 1 PLOT TO SHOW LINEAR CORRELATION BETWEEN TWO VARIABLES;
PROC SGSCATTER DATA = C;
* Y FIRST THEN X IN SPECIFY PLOT;
PLOT SYSTBP * SMKYRS;
RUN;

** 2 LINEAR CORRELATION ANALYSIS OF SYSTOLIC BLOOD PRESSURE;
*  A. ANALYSIS FOR THE TOTAL SAMPLE;
PROC CORR DATA = C;
VAR SYSTBP SMKYRS SMKDAYS SMKNUMS COTININE H_COTININE;
RUN;
* B. ANALYSIS FOR SUBJECTS NOT ON HYPERTENSION MEDICATION;
PROC CORR DATA = C;
VAR SYSTBP SMKYRS SMKDAYS SMKNUMS COTININE H_COTININE;
WHERE HBP_MED NE 1;
RUN;
* C. ADD CORRELATION MATRIX PLOT FOR VISUALIZATION;
PROC CORR DATA = C PLOTS=MATRIX (HISTOGRAM) PLOTS(MAXPOINTS=NONE);
VAR SYSTBP SMKYRS SMKDAYS SMKNUMS COTININE H_COTININE;
WHERE HBPMED NE 1;
RUN;
** 3 LINEAR CORRELATION ANALYSIS OF DIASTOLIC BLOOD PRESSUE;
*  A. ANALYSIS FOR TOTAL SAMPLE;
PROC CORR DATA = C PLOTS=MATRIX (HISTOGRAM) PLOTS(MAXPOINTS=NONE);
VAR DIASBP SMKYRS SMKDAYS SMKNUMS COTININE H_COTININE;

RUN;
* B. ANALYSIS FOR SUBJECTS NOT ON HYPERTENSION MEDICATION;
PROC CORR DATA = C;
VAR DIASBP SMKYRS SMKDAYS SMKNUMS COTININE H_COTININE;
WHERE HBP_MED NE 1;
RUN;
* C. ADD CORRELATION MATRIX PLOT FOR VISUALIZATION;
PROC CORR DATA = C PLOTS=MATRIX (HISTOGRAM) PLOTS(MAXPOINTS=NONE);
VAR DIASBP SMKYRS SMKDAYS SMKNUMS COTININE H_COTININE;
WHERE HBP_MED NE 1;
RUN;
*********************************************************************************;
```

The first analysis included in SAS Program 4.7 is a scatter plot to visualize the correlation between the two continuous variables. This is achieved using the SAS Procedure **PROC SGSCATTER**. As a demonstration, we plot the two variables: SYSTBP (systolic blood pressure) and SMKYRS (years of smoking). Figure 4.11 shows the SMKYRS and SYSTBP plot.

In the figure, each dot represents one participant with two values, one for SYSTBP (systolic blood pressure) and another for SMKYRS (years of smoking). These dots distribute roughly along with an upward line (dashed red line), showing a positive correlation between the two. That is as years of smoking increases, systolic blood pressure increases. Further, most data points are located around the dashed red line, suggesting a significant positive correlation. However, the correlation coefficient would not be very high since many data points are scattered off the line.

Interested students can use the same method to plot other variables in the dataset.

Fig. 4.11 X ~ Y plot for a linear correlation between a continuous X (years of smoking) and a continuous Y (systolic blood pressure)

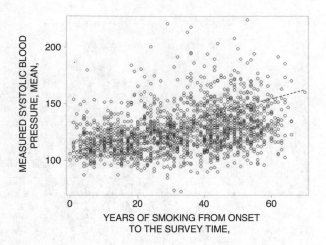

4.8.4 Results from the First Correlation Analysis

Figure 4.12 presents the main outputs from the linear correlation analysis in SAS Program 4.7, Section 2A. It contains two parts, one for sample descriptive statistics and one for correlation analysis. The descriptive statistics include sample size N, mean, SD, min, max, and label for all variables.

The second part is a correlation matrix. What important for an exploratory analysis are the results in the first row that assess the correlation of systolic blood pressure with the five X measures, including SMKYRS (years of smoking), SMKDAYS (days of smoking), SMKNUMS (number of cigarettes smoked per day), COTININE (levels of cotinine in serum), and H_COTININE (level of hydroxycotinine in serum).

In this second part, there are 3 numbers in each cell; the first one is correlation coefficient r, second one is p-value, and third one is sample size. Sample size (n = 1705) was the smallest for years of smoking. This is because this smoking variable was defined for lifetime smokers and non-smokers were excluded. Of the five smoking measures, only this one (r = 0.3434, $p < 0.001$) was seen to be statistically significant. This result is also consistent with the scatter plot as shown in Fig. 4.11.

Interested students can plot other variables and compare the plots with the estimated r from the correlation analysis. This is one of the most practical approaches to gain a solid understanding of the linear correlation between two variables.

The CORR Procedure

6 Variables:	SYSTBP SMKYRS SMKDAYS SMKNUMS COTININE H_COTININE

Simple Statistics							
Variable	N	Mean	Std Dev	Sum	Minimum	Maximum	Label
SYSTBP	4187	124.94467	18.66920	523143	72.66667	224.66667	MEASURED SYSTOLIC BLOOD PRESSURE, MEAN,
SMKYRS	2063	33.50606	16.46546	69123	0	70.00000	YEARS OF SMOKING FROM ONSET TO THE SURVEY TIME,
SMKDAYS	3973	6.31286	11.81666	25081	0	30.00000	DAYS SMOKED IN THE PAST 30 DAYS 0-30,
SMKNUMS	3970	2.71310	6.30948	10771	0	60.00000	AVERAGE # CIGARETTES SMOKED PER DAY 1-60
COTININE	4591	58.17481	129.26590	267081	0.01100	924.00000	COTININE LEVEL IN SERUM >0.015=SMOKING,
H_COTININE	4591	23.04388	58.49945	105794	0.01100	816.00000	HYDROXYCOTININE IN SERUM >0.015=SMOKING

Pearson Correlation Coefficients Prob > |r| under H0: Rho=0 Number of Observations						
	SYSTBP	SMKYRS	SMKDAYS	SMKNUMS	COTININE	H_COTININE
SYSTBP MEASURED SYSTOLIC BLOOD PRESSURE, MEAN,	1.00000 4187	0.34338 <.0001 1705	0.02385 0.1756 3225	0.02661 0.1309 3224	-0.00250 0.8753 3952	-0.01496 0.3471 3952
SMKYRS YEARS OF SMOKING FROM ONSET TO THE SURVEY TIME,	0.34338 <.0001 1705	1.00000 2063	0.06456 0.0468 949	0.20296 <.0001 947	-0.14509 <.0001 1856	-0.06311 0.0065 1856
SMKDAYS DAYS SMOKED IN THE PAST 30 DAYS 0-30,	0.02385 0.1756 3225	0.06456 0.0468 949	1.00000 3973	0.80436 <.0001 3970	0.77312 <.0001 3531	0.68315 <.0001 3531
SMKNUMS AVERAGE # CIGARETTES SMOKED PER DAY 1-60	0.02661 0.1309 3224	0.20296 <.0001 947	0.80436 <.0001 3970	1.00000 3970	0.70473 <.0001 3529	0.67441 <.0001 3529
COTININE COTININE LEVEL IN SERUM >0.015=SMOKING,	-0.00250 0.8753 3952	-0.14509 <.0001 1856	0.77312 <.0001 3531	0.70473 <.0001 3529	1.00000 4591	0.85242 <.0001 4591
H_COTININE HYDROXYCOTININE IN SERUM >0.015=SMOKING	-0.01496 0.3471 3952	-0.06311 0.0065 1856	0.68315 <.0001 3531	0.67441 <.0001 3529	0.85242 <.0001 4591	1.00000 4591

Fig. 4.12 Typical Output from SAS Program 4.7

4.8.5 *Correlation and Scatter Plots for all Correlation Analyses*

Table 4.4 summarizes the key findings from all linear correlation (bivariate) analyses included in SAS Program 4.7 for both systolic and diastolic blood pressure. By using measured blood pressure as a continuous variable for subjects and by excluding subjects who are on medication, three reported smoking measures were found to be positively correlated with systolic blood pressure and one was significantly associated with diastolic blood pressure. On the other hand, the two biomarkers of tobacco exposure were not significantly correlated with blood pressure.

To gain a better understanding of the data, Fig. 4.13 presents results from SAS Program 4.7 Sections 2C and 3C for systolic and diastolic blood pressure, respectively. The bar charts show the distribution of the two blood pressure measures, which is approximately normal. The four scatter plots show the relationships between individual smoking measures and the two blood pressure measures, respectively. Results for hydroxycotinine are not shown because SAS program only allows for five columns of plots in one chart.

Table 4.4 Results from Simple Linear Correlation between Measured Mean Systolic and Diastolic Blood Pressure (mmHg) and five smoking measures stratified by anti-hypertension medication

Influential factor	Total sample			Not on HBP medication		
	N	Mean (SD)	Corr	N	Mean (SD)	Corr
Systolic blood pressure (mmHg)						
Years of smoking	2063	33.51 (16.47)	0.343**	1412	29.04 (15.99)	0.344**
Days of smoking	3973	6.31 (11.82)	0.024	3014	6.48 (11.93)	0.066**
No. cigarettes smoked	3970	2.71 (6.31)	0.027	3011	2.69 (6.17)	0.059**
Cotinine level	4591	58.17 (129.27)	−0.003	3316	58.77(127.71)	0.019
Hydroxycotinine	4591	23.04 (58.50)	−0.015	3316	21.91 (52.87)	0.013
Diastolic blood pressure (mmHg)						
Years of smoking	2063	33.51 (16.47)	−0.022	1412	29.04 (15.99)	0.098**
Days of smoking	3973	6.31 (11.82)	0.022	3014	6.48 (11.93)	0.015
No. cigarettes smoked	3970	2.71 (6.31)	0.013	3011	2.69 (6.17)	−0.002
Cotinine level	4591	58.17(129.26)	0.010	3316	58.77 (127.71)	−0.007
Hydroxycotinine	4591	23.04 (58.50)	−0.018	3316	21.91 (52.87)	−0.016

Data source: US Adults 20–69, the 2017–2018 National Health and Nutrition Examination Survey

Although no clear correlation is revealed from these plots except a few (i.e., years of smoking), such results are anticipated. Since data for this analysis was derived from a population-based survey study with a large sample, the complex tobacco-hypertension relation is thus embedded in the complex network relationship between many factors and hypertension in addition to tobacco exposure. This is also one reason for the need of multivariate analysis to verify an observed relationship from bivariate analysis.

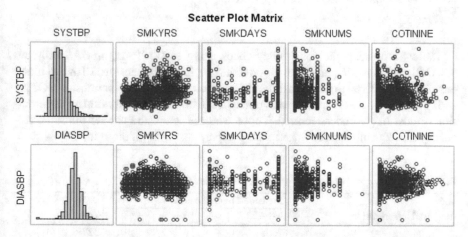

Fig. 4.13 Correlation matrix plotting to enhance mastery of data: Output of SAS Program 4.7, 2C and 3C

Here we only show results for the computed mean blood pressures of three repeated measurements. Analysis of the 3 pairs of individual measures of blood pressure will be conducted in practice.

4.8.6   Student T-Test as Correlation Measure
for a Continuous Outcome

Lastly, SAS 4.8 shows the procedure to compare results of the same tobacco use measures in predicting two binary outcome measures: HBP from self-report and HBPX from measured blood pressure through physical examination in clinical settings.

The program first checks discrepancies between HBP and HBPX. The program then moves to create a new dataset C by excluding all subjects who were on antihypertensive medication at the time of survey. With the newly created dataset C, Student-t test, as introduced in Sect. 4.5, is used to measure the continuous Xs between participants with and without hypertension and to test if any observed difference is real or due to sampling error.

```
*********************************************************************************
* SAS PROGRAM 4.8 BIVARIATE ANALYSIS OF CONTINUOUS OUTCOME VARIABLE
*******************************************************************************;
** 1 CHECK DISCREPENCY BETWEEN REPORTED AND MEASURED HBP;
PROC FREQ DATA = C;
TABLES HBP * HBPX/NOPERCENT CHISQ;
RUN;
** 2 CREATE NEW DATA EXCLUDING SUBJECTS ON MEDICATION;
DATA D; SET C; IF HBPMED NE 1; PROC CONTENTS; RUN;
** 3 ANALYSIS FOR REPORTED HYPERTENSION;
PROC TTEST DATA = D;
CLASS HBP;
VAR SMKYRS SMKDAYS SMKNUMS COTININE H_COTININE;
RUN;
** 4 ANALYSIS FOR MEASURED HYPERTENSION;
PROC TTEST DATA = D;
CLASS HBPX;
VAR SMKYRS SMKDAYS SMKNUMS COTININE H_COTININE;
RUN;
*******************************************************************************;
```

Table 4.5 presents the consistency check using **PROC FREQ** in SAS Program 4.8. Of the 1861 participants who reported having had hypertension, 1016 had blood pressures considered to be normal (could be those who are on hypertension). Of the 1463 subjects who were measured hypotensive, 618 (18.88%) reported no hypertension – most likely under-reported. Those who are interested can do the same frequency check using dataset C; and then compare results with those in Table 4.5.

Table 4.5   Consistency between Reported and Measured Hypertension

Reported hypertension	Measured hypertension		Total
	No	Yes	
No	2665	618	3273
Yes	1016	845	1861
Total	3671	1463	5134

Table 4.6 Differences in tobacco exposure – high blood pressure between self-reports and lab-measured blood pressure, US Adults 20–69

Tobacco exposure	Reported hypertension			Measured hypertension		
	Yes (SD)	No (SD)	Diff (SD)	Yes (SD)	No (SD)	Diff (SD)
Years of smoking	31.2 (15.4)	28.6(16.1)	2.6 (16.0)*	36.4 (14.5)	26.6 (15.7)	9.8 (15.4) **
Days of smoking	10.0 (13.7)	6.0 (11.6)	4.0 (11.9)**	8.0 (12.9)	6.1 (11.6)	2.0 (11.9) **
# Cigarettes smoked per day	4.2 (7.6)	2.5 (5.9)	1.7 (6.1)**	3.4 (6.6)	2.5 (6.0)	0.9 (6.2) **
Cotinine, ng/ml	81.2 (146)	55.7(125)	25.5(127) **	67.3 (136)	56.3(125)	11.0 (128) *
Hydroxycotinine	30.1 (59.8)	20.8(51.8)	9.4(52.8) **	24.6 (55.7)	21.1 (52.0)	3.5 (52.9)

Note: *: $p < 0.05$ and **: $p < .01$ from Student t-test. See SAS Program 4.8 for analysis. Data source: the 2017–2018 National Health and Nutrition Examination Survey (NHANES)

Table 4.6 summarizes results from SAS Program 4.8. The same measure of tobacco exposure X performed differently for different outcome measures of Y for hypertension. Of the five continuous measures of tobacco exposure, four (days of smoking, number of cigarettes smoked per day, and the two biomarker measures) performed better for hypertension from self-reports than for measured blood pressure (greater differences and smaller v-values).

Furthermore, the two biomarkers were better associated with the reported hypertension than measured hypertension using the same criteria of a larger between-group difference and a smaller p value.

Different results for different measures of smoking as X and high blood pressure as Y provide evidence supporting the selection of best or most suitable data for further analysis.

4.9   Presentation and Interpretation of Bivariate Results

Bivariate analysis with various alternative measures of both X and Y will produce a large set of results supporting variable selection for further analysis. Several guidelines are outlined to assist in presenting and interpreting the findings from the bivariate analyses and planning for the next step of a research study.

4.9.1   Select Results with Strong Association for Further Analysis

Selecting the X ~ Y measures with the strongest association for further analysis is the common practice in research. In the examples included in this chapter, if reported high blood pressure is used as Y, results for the five measures in Table 4.3 can be used for further analysis, including years of smoking measuring cumulative exposure; days and number of cigarettes smoked per day measuring frequency and amount of smoking; and the two biomarkers (serum cotinine and hydroxycotinine) measuring recent smoking with an objective measure.

If a proposed X ~ Y relation is theory-based, all of the measures for X and Y are from a reliable data source; the approach to select variables for further analysis will be based on the strength of association using different measures. Obviously, a pair of X ~ Y measures with the strongest effect will be selected for further analysis, including the ones with highest values of chi-square for categorical X and categorical Y, largest differences for continuous X and categorical Y, and the largest linear correlation coefficient for continuous X and continuous Y. With the same effect, the X ~ Y measures with the smallest p-values will also be selected.

It is worth noting that in practice, a weak X ~ Y association from bivariate analysis may not be adequate to exclude a theory-based X ~ Y relation from entering further analyses because results from bivariate analysis are likely to be biased. The relationship between tobacco exposure and heart disease can be used as an example. There are many steps from exposure to tobacco to the development of heart disease. A weak association between serum cotinine and the risk of heart disease may not be adequate to exclude this biomarker from further analysis.

4.9.2   Presentation of Results from Bivariate Analysis Using Table 2

Results from bivariate analysis are often reported as Table 2 in a manuscript in etiological studies for publication consideration. Selection of a table format to present bivariate results is easy in most cases. For example, if the outcome Y is binary and influential factors are categorical, the format of Table 4.2 can be adapted; if Y is binary, but X is continuous, the format of Table 4.3 can be used; and if both X and Y are continuous, the format of Table 4.4 can be used as a reference.

However, it is somewhat challenging to create a table to present bivariate results with a mixture of both categorical and continuous measures of X, which is most often the case in practice. Using findings from the analyses described in this chapter, Table 4.7 presents a template of Table 2 that can be used in practice to present results from bivariate analysis with a binary Y.

Table 4.7 A Template of Table 2 in Manuscripts – Results from Bivariate Analysis of Associations between Cigarette Smoking and High Blood Pressure among US Adults 20–69, 2017–2018 NHANES data

Influential factor	Hypertension	No hypertension	T/chi-sq (p-value)
Lifetime smoking, n (%)			
Yes	902 (42.4)	1227 (57.6)	58.93(<.001)
No	959 (31.9)	2046 (68.1)	
Years of smoking			
Mean (SD)	40.11 (14.6)	28.6 (16.1)	16.93 (<0.001)
If smoked in the past 30 days			
Yes	348 (26.6)	620 (23.3)	5.45 (0.020)
No	959 (73.4)	2046 (76.7)	
Days of smoking in past 30 days			
Mean (SD	6.9 (12.2)	6.0 (11.6)	3.01 (0.0245)
# Cigarettes smoked per day			
Mean (SD)	3.2 (7.0)	2.5(5.9)	3.01 (0.001)
If currently smoking (cotinine>0.015 ng/ml)			
Yes	1049 (62.7)	1943 (66.6)	7.21 (0.007)
No	625 (37.3)	975 (33.4)	
Hydroxycotinine (ng/ml)			
Mean (SD)	1510 (80.8)	2643 (80.8)	0.41 (0.813)

Data source: the National Health and Nutrition Examination Survey (NHANES)

As a last point, in preparing Table 2 to report results from bivariate analysis, differences in key demographic and socioeconomic factors between the disease and non-disease group are often included first. These results provide useful information about heterogeneity of the same between the two comparison groups. Such results are the basis supporting inclusion of these variables in multivariate analysis as covariates.

4.9.3 Interpretation

Results from bivariate analysis indicates a significant and positive association between exposure to tobacco, including cigarette smoking and biomarkers of tobacco exposure (nicotine), and high blood pressure among US adults. Measures of current and cumulative exposure, frequency, and amount were all associated with self-reported high blood pressure. These results provide preliminary data supporting the hypothetical relationship between tobacco use and high blood pressure. Further analysis with multivariate models is needed to confirm the results by adjusting for demographic factors and controlling for confounders.

4.9.4   Caveat – Avoidance of Fishing in Bivariate Analysis

Bivariate analysis must be hypothesis-driving. The purpose of the analysis is simply to identify the most relevant measures of X and Y to support a hypothetic relation. As we described in this chapter, all analyses are conducted to test different measures of tobacco exposure X and hypertension Y. The goal is to identify measures of X and measures of Y that show the strongest correlation between smoking and hypertension – the hypothetic relation.

With the statistical software and widely available data, a malpractice of bivariate analysis is to screen all variables in the data to generate a hypothetic relation. This fishing approach is not allowed in epidemiology for high quality research. The main problem associated with this approach is that p-values from such fishing bivariate testing will be inflated, increasing the likelihood of drawing false conclusions.

4.10   Practice

4.10.1   Statistical analysis and computing

1. Further practice to enhance skills for data processing and variable recoding using SAS Program 4.1.
2. Practice bivariate analysis for different types of X and Y (i.e., continuous and categorical) using student t-test, chi-square test, simple linear correlation, correlation plot, and SAS Programs 4.2 to 4.8).
3. Complete the remaining bivariate analyses as indicated in different sections of this chapter.
4. Repeat practice to become skillful in using the three key SAS Procedures (**PROC FREQ, PROC TTEST** and **PROC FCORR**) covered in this chapter for bivariate analysis.

4.10.2   Update Your Research Project

1. Conduct bivariate analysis for your own project. This can be done in several ways. One approach is to select an influential factor X and an outcome Y based on the study question you proposed, then conduct bivariate analysis to check if your hypothesis is supported by any data. Another approach is that you already have some idea that the X (i.e., smoking) and Y (i.e., high blood pressure) you selected are related, and you are now seeking for one variable (i.e., days of smoking or cotinine level) best suitable to test the hypothetical relationship. Bivariate analysis can be used to help you make the decision as shown in this chapter.

2. Create/update Table 2 of your study to report the results from bivariate analysis.
3. Update/revise all parts of your own study, including title, abstract, Sections of Introduction, Materials and Methods, Results, Interpretation and Temporary Conclusions.
4. If you want to select different variables or even change the study topic to address another issue supported by the findings from the exploratory bivariate analysis, this is the right time to do so. Simply update everything after you make the change.

4.10.3 Study Questions

1. What are the characteristics of a hypothetic X ~ Y relation, and how does it relate to the connected universe in the real world?
2. Use examples to describe that a character can be measured using different variables. What does this mean for an epidemiologist in studies to examine a hypothetic X ~ Y relationship?
3. Use examples to illustrate that one variable can provide information about multiple characters and discuss the importance of this phenomenon in epidemiological research to examine an X ~ Y relationship for causal inference.
4. Bivariate analysis is the first step to provide empirical data supporting our thoughts or hypothesis about an X ~ Y relationship. Please discuss the exploratory nature of bivariate analysis and cautions in interpreting bivariate analysis results, as well as the need for further analysis?

References

Chen, X., Stanton, B., Gong, J., Fang, X., Li, X.: Personal social capital scale: an instrument for health and behavioral research. Health Educ. Res. 24(2), 306–317 (2009)
Chen, X., Wang, P., Wegner, R., Gong, J., Fang, X., Kaljee, L.: Measuring social capital investment: scale development and examination of links to social capital and perceived stress. Soc. Indic. Res. 120(3), 339–687 (2015)
Golden, S.D., Earp, J.A.: Social ecological approaches to individuals and their contexts: twenty years of health education & behavior health promotion intervention. Health Educ. Behav. 39(3), 364–372 (2012)
Higgins, C., Hodges, C.: Studies on prostatic cancer. 1. The effect of castration, of estrogen and of androgen injection on serum phosphatases in metastatic carcinoma of the prostate. Cancer Res. 1, 293–297 (1941)
Hu, J., Jiao, R., Jin, L., Xiong, M.: Application of causal inference to genomic analysis: advance in methodology. Front. Genet. 9, 238 (2018). https://doi.org/10.3389/fgene.2018.00238
Nishiura, H., Kobayasgu, T., Miyama, T., et al.: Estimation of the asymptomatic ratio of novel coronavirus infections (COVID-19). Int. J. Infect. Dis. 94, 154–155 (2020)
Omran, A.R.: The epidemiological transition: a theory of the epidemiology of population change. Milbank Q. 83(4), 731–757 (2005)

Patel, C.J.: Introduction to environment and exposome-wide association studies: a data-driven
    method to identify multiple environmental factors associated with phenotypes in human pop-
    ulation. In: Rider, C.V., Simmons, J.E. (eds.) Chemical Mixtures and Combined Chemical
    and Nonchemical Stressors: Exposure, Toxicity, Analysis, and Risk, pp. 129–149. Springer,
    Cham (2018)
Paul, D.S., Beck, S.: Advances in epigenome-wide association studies for common diseases.
    Trends Mol. Med. **20**(10), 541–543 (2014)
Wang, K., Chen, X., Bird, V., Gerke, T.A., Manini, T.M., Prosperi, M.: Association between age-
    related reductions in testosterone and risk of prostate cancer – an analysis of patients' data with
    prostate diseases. Int. J. Cancer. **141**(9), 1783–1793 (2017)

Chapter 5
Confirmation with Multiple Regression Analysis

Sort out the truth from smoke and mirrors.

In Chap. 4, we learned how to find data and conduct simple bivariate analysis to test hypothetical X ~ Y relationships with multi-measurements of the same character. In this chapter, we will continue the research to verify or confirm a promising X ~ Y relationship with the most suitable variables detected through bivariate analysis. As described in Chap. 4, an X ~ Y relation is what we assumed. We use it as a reflection of the true relationship in the real world. Nevertheless, the actual relationship could be much more complex than we thought. Thus, an X ~ Y relation revealed through bivariate analysis may not be true without further verification by considering factors that may affect the X ~ Y relation, including known and unknown factors.

The potential smoking-blood pressure relationship identified through bivariate analysis in the previous chapter presents as a typical example. With multiple measures of smoking behavior as X and blood pressure as Y, we observed that years of smoking (X) and systolic blood pressure (Y) can be used to test the hypothetic X ~ Y relation. However, the estimated result from the bivariate analysis could be biased (either over-estimated or underestimated) due to other factors. For example, we know that hypertension is more prevalent in males than in females (Ramirez and Sullivan 2018); the smoking-blood pressure relationship could be biased without considering this gender difference (Alhawari et al. 2018). Furthermore, psychological factors, such as stress and depression, can affect both smoking and hypertension, thus they can confound the smoking-blood pressure relationship.

Multiple linear regression provides a tool to verify a potential X ~ Y relation by inclusion of other potentially influential factors. This method is suitable for analyzing an X ~ Y relation *when Y is measured using a continuous variable*. Multiple linear regression is a multivariate method commonly used in research to investigate the relation of more than one influential factor with an outcome. This approach is valid only if all Xs each are associated with Y independently, which can hardly be found in the real world. In this chapter, we use it only to verify an X ~ Y relation with one X, while considering all other factors as covariates. This is the goal when multiple linear regression is used in etiological research.

© The Author(s), under exclusive license to Springer Nature Switzerland AG 2021   125
X. Chen, *Quantitative Epidemiology*, Emerging Topics in Statistics and
Biostatistics, https://doi.org/10.1007/978-3-030-83852-2_5

To master this approach, in this chapter we will focus on:

1. Understanding the concept of simple and multiple regression as well as covariates and confounders;
2. Selecting covariates, including demographic factors and confounders for analysis;
3. Conducting multiple regression analysis to verify a potential X ~ Y relation from bivariate analysis by adjusting demographic factors and controlling for confounders;
4. Interpreting and reporting the results from regression analysis and drawing conclusions.

5.1   An X ~ Y Relationship in a Multivariate Framework

As discussed in Chap. 4, all things in the universe are connected with each other, forming complex causal correlation network systems in a 3D format. It is thus impossible to investigate all the relationships with the multivariate methods available to date. We take a different approach by working on one hypothetic X ~ Y relation as an approximation of the true relation in the real world. We are aware that this approximated relation consists of only a tiny part of the 3D complex network relationships in the universe.

5.1.1   Concepts of Single and Multivariate Models

To confirm a hypothetical X ~ Y relation from bivariate analysis, interrelationships between an influential factor X of interest with other influential factors, termed as CovX must be considered. If the X ~ Y relation remains significant after controlling for CovX's that are known to be associated with either X, or Y, or both, such relationship is likely to be valid.

Multiple linear regression provides a statistical tool to control for multiple CovX's while verifying an X ~ Y relationship. To prepare for the regression analysis, we first introduce two conceptual models for an X ~ Y relationship: (i) single X single Y model and (ii) multiple X's and single Y model (Fig. 5.1).

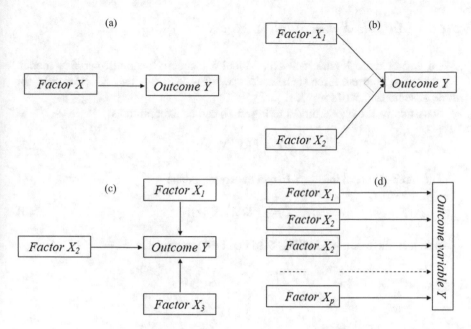

Fig. 5.1 Geometric Presentation of the Typology of Simple Causal Mechanisms. Note: (**a**) Single cause and single outcome; (**b**) dual causes and single outcome; (**c**) triple causes and one outcome; and (**d**) quadruple causes and one outcome. In all models, the influential factors Xs are independently (at 90 degree from each other) associated the outcome Y

5.1.2 Single X – Single Y Regression Model

As shown in Fig. 5.1a, one X is assumed to be associated with one Y. Statistically, this model can be written as:

$$Y = f(X,e). \tag{5.1}$$

where $f()$ represents the function that links X with Y, and e represents the residuals that remain after the X ~ Y relationship is extracted from the data using the model.

Although the simplest, Model 5.1 is essentially a bivariate model for an etiological study. In this model, only one influential factor X (known as an independent variable or IV in statistics) is associated with the outcome Y (known dependent variable or DV in statistics). This model is very useful to quantify linear relationships with data from laboratory-based experimental studies in which many other potential influential factors have been controlled through strict experimental designs.

Different from correlation analysis in Chap. 4, with Model 5.1, the X ~ Y association is characterized by a link function $f()$, while the link function $f()$ is determined by the type of Y, the DV. When Y is continuous and assumed to be distributed normally, as in this chapter, a linear function can be used for $f()$; Model 5.1 then becomes a simple linear regression.

5.1.3   Multiple-X and Single Y Model

When two or more Xs are included, Model 5.1 becomes a multi-variable model. Figure 5.1b–d present three such models with Fig. 5.1b for two X's, Fig. 5.1c for three X's and Fig. 5.1d for p X's.

Statistically, the two-X model in Fig. 5.1b can be expressed as:

$$Y = f(X_1, X_2, e); \tag{5.2}$$

The three-X model in Fig. 5.1c can be expressed as:

$$Y = f(X_1, X_2, X_3, e); \tag{5.3}$$

And last, the p-X model in Fig. 5.1d can be expressed as:

$$Y = f(X_1, X_2, X_3, \ldots X_p, e). \tag{5.4}$$

5.1.4   Multivariate Covariate Model for Verification Analysis

When multivariate model 5.4 is used to verify an X ~ Y relation by controlling for other factors, X_1 in the model is used as the influential factor of interest, while the remaining (1-p) Xs are covariates (see Fig. 5.2). Throughout the text, CovX is used to represent all types of covariates, including demographic factors and confounders.

Fig. 5.2 Multivariate model with p-1 covariates to confirm an X ~ Y relationship using regression analysis

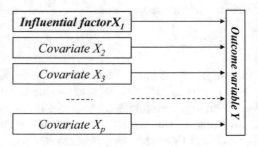

Following Fig. 5.2, we will express a multivariate regression analysis using Model 5.5 as shown below:

$$Y = f(X_1, CovX_2, CovX_3, \ldots CovX_p, e); \tag{5.5}$$

With a continuous outcome Y, a linear function is used for $f()$. In this case, Model 5.5 becomes the typical multiple linear regression:

$$Y = \alpha + \beta_1 X_1 + \beta_2 covX_2 + \beta_3 covX_3 + \ldots \beta_p covX_p + e \qquad (5.6)$$

In Model 5.6, β_1 quantifies the association between X_1 and Y, or the independent effect of the influential factor IV on the outcome DV after the effects from $CovX_2$ to $CovX_p$ on Y are adjusted. The regression coefficients β_2 to β_p are byproducts measuring, individually, the relationships of these (1-p) CovX with Y.

Model 5.6 is the analytical tool used in this text to confirm an X ~ Y relationship for any Y that is measured continuously. For example, to study the smoking (X_1) ~ lung cancer (Y) relationship, many other factors (CovXs) that are known to be associated with Y and/or X_1 can be included, such as age, education, income, marital status, dietary habit, and physical activities $(X_2$ to $X_p)$. If β_1 for X_1 remains statistically significant after inclusion of all the CovXs, such results can be used as evidence to support the conclusion that the smoking ~ lung cancer relationship from bivariate analysis is likely to be true. In this case, the estimated β_1 is termed as the *adjusted effect* or *net effect* after potential effects from covariates are considered.

5.1.5   Statistical Requirements for Linear Regression

Linear regression is commonly used in medical, health, and behavioral studies to verify results from exploratory bivariate analysis, such as Student t-test, chi-square test, ANOVA, and linear correlation. A linear regression requests that Y, the DV must be continuous and follow the *normal distribution* with mean and standard deviation (SD). This is the statistical foundation for regression analysis.

Although linear regression requires the outcome Y to be continuous, the influential factor X_1 and all (1-p) CovXs can be non-continuous, including binary (e.g., male/female, migrant or non-migrant, smokers vs. nonsmokers), ordered (e.g., levels of education from less than high school, to high school, and further to college+), or simply categorical (e.g., racial groups, migration status).

5.2   Simple Linear Regression

5.2.1   An Introductory to Simple Linear Regression

The word regression means "return to a former status"; literally, it is a bad term for epidemiologists since we do not use this method to assess if something will return to its former status. A simple linear regression is essentially a linear equation (model) with one Y as DV and one X as IV. X can vary freely; but variations in Y depend on, or are determined by X. It is in this regard the variable X in statistics is used to replace an *influential factor* in epidemiology. A multiple linear regression is simply an extension of a simple linear regression model to include multiple X's.

As an introduction to the application of multivariate regression analysis in confirming results from bivariate analysis, let us start by conducting a simple linear regression with a hypothetic dataset using SAS Program 5.1. In the program, 8 observations with three variables are generated, the dependent variable Y, an independent variable X, and another independent variable **SEX**. Students can run the program yourself and compare your results with those reported next.

```
*******************************************************************************
SAS Program 5.1. UNDERSTANDING OF A REGRESSION COEFFICIENT
*******************************************************************************;
* STEP 1: CREATE A WORK DATASET NAMED A WITH 3 VARIABLES Y X AND SEX;
DATA A; INPUT Y X SEX; CARDS;
2   2   0
8   5   0
12  6   1
4   3   1
10  7   1
7   4   0
9   6   1
6   4   0
;
RUN;
* STEP 2: CHECK THE DATASET JUST CREATED;
PROC PRINT DATA = A; RUN;
* STEP 3: CONDUCT STUDENT T-TEST TO CHECK SEX DIFFERENCE IN Y;
PROC TTEST DATA = A ALPHA =0.5 PLOTS=(NONE);
VAR Y;
CLASS SEX;
RUN;
* STEP 4: CONDUCT REGRESSION ANALYSIS FOR BINARY X-Y RELATION;
PROC REG DATA = A;
MODEL Y = SEX;
RUN;
* STEP 5: CONDUCT REGRESSION ANALYSIS FOR ANY X-Y RELATION;
PROC REG DATA = A;
MODEL Y = X;
RUN;
*******************************************************************************;
```

5.2.2 Regression Coefficient – X with a 2-Level Measure

Results from Student t-test in SAS Program 5.1 Step 3 indicate the mean of Y = 8.75 for male and 5.75 for female with sex difference in Y = 3.00.

SAS Program 5.1 Step 4 runs a simple linear regression $Y = \alpha + \beta(SEX)$ using the same data. In the regression analysis, the intercept α and the slope β are estimated using the ordinary least square (OLS) method. Results from the analysis indicate that the estimated $\alpha = 5.75$ and $\beta = 3.00$.

What a surprise, the estimated $\beta = 3.0$ from the regression exactly equals the sex difference in Y from Student t-test and $\alpha + \beta = 5.75 + 3.00 = 8.75$, the mean for males from Student t-test. Why are the results from regression analysis consistent with those from Student t-test?

This can be further understood by putting the regression results into the linear equation:

$$Y = 5.75 + 3.00(SEX).$$

Note that the variable **SEX** was coded as 0 and 1(two levels). The estimated intercept α is the measurement of **Y** when **SEX** = 0 (female); the estimated β slope equals the difference in the mean of Y between male and female since the mean for male = mean of female (5.75) plus 3.00, the difference in the mean of **Y** between male and female.

Figure 5.3a plots the results from the regression analysis. Relative to the Student t-test that simply compares the sex difference in Y, *the estimated slope β from regression provides a number to quantify the "impact" of the independent variable X (here SEX) on Y using the difference or the <u>shortest (vertical) geometrical distance in Y</u> between the two measured levels of X under a linear equation model.*

The regression result presented above indicates that a one-unit change in X (here from female to male) is associated with 3.00-unit changes in Y; thus regression analysis uses <u>one number</u> to quantify the X ~ Y relationship.

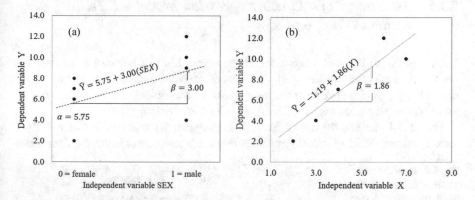

Fig. 5.3 Regression quantifies the relation between X and Y using the distance: (**a**) for a 2-level X and (**b**) for a continuous X (hypothetic data; analyses are in SAS Program 5.1)

5.2.3   Regression Coefficient – Continuous X with Countless Levels

By extending the IV from a two-level measure like **SEX** to a continuous measure of any X with countless levels, results from SAS program 5.1 Step 5 shows that with the same OLS method, the estimated intercept $\alpha = -1.19$ and slope $\beta = 1.86$. The results are plotted in Fig. 5.3b. From the figure it can be seen that the estimated $\beta = 1.86$, this is the vertical distance for change in Y, the DV for each unit change in X, the IV. With every unit increase in X, Y will move up 1.86 units; and vice versa.

5.2.4 Regression Coefficient – The Effect of X on Y with Geometric Distance

In conclusion, results in Fig. 5.3a, b indicate that in linear regression analysis, *the estimated regression slope β quantifies the impact of X on Y using the shortest geometric distance. It tells the changes in Y in response to as every unit change in X.* In this book, we consider the regression coefficient β as a distance measure and use it to help understand the changes in an estimated β coefficient after inclusion of CovXs, and why a multiple linear regression is needed to confirm/verify an X ~ Y relationship revealed from exploratory bivariate analysis.

It is worth noting that although regression provides an analytical tool to quantitatively assess an X ~ Y relationship, *it does not by any means warrant the relation as causal* (Bordacconi and Larsen 2014). We will discuss more about the causal inference toward the end of this chapter.

5.2.5 Assessment of a Linear Regression Model – F Test, Student T-Test, and R^2

Three tests from the SAS output for linear regression can be used to assess if a regression model fits the data well: (i) F test or variance analysis for overall data – model fit; (ii) Student t-test for testing regression coefficients α and β, and (iii) R^2 for assessing variances explained by the model with the IVs.

Figure 5.4 presents the output from SAS Program 5.1 that consists of the three tests. F value = 41.96 (p < 0.01) indicates that the linear model is valid for the data;

Fig. 5.4 Data-model fit and significance test for linear regression, output from SAS Program 5.1 Step 5

Analysis of Variance					
Source	DF	Sum of Squares	Mean Square	F Value	Pr > F
Model	1	64.30503	64.30503	41.96	0.0006
Error	6	9.19497	1.53249		
Corrected Total	7	73.50000			

Root MSE	1.23794	R-Square	0.8749
Dependent Mean	7.25000	Adj R-Sq	0.8540
Coeff Var	17.07503		

Parameter Estimates					
Variable	DF	Parameter Estimate	Standard Error	t Value	Pr > |t|
Intercept	1	-1.06918	1.35681	-0.79	0.4607
X	1	1.79874	0.27768	6.48	0.0006

the t = 6.48 (p < 0.01) from Student t-test for the slope of X suggests the estimated $\beta = 1.7987$ is statistically extremely significant. The estimated $R^2 = 0.87$, indicates that 87% of the variations in Y can be explained by X.

In practice, the F-test must be significant for any linear regression model to be meaningful. If the F-test is not significant, the estimated regression coefficients will be meaningless even if significant. In etiological studies, researchers often pay attention to the significance of β for an X; while in prediction modeling, a larger R^2 is very important in addition to the significance of individual β coefficient. Coefficient α (intercept) is often ignored in etiological studies.

5.3   Covariates in Multiple Linear Regression

Despite wide acceptance and frequent applications of multiple linear regression in research, several questions remain to be clarified. In practice, a β coefficient for the same X (e.g., the variable of interest) often varies (increases or declines) in a multiple regression model depending on the covariate added to the model. How does this happen? Can we tell in advance the direction of change by adding a covariate? Using a simple linear regression in Sect. 5.2, we already demonstrated that a β coefficient is a distance measure to quantify an X ~ Y relationship, but how can we understand the same β coefficient in a multiple regression model?

5.3.1   Covariance of X's and the Independent Effect of Multi-Xs on Y

Statistically, multiple linear regression is used to assess the independent effect of more than one X on Y. For example, the regression model 5.2 in Sect. 5.1.3 can assess the independent effect of X_1 and X_2 on Y (Fig. 5.1b), and the regression model 5.4 also in Sect. 5.1.3 can assess independent effect of an influential factor of interest X_1 on Y after considering the effect of (1-p) covariates X_2 to X_p (Fig. 5.1d).

However, from the discussion in Chap. 4, we already know that connections among all variables in the universe are network-like in a 3D format, suggesting few relationships between two variables are vertical or independent (mathematically known as orthogonal). How can we say that the estimated β coefficients for multiple X's are vertically distant between individual X's and Y? Let us consider a situation with n participants (observations), two independent variable X's and one dependent variable Y:

$$\text{Let } Y = [Y_1, Y_2, \dots Y_n], \ X = \begin{bmatrix} X_{1,1}, X_{2,1} \\ X_{1,2}, X_{2,2} \\ \dots \\ X_{1,n}, X_{2,n} \end{bmatrix}, \text{ and } \beta = [\beta_1, \beta_2].$$

With the notation, a regression model can be written as:

$$Y = X\beta \tag{5.7}$$

To solve for β, multiply both sides of model (5.7) by X: $XY = XX'\beta$. In this model, XX' is known as the *covariance matrix*. In current case, XX' is the variance and covariate matrix of X_1 and X_2:

$$cov(X) = \begin{bmatrix} \sigma_{11}, \sigma_{12} \\ \sigma_{21}, \sigma_{22} \end{bmatrix}. \tag{5.8}$$

Where σ_{11} and σ_{22} on the diagonal place are the variances of X_1 and X_2, respectively. The other two elements off the diagonal are σ_{12} and σ_{21}, the covariances between X_1 and X_2.

The covariance σ_{12} and σ_{21} will be zero if X_1 and X_2 are independent from each other. Mathematically, to solve a multiple linear regression, the σ_{12} and σ_{21} off the diagonal are set to zero regardless of the true relationship between X_1 and X_2. This is why a multivariate linear regression model is said to measure the independent effect of all Xs included in a regression model. If some Xs are correlated with each other, such correlation is forced to zero or totally ignored.

Knowing the characteristics of a regression model in statistics makes it possible to think of the impact by adding a covariate on the beta coefficient of the influential factor X of interest. If a covariate CovX is independent of X, adding the CovX will not alter the β coefficient for X since there is no ignorance of any correlation between X and CovX. However, if a CovX is not independent but correlated with X, the β coefficient for X will change after the CovX is added to the regression model. This is because a regression model can only capture the independent part (vertical distance) of the X (as well as that for the CovX).

5.3.2 Monte Carlo Simulation Studies with Both X and CovX Being Positively Associated with Y

To demonstrate the impact of a covariate CovX on the effect of the main influential factor X on Y, 3 scenarios are simulated: (i) CovX is independent of X, (ii) CovX is positively associated with X (r = 0.7), and (iii) CovX is negatively associated with X (r = −0.4). In addition, both X and CovX are positively associated with Y. In the simulation studies, the sample size was set at n = 500, a normal distribution was used for X and CovX; Y was generated using the simulated X and CovX by imposing the two known β-coefficients, one for X and one for CovX. For each scenario, 3 regression models were used, one containing both X and CovX, one for X only, and one for CovX only. Results from the simulation studies are summarized in Table 5.1.

Table 5.1 Simulation results indicating different impacts of a CovX on the X ~ Y relationship in multiple regression with Y = $\alpha + \beta_1 X + \beta_2$ CovX

Simulated CovX-X relation	β_1 for X (true=1)	β_2 for CovX (true=2)	F-value (p)	R^2
Independent				
X & CovX	1.1167**	1.9075**	102.3 (0.000)	0.63
X only	1.1172**	n/a	26.4 (0.000)	0.18
CovX	–	1.9709 **	97.9 (0.000)	0.45
Correlated, r = 0.7				
X & CovX	1.1090**	1.7820**	112.7 (0.000)	070
X only	2.2357**	n/a	118.7 (0.000)	0.55
CovX	–	2.6219**	166.0 (0.000)	0.63
Correlated, r = −0.4				
X & CovX	1.1618**	2.01512**	84.09 (0.000)	0.59
X only	0.4852*		4.26 (0.041)	0.03
CovX		1.6683**	82.6 (0.000)	0.41

Note: X: the factor of interest, CovX: Covariate, sample size n = 500. X and CovX ~ N (mean, SD). True value $\beta_1 = 1$ for X and $\beta_2 = 2$ for CovX. Differences between the simulated and the true values are due to random error in the Monte Carlo simulation. *: $p<0.05$ and **: $p<0.01$

5.3.3 Adding an Independent Covariate Not Affecting the Estimated X ~ Y Relation

The top three rows of Table 5.1 are results from the simulated study of Scenario 1 in which CovX was independent of X_1. Results in row 1 show that the estimated $\beta_1 = 1.1167$ (p < 0.001) for X_1. This result is an adjusted measure of the X_1 ~ Y relationship after the impact of *CovX* is controlled.

Results in row 2 present the estimated β'_1 with a regression model containing only X_1. In other words, this is the raw and unadjusted effect equivalent to a bivariate result as introduced in Chap. 4. The estimated $\beta'_1 = 1.1172$ (p < 0.001) for X, slightly greater than but very close to the adjusted β_1 (1.1167) when the *CovX* was controlled. The difference is primarily due to random error. For informational purpose, β'_2 for *CovX* was presented in row 3 of the table.

Figure 5.5a depicts the difference in the estimated β coefficients using the multiple and simple (bivariate) regression analyses. Since the X_1 and *CovX* are independent, they are parallel to each other with regard to their impact on Y. No matter only if X_1 or both X_1 and *CovX* are included, the estimated β_1 for X_1 will be similar to each other as shown by a vertical distance from X_1 to Y.

With these results, we can conclude that *the main effect of X on Y will not be altered by adding a CovX that is independent of X_1.*

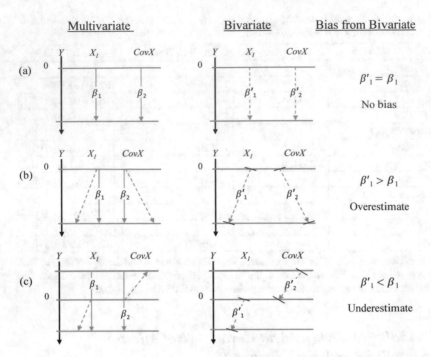

Fig. 5.5 Multivariate analysis to correct biased β from bivariate analysis: (**a**) X and CovX independent, (**b**) X and CovX positively correlated, and (**c**) X and CovX negatively associated. (Note: CovX: covariate variable X; β_1: regression coefficient for X in multivariate regression, and β'_1: regression coefficient from simple linear regression (bivariate) analysis)

5.3.4 Adding Positively Correlated Covariates Reducing (Correcting) the Overestimated Effect

The three rows in the middle panel of Table 5.1 contain the results for Scenario 2 in which X_1 and $CovX$ were positively correlated ($r = 0.7$) with each other. Results in row 1 show the estimated $\beta_1 = 1.1090$ ($p < 0.01$) for X_1 (close to the true value of 1), after adjusting $CovX$. Results in row 2 indicate that the estimated $\beta'_1 = 2.2357$ ($p < 0.01$), the regression coefficient for the same X_1 when $CovX$ was not included. This β'_1 is eventually a bivariate estimate that is biased. For informational purposes, β'_2 for $CovX$ only was included in row 3.

Figure 5.5b further illustrates the impact of a positive $CovX$ from Scenario 2. When X_1 and $CovX$ are not independent but positively correlated, the $X_1 \sim Y$ and $CovX$ and Y relations are not vertical but tilted (dashed line). When the $X_1 \sim Y$ relation was quantified using a simple linear regression (bivariate), the regression model treats the tilted relationship as vertical, leading to positive bias (overestimation). To obtain the independent effect of X_1 on Y (i.e., the shortest distance from X_1 to Y, the solid vertical line), $CovX$ must be included.

In conclusion, different from Scenario 1, ignorance of a positively correlated *CovX* will lead to an overestimate of the true $X_1 \sim Y$ relationship. To correct for the bias, positively correlated *CovX*'s must be included.

5.3.5   Adding a Negatively Correlated Covariate Bringing Up (Correcting) the Underestimated Effect

The last three rows in Table 5.1 present the results for Scenario 3 in which X_1 and *CovX* were set to be negatively correlated (r = −0.4). As in the previous two scenarios, results with both X_1 and *CovX* included in one regression model, the estimated $\beta_1 = 1.1618$ (p < 0.01), close to the true value of 1. However, when *CovX* was excluded, the estimated $\beta'_1 = 0.4852$ (p < 0.01), which is much smaller than the true value 1.00. For informational purposes, β'_2 for CovX was also presented in the table.

Likewise, Fig. 5.5c demonstrates the mechanisms by which the inclusion of negatively correlated *CovX* can help correct the underestimation of the impact of X_1 on Y. A negatively correlated *CovX* acts on a direction opposite of that for the influential factor X_1, in addition to a tilted relationship with Y. When X_1 is analyzed alone, only the tilted part from X_1 will be captured, leading to an underestimated regression coefficient β'_1. When both X_1 and *CovX* are included, it will help to obtain the adjusted, thus vertical relationship between X and Y (the solid line in multivariate regression).

In conclusion, different from Scenarios 1 and 2, ignorance of a negatively correlated *CovX* will lead to an underestimate of the true $X_1 - Y$ relation. Negatively correlated *CovXs* thus need to be included.

5.3.6   Summary for All Eight Scenarios

Findings from our simulation of all eight possible scenarios for one Y, one X, and one *CovX* are summarized in Table 5.2. Results in this table will be used as guidance to understanding results from multivariate regression analyses to confirm $X \sim Y$ relations revealed from bivariate analysis.

So far, results in eight possible scenarios with one *CovX* are clear. The impact, however, will become rapidly more complex as the number of *CovXs* increases. For one *CovX*, we only need to consider one X-*CovX* relation; for two $CovX_1$ and $CovX_2$, three relations must be considered, including $CovX_1$-X, $CovX_2$-X and $CovX_1$-$CovX_2$. Additional methodological research is needed to examine these more complex scenarios.

Table 5.2 Bias from bivariate analysis for eight different scenarios with one dependent variable Y, one independent variable X, and one CovX: Results from simulation analysis

Scenario	X and Y relation	CovX and X	CovX and Y	Bivariate estimate
Scenario 1	Positive (+)	Positive (+)	Positive (+)	Overestimate (+)
Scenario 2	Positive (+)	Positive (+)	Negative (−)	Underestimate (−)
Scenario 3	Positive (+)	Negative (−)	Positive (+)	Underestimate (−)
Scenario 4	Positive (+)	Negative (−)	Negative (−)	Overestimate(+)
Scenario 5	Negative (−)	Positive (+)	Positive (+)	Overestimate (+)
Scenario 6	Negative (−)	Positive (+)	Negative (−)	Underestimate (−)
Scenario 7	Negative (−)	Negative (−)	Positive (+)	Underestimate (−)
Scenario 8	Negative (−)	Negative (−)	Negative (−)	Overestimate (+)

5.4   Demographic Factors as Covariates

With knowledge gained in the previous sections, we are now planning to use the methods and concepts to analyze real data. The purpose is to show how to verify a promising X ~ Y relationship revealed from bivariate analysis using multiple regression to include covariates. In this section, we will focus on demographic factors. Influential factors as confounders will be addressed in Sect. 5.5.

5.4.1   Importance of Controlling Demographic Factors

In quantitative analysis of observational data, demographic factors reflect the *heterogeneity* of a study sample (or the study population). It is well known that homogeneity is a key to ensuring internal validity for etiological studies. However, study samples from observational studies are often highly heterogeneous. For example, survey studies often recruit participants to represent a population with different genders at different age ranges and coming from different racial/ethnic groups with different levels of education.

Further, it has been well-established that a medical, health, and/or behavioral problem often differs for subgroups with different demographic and socioeconomic conditions. For example, males are more likely than females to suffer from cardiovascular problems; youth are more likely than adults to explore new drugs, cancer often occurs in older individuals, not to mention substantial racial/ethnic differences in quality of life, substance use, mental health, incidence and prevalence of diseases, and access to healthcare.

In this section, we will use real data to demonstrate how to include demographic factors as covariates to assist in etiological studies and discuss why it is needed to include them to confirm a hypothetic X ~ Y relationship.

5.4.2   An Example of Tobacco Smoking and High Blood Pressure Relationship

In Chap. 4, we demonstrated a significant relation between tobacco use X and high blood pressure Y using a set of measures for both X and Y. In this section, we will use years of smoking as X and measured systolic blood pressure as Y. The bivariate analysis in Chap. 4 indicated both the X and the Y are a good selection for further analysis.

Blood pressure Y will be assessed using the mean of three repeated measures. This variable is selected for several reasons. First, this measure is continuous, making it suitable for linear regression analysis. Second, this measure was computed by taking the average of three consecutive measures, which is highly valid and reliable. Last, this variable has been demonstrated from bivariate analysis in Chap. 4 as a good outcome measure.

As a demonstration, two demographic factors were included as covariates, gender (male/female) and race (White vs. other). These two variables are used in almost all observational studies. Knowledge and skills gained using these two variables provide a method to assist in selecting other demographic and socioeconomic factors. It is worth noting that age as a demographic factor is not included for demonstration. This is because the variable age may be highly correlated with X – years of smoking. Adding age may cause a collinearity problem (see Sect. 5.5 for more detailed discussion on highly correlated covariates).

5.4.3   Data Sources and SAS Program

Data were derived from the 2017–18 NHANES. Participants 20 years of age and older are included. The final sample contains 3148 participants after exclusion of those with missing data (1971 with no data on gender and 2495 with no blood pressure data). Participants who reported to be on antihypertensive medication (n = 3148) were also excluded. Use of medicine to treat hypertension is an confounder that will interfere with the analysis to determine the smoking and blood pressure relationship.

Data for this part of analysis are generated from the dataset DATCH4 used in Chap. 4. Sections 1 and 2 of the SAS Program show how to create DATCH5 for this chapter by accessing the DATCH4, create and label new variables, and check data for analysis; and Sections 3–6 show how to conduct analysis to verify bivariate results that smoking is a risk factor for high blood pressure. Three demographic variables (age, gender, and race) were included and two (gender and race) were used in analysis.

The program can easily be extended to include other covariates.

```
*********************************************************************************
* SAS PROGRAM 5.2. DATA PREPARATON AND ANALYSIS TO ADJUST DEMOGRAPHIC FACTORS
*********************************************************************************;
** PART 1 DATA PREPARATION;
* 1 CREATE DATCH5 FROM DATCH4 FOR THE FIRST SET OF ANALYSIS;
LIBNAME SASDATA "C:\QUANTLAB\A_DATA\";
* READ IN AND CHECK DATA;
DATA SASDATA.DATCH5; SET SASDATA.DATCH4;
* CREATE AND LABEL A TWO-LEVEL RACIAL GROUP FOR USE TO ADJUST DEMOGRAPHIC FACTOR;
IF RACE5 NE . THEN RACE2   = (RACE5 EQ 1);
LABEL RACE2  = "WHITE = 1 OTHER = 0";
* KEEP NEWLY CRREATED AND SELECTED VARIABLES CREATED FOR CHAPTER FOUR FOR ANLAYSIS;
KEEP AGE GENDER RACE5 RACE2 EDUCATION MARRIAGE DIASBP SYSTBP HBP HBPX HBPMED SMKYRS
SMKDAYS SMKNOW COTININE H_COTININE SEQN; RUN;
** 2 CHECK DATA
* CHECK VARIABLES AND OBSERVATIONS;
PROC CONTENTS DATA = SASDATA.DATCH5; RUN;
* CHECK DATA FOR MISSING;
PROC FREQ DATA = SASDATA.DATCH5; TABLES SYSTBP RACE2; RUN;
** 3 CREATE WORK DATASET A FOR USE N=3033;
DATA A; SET SASDATA.DATCH5;
* INCLUSION OF 4187 OBSERVATIONS WITH NO MISSING ON SYSTBP;
IF SYSTBP NE .;
* EXCLUDE 3033 PARTICIPANTS ON ANTI-HBP MEDICATION, A CONFOUNDER FOR SMOKING-SYSTBP;
IF HBPMED NE 1; * HBPMED = 1 FOR PARTICIPANTS ON ANTIHYPERTENSIVE DRUGS;
IF SMKYRS EQ . THEN SMKYRS = 0; * CODE PARTICIPANTS WITH MISSING TO ZERO (NO SMOKING);
RUN;
** PART 2. REGRESSION MODELING ANALYSIS
* 1 CORRELATION ANALYSIS WITH GENDER AND RACE2 AS COVARIATES;
PROC CORR DATA =A;
VAR SYSTBP SMKYRS GENDER RACE2 AGE;
RUN;
** 2 REGRESSION CONSIDERING GENDER AS COVARIATE
* ADJUSTED EFFECT FOR SMKYRS ON SYSTBP AFTER GENDER DIFFERENCE IS CONSIDERED;
PROC REG DATA = A;
MODEL SYSTBP = SMKYRS GENDER;
RUN;
* 3 BIASED BETA WITHOUT ADJUSTING GENDER DIFFERENCES;
PROC REG DATA = A;
MODEL SYSTBP = SMKYRS;
RUN;
** 4 ANALYSIS WITH RACE2 AS COVARIATE;
* ADJUSTED EFFECT FOR SMKYRS ON SYSTBP AFTER RACIAL DIFFERENCE IS CONSIDERED;
PROC REG DATA = A;
MODEL SYSTBP = SMKYRS RACE2;
RUN;
** 5 ADJUSTED EFFECT OF SMKYRS ON SYSTBP AFTER GENDER AND RACE ARE CONSIDERED;
PROC REG DATA = A;
MODEL SYSTBP = SMKYRS GENDER RACE2;
RUN;
*********************************************************************************;
```

5.4.4 Correlation Analysis

Based on our simulations in Sect. 5.3, the verification analysis started by checking
the correlation among all related variables, including Y (systolic blood pressure), X
(years of smoking), CovX's (gender and race). In general, age is included as a
covariate. However, in this analysis, by knowledge the variable AGE is closely correlated with X (SMKYRS). Relative to younger participants, older participants are
more likely to smoke for longer periods. In addition, the purpose of the study is to
determine if more years of smoking is associated with high blood pressure; therefore, age will no longer be an indicator of sample diversity.

Correlation analysis was completed with SAS Program 5.2, Part 2.1. First, descriptive statistics for all five variables are estimated in the correlation analysis (results not shown). Second, correlations between the five variables were computed and presented using a correlation coefficient matrix as shown in Fig. 5.6. According to the results, X (SMKYRS) was positively associated with Y (SYSTBP, r = 0.1968). This is also the bivariate result we observed in Chap. 4.

Pearson Correlation Coefficients, N = 3033 Prob > |r| under H0: Rho=0					
	SYSTBP	SMKYRS	GENDER	RACE2	AGE
SYSTBP MEASURED SYSTOLIC BLOOD PRESSURE, MEAN,	1.00000	0.19675 <.0001	-0.15376 <.0001	-0.05686 0.0017	0.40619 <.0001
SMKYRS YEARS OF SMOKING FROM ONSET TO THE SURVEY TIME,	0.19675 <.0001	1.00000	-0.20201 <.0001	0.16808 <.0001	0.44463 <.0001
GENDER GENDER 1=MALE 2=FEMALE,	-0.15376 <.0001	-0.20201 <.0001	1.00000	0.00164 0.9279	-0.04602 0.0112
RACE2 WHITE = 1 OTHER = 0	-0.05686 0.0017	0.16808 <.0001	0.00164 0.9279	1.00000	0.05549 0.0022
AGE AGE IN YEAR,	0.40619 <.0001	0.44463 <.0001	-0.04602 0.0112	0.05549 0.0022	1.00000

Fig. 5.6 Pearson correlation between outcome Y (SYSTBP), influential factor X (SMKYRS) and covariates GENDER, RACE2 and AGE; output of SAS Program 5.2 Part 2

Of the three CovX's, the first one (GENDER) was negatively associated with X (r = −0.2020. p < 0.01), as well as Y (r = −0.1538, p < 0.01). This correlation pattern corresponds to Scenario 4 in Table 5.2; therefore, results from bivariate analysis about effect of smoking may be biased toward underestimation.

The second one (RACE2) was positively correlated with X (SMKYRS) with r = 0.1681 (p < 0.01) and negatively associated with Y (SYSTBP) with r = −0.0569 (p < 0.01). This correlation pattern corresponds to Scenario 2 in Table 5.2; thus, results from bivariate analysis could be biased toward overestimation.

Likewise, the estimated r = 0.4493 (p < 0.01) for the correlation between AGE and X (SMKYRS), the highest among all 10 pairs of correlations. This high correlation supports our decision at the beginning to exclude this variable as a covariate. We will revisit it in Sect. 5.5 when dealing with confounders.

5.4.5   Analysis with Gender Included as Covariate

Figure 5.7 displays the SAS output from the regression analysis part in SAS program 5.2.2. Results in the top part indicate the estimated $\beta_1 = 0.1756$ (p < .0001) for X (SMKYRS). This would be the effect of X on Y (SYSTBP) after considering gender differences in the X ~ Y relation; therefore, it is an adjusted estimate that is closer to the true relation. This finding is consistent with the knowledge in the

Parameter Estimates						
Variable	Label	DF	Parameter Estimate	Standard Error	t Value	Pr > |t|
Intercept	Intercept	1	125.67337	1.05658	118.94	<.0001
SMKYRS	YEARS OF SMOKING FROM ONSET TO THE SURVEY TIME,	1	0.17563	0.01836	9.57	<.0001
GENDER	GENDER 1=MALE 2=FEMALE,	1	-4.12192	0.62622	-6.58	<.0001

Parameter Estimates						
Variable	Label	DF	Parameter Estimate	Standard Error	t Value	Pr > |t|
Intercept	Intercept	1	119.14709	0.36760	324.12	<.0001
SMKYRS	YEARS OF SMOKING FROM ONSET TO THE SURVEY TIME,	1	0.20004	0.01811	11.05	<.0001

Fig. 5.7 Smoking (X) and systolic blood pressure (Y) relation with (top) and without (bottom) adjusting for gender, output of regressions 2 & 3 from SAS Program 5.2.2-2.3

literature about heterogeneity and the significant gender-smoking and gender –systolic blood pressure relationship from the previous step of analysis.

Results in the bottom part show that the unadjusted coefficient (β'_1) for the same X on Y. In this case, the unadjusted $\beta'_1 = 0.2000$, greater than 0.1756, the adjusted β_1. In another words, the X ~ Y association would be *overestimated* by 14% (0.2000–0.1756) if gender were not considered. This result is consistent with the rule for Scenario 4 in Table 5.2: positive X ~ Y relation, and negative CovX~X and CovX~Y relation will lead to a bias (overestimate) of the X ~ Y relationship.

Figure 5.8 is a geometric presentation showing the estimated beta for the X ~ Y relationship with and without considering CovX (GENDER). Left part of the figure shows, if only bivariate analysis is used, the regression model will treat the slanted X ~ Y relation as vertical, leading to an overestimated β'_1 (dashed line). The right part of Fig. 5.8 shows the adjusted β_1 (the solid vertical line) after adding CovX (GENDER) with the adjusted part = (0.2000–0.1756).

Fig. 5.8 Compare unadjusted and adjusted beta coefficients – bias toward overestimate if gender was not considered

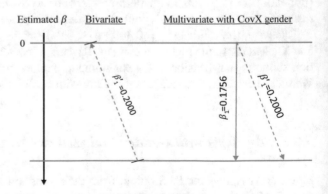

Another piece of information from the figure is that it is also possible to determine the angle between X and CovX with the vertical triangle sum theorem – solving for an angle knowing the length of the two sides. Interested students can give it a try.

5.4.6   Analysis with Race Included as Covariate

Correlation analysis results in Fig. 5.6 indicate that CovX race (RACE2) was positively associated with X (SMKYRS) and negatively associated with Y (SYSTBP), which corresponds to Scenario 2 listed in Table 5.2. If this is the case, bivariate analysis will lead to an *underestimated* beta coefficient. This is just what we observed from our data. Results from bivariate analysis (Fig. 5.7) indicated $\beta'_1 = 0.2000$ for X (smoking); results from multivariate analysis in Fig. 5.9 indicate the adjusted β_1 (X | race) = 0.2159 (rounded up from 0.24586). There was a 0.0115 (7%) increase in the estimated beta after race is considered as CovX. Interested students may try to present the results geometrically following the method in Fig. 5.8.

By considering results presented above for gender and race, we can conclude that if the demographic compositions (i.e., gender and race) are not adjusted, the X ~ Y relationship can either be overestimated or underestimated, depending on the influences of specific demographic factors.

Parameter Estimates						
Variable	Label	DF	Parameter Estimate	Standard Error	t Value	Pr > |t|
Intercept	Intercept	1	120.06809	0.40750	294.64	<.0001
SMKYRS	YEARS OF SMOKING FROM ONSET TO THE SURVEY TIME,	1	0.21586	0.01829	11.80	<.0001
RACE2	WHITE = 1 OTHER = 0	1	-3.44312	0.66930	-5.14	<.0001

Fig. 5.9 Smoking(X) and systolic blood pressure (Y) relation after adjusting for differences in racial composition, output of SAS Program 5.2.4

5.4.7   Analysis with Both Gender and Race Included

A natural extension of the previous two analyses would be to include both gender and race in one model as covariates. This model will thus adjust population composition with regard to both gender and race: a broader conceptual framework than either the gender or race alone in the previous analyses. This step of analysis was completed using SAS Program 5.2.5 and the output is presented in Fig. 5.10.

When both gender and race are considered, the estimated β_1 (X | gender, race) = 0.1914. This is the adjusted regression coefficient. Relative to the unadjusted, this adjusted estimate of β_1 better reflects the association between cigarette smoking and high blood pressure among adults in the United States. More detailed interpretation will be presented in the next section.

Parameter Estimates						
Variable	Label	DF	Parameter Estimate	Standard Error	t Value	Pr > |t|
Intercept	Intercept	1	126.37227	1.06200	119.00	<.0001
SMKYRS	YEARS OF SMOKING FROM ONSET TO THE SURVEY TIME,	1	0.19139	0.01857	10.31	<.0001
GENDER	GENDER 1=MALE 2=FEMALE,	1	-4.00826	0.62425	-6.42	<.0001
RACE2	WHITE = 1 OTHER = 0	1	-3.28560	0.66536	-4.94	<.0001

Fig. 5.10 Smoking was positively associated with systolic blood pressure after adjusting for both gender and race, output of SAS Program 5.2.5

5.4.8   Interpreting Results with Inclusion of Demographic Factors as Covariates

In quantitative epidemiology, results obtained by including one demographic factor can be interpreted as the X ~ Y relationship after removing the difference caused by the demographic factor. For example, in our first analysis for gender, β_1 (X | gender) = 0.1756. This means that the detected positive relationship between smoking and blood pressure can be generalized to any population regardless of gender; or the X ~ Y relationship with adjusted β_1 = 0.1756 is independent of gender.

Likewise, β_1 (X | race) = 0.2159 from the second analysis indicate this strong smoking-high blood pressure is independent of race. It can be generalized to any population regardless of racial differences. Certainly, when both gender and race are included, the adjusted result can be interpreted as a measure of smoking-blood pressure regardless of the heterogeneity in the gender and racial composition of a population.

In epidemiology, researchers often select a set of commonly used demographic and socioeconomic factors as covariates, such as age, gender, race, education, income, etc. After a set of covariates is selected, it places the multiple regression analysis of an X ~ Y relationship in a space, or conceptual framework defined by these factors. With the assistance of this framework, the adjusted effect of X on Y can be estimated to remove the bias and the results can thus be generalized to a population regardless of diversities of the study sample (and so does the population) defined by these covariates.

Demographic factors are included in almost all observational studies to examine factors associated with a health outcome. The following presents a template for beginners to write up such findings:

"After adjusting for the demographic factors gender and race, findings from multiple regression analysis confirmed the bivariate result that smoking was positively associated with blood pressure."

5.5   Confounders as Covariates

To confirm an X ~ Y relationship revealed from exploratory bivariate analysis, confounders must be considered in addition to demographic and socioeconomic factors described in Sect. 5.4. In this section, we will (i) introduce the concept of confounders analytically, (ii) discuss methods for analyzing confounding variables, (iii) demonstrate the application of regression analysis with real data to control for confounders, and (iv) interpret the results.

5.5.1   Confounders

By definition, confounders are variables that are *known* to be associated with both the independent variable X and the dependent variable Y. Furthermore, the association is not determined by the data at hand alone, and it *must be based on the prior knowledge*, including theoretical analysis, or published data (VanderWell 2019). These types of variables are named as confounders because they may lead to a biased estimate of the X ~ Y relationship if not considered in statistical analysis.

Like demographic factors, confounders represent another type of covariates. The impact of a confounder can be understood using the analytical methods and scatter plots as discussed in Chap. 4 and applied in Sect. 5.4. In this section, we introduce another concept: **Vectors** to help understand confounders. Vector is an indictor used in physics to describe force that contains both magnitude and direction. This concept was implied in Sect. 5.4 for multivariate regression by controlling for demographic factors as in Fig. 5.8.

Figure 5.11 illustrates correlations between two variables CovX and X using vectors. Different from the scatter X ~ Y plot, two vectors (arrowed lines) are used to represent two variables and correlations between the two variables are measured

Fig. 5.11 Understanding correlation using the concept of vector: (**a**) Two vectors X and CovX independent from each other (r = 0), (**b**) the CovX- X angle >45 degree (r < 0.5); (**c**) the CovX – X angle <45degree (r > 0.5); and (**d**): CovX-X angle = 0 (r = 1)

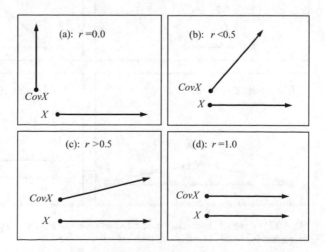

using the angle between the two vectors. Figure 5.11a shows a zero correlation between CovX and X. These two variables point to two different directions with an angle of 90°. It tells us that changes in X are totally independent of CovX; quantitatively, r = 0.0.

Different from Fig. 5.11a, b, c, present two typical cases in which CovX is associated with X with r varying between 0 and 1. The correlation will be 0 < r < 0.5 if the angle between the two variables are in the range of 45°< angle <90° as in Fig. 5.11b; and the correlation will be 0.5 r < 1.0, if the angle between the two variables are in the range of 0°< angle <45° as in Fig. 5.11c. Last, Fig. 5.11d depicts a complete correlation between CovX and X. In this case, any changes in X are completed related to CovX. This is a visual presentation of the concept of ***collinearity*** in statistics. In this case, the correlation coefficient = 1.0 for CovX and X.

The relationships presented in Fig. 5.11 can easily be extended to show negative correlations by switching the two vectors to be in opposite directions, against each other. Levels of correlation between the two variables can still be measured using the angle between the two vectors.

With the knowledge of correlation described using vectors, Fig. 5.12 depicts the concept of a CovX in confounding a potential X ~ Y relationship for four different conditions. Figure 5.12a shows a weak confounding of CovX on the X ~ Y relationship. Although CovX is associated with both X and Y, the CovX-X angle and CovX~Y angle are close to 90°, indicating a weak impact of this CovX on the X ~ Y relationship.

Likewise, Fig. 5.12b presents a case in which CovX is a moderate confounder and Fig. 5.12c, a stronger confounder. The difference between the two is the angle

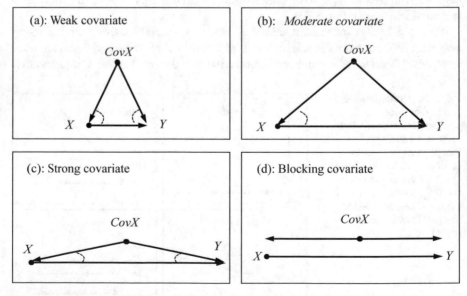

Fig. 5.12 Geometric presentation of different levels of confounding: (**a**) Weak, (**b**) moderate, (**c**) strong and (**d**) totally block X ~ Y relation

between CovX and X and CovX and Y; a smaller angle means stronger correlation and a larger angle means weaker correlation.

Last, Fig. 5.12d indicates a special case in which CovX and X and CovX and Y are both fully correlated – *collinearity*. In this case, CovX can totally block (or replace) the X ~ Y relationship if this variable is included together with X in a multivariate regression analysis, regardless of if the X ~ Y relationship is theory-based or supported by data or both.

5.5.2 Guidance for Confounder Selection

A challenge for many researchers is the selection of variables as confounders to verify a potential X ~ Y relationship with multivariate regression. Discussions in the previous section provide some theoretical knowledge; however, *the selection of variables as CovX is both an art and science* and there is no standard procedure to follow. The following are some methods commonly used in practice.

Method I: *Knowledge-based selection.* This method is based on the definition that a confounder is known to be associated with both X and Y. The method relies heavily on the previous knowledge and experience, intensive literature review, and even some pilot studies. With adequate knowledge, confounders often automatically come into play when thinking of an X ~ Y relation. Use the same example of smoking – high blood pressure. In this case, bodyweight immediately comes up as a confounder since numerous studies repeatedly report a positive relationship between the variable overweight and the variable high blood pressure (Dua et al. 2014); and studies also found that people purposefully smoke to control body weight (Seeley and Sandoval 2011).

Method II: *Logic analysis.* For example, to confirm the relationship between physical activity X and bodyweight Y, any factors that may affect X and Y should be considered, such as socioeconomic status since people with better education and higher income are more likely to engage in physical activities, and socioeconomic status is often negatively associated with the prevalence of overweight and obesity. To confirm if keeping physical distance X is protective against a COVID-19 infection Y, all factors that affect facemask wearing and COVID-19 infections should be considered. A typical factor is residential housing. People who live in a single-family house in the better off communities are physically distanced from others by nature, compared to those living in rental apartments; furthermore, residential settings can also be a risk factor for COVID-19 infection.

Method III: *Preliminary analysis.* If you have no idea whether to include a variable as a confounder, a last approach would be to conduct some analysis by associating a potential confounder with both X and Y, such as correlation analysis as being used in examining demographic factors in Sect. 5.4. If a variable is significantly associated with both X and Y, this variable is likely to be a confounder.

When Method III is used, two points must be kept in mind. First, no significant relationship cannot rule out the role of a variable as a confounder if existing knowledge suggests otherwise. This is because many other factors can affect the significance level in testing a relationship between any two variables. Second, relative to the correlation of a confounder with X, the correlation of a confounder with Y is more important.

5.5.3 Avoid Overcontrolling of Confounders

Graduate students as well as many junior investigators often like to include a large number of confounders as covariates using multiple regression models as if this is the means to ensure the validity of their research findings. In most cases, inclusion a long list of covariates may jerpodize the analysis given the complex, mostly unknown relationship among these variables as discussed in Chaps. 2 and 3. Inclusion of confounders is primarily a make-up procedure if the validity of a study cannot be ensured through research design. The following are several examples of incorrect use of confounders by medical and graduate students.

To examine the relationship between tobacco smoking and high blood pressure, the reported cigarette smoking in the past month is used as a measure of X; and a diagnosed high blood pressure is used as the outcome. In addition to smokers, non-smokers may also be exposed to secondhand smoking which can be assessed using biomarkers (i.e., cotinine in the blood). By definition, secondhand smoking is associated with smoking and high blood pressure, therefore this variable (cotinine in the blood) should be included as a CovX to verify the X ~ Y relationship. However, when the blood cotinine is included in the model, a significant X ~ Y relation revealed from a bivariate analysis become non-significant except the CovX – blood cotinine.

The fundamental error in this example is that there is a chained relation from smoking to blood cotinine and further to high blood pressure. When blood cotinine is analyzed like a variable independent from tobacco smoking, it blocks the smoking – high blood pressure relationship. Other typical examples include: Examining the association of small dosage of aspirin use (X) and chest Pain (Y) while adding frequency and dosage of aspirin use as CovX or confounders; associating age of smoking onset (X) with depression (Y) while adding age as a CovX or a confounder; and quantifying the relationship between citizenship (X) and substance use (Y) while considering years of staying in the US as a CovX or a confounder. More detailed discussions on covariates and confounders can be found in Chap. 8.

One characteristic common to the three examples described in the previous paragraph is that in each sample, both the X and the CovX provide data measuring the same character (see more discussion about this topic in Chap. 2). Using aspirin (yes/no), frequency and dosage of use all measure the same character – aspirin usage; age of smoking onset and age both provide information about years of living (age is an exact measure while age of onset is an approximate); citizenship and years staying in the US both measure the levels of acculturation to the American culture. As long as one is used as the X, the other cannot be included as CoX or confounder.

5.5.4 Measured and Unmeasured Confounders

As described above, selection of factors as confounders depends to a great extent on our knowledge about the study question. Therefore, there is no way to determine if all potential factors are included. This led to the concept of measured and unmeasured confounders (Fig. 5.13).

Fig. 5.13 Unmeasured confounders cannot be fully ruled out in etiological studies with multivariate analysis

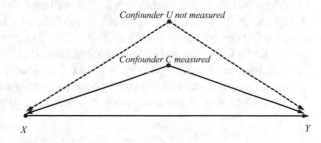

When conducting multiple regression analysis to confirm a hypothetic X ~ Y relationship by inclusion of a number of selected confounders, we must be aware of the potential omission of significant confounders.

5.5.5 Differences Between Confounders and Demographic Factors

In Sect. 5.4, demographic factors as covariates were systematically discussed and empirically tested. In the analyses, demographic factors were used simply as covariates, not confounders. After discussion about confounders above, it can be seen that a demographic factor can also be a confounder if it is significantly associated with both X and Y. The difference lies in the purpose of an analysis. When a demographic factor (i.e., gender) is used as a covariate, the purpose is NOT to detect if an X ~ Y relationship is confounded by the variable but to improve the generalizability of the findings – *external validity*. However, when a variable is used a confounder, the purpose is to ensure if an estimated X ~ Y relationship is biased – *internal validity*. Although the difference is more conceptual than analytical, it is very important to make this distinction.

5.6 Demonstration of Confounders with Empirical Data

In this section, we will conduct analysis with real data utilizing the knowledge and principles described above. The dataset DATCH5 will be expanded to add new variables. This step will be completed using SAS Program 5.3. With the expanded dataset, a series of analyses will be conducted using SAS Program 5.4.

5.6.1 Data Processing

SAS Program 5.3 below shows how to expand dataset DATCH5 by adding two new variables DEPRESS (for depressive symptoms) and BMI (for body mass index) as confounders. Before executing this program, please make sure you have the datasets DPQ_J.XPT and WHQ_J.XPT downloaded from NHANES and saved in the folder C:\QUANTLAB\A_DATA\ORIGINAL\. It will take 4 steps to complete the dataset expansion: Step 1. Read in DATCH5 as TEMP1; step 2. Create TEMP2 by reading and processing the original dataset DPQ_J.XPT to create the variable DEPRESS using 9 items from Patient Health Questionnaire (PHQ-9); step 3. Create TEMP3 from the original data WHQ_J.XPT to create the variable BMI, including the conversion of height in inch and weight in pound into meter and kg; and step 4. Expand the DATCH5 by sorting and combining the three temp datasets.

```
*******************************************************************************;
* SAS PROGRAM 5.3. EXPAND DATCH5 BY ADDING DEPRESS FROM DPQ_J AND BMI FROM WHQ_J
*******************************************************************************;
** 1 SPECIFIY DATA FILE LOCATION;
LIBNAME SASDATA "C:\QUANTLAB\A_DATA\";
** 2 PROCESS DEPRESSION DATA AS A CONFOUNDER
* READ, CONVERT AND PROCESS THE ORIGINAL DPQ_J TO OBTAIN DEPRESSION MEASURES AND
CREATE TEMP1;
LIBNAME XPTDATA XPORT "C:\QUANTLAB\A_DATA\ORIGINAL\DPQ_J.XPT" ACCESS=READONLY;
PROC COPY INLIB=XPTDATA OUTLIB=SASDATA; PROC CONTENTS; RUN;
DATA SASDATA.DPQ_J; SET SASDATA.DPQ_J;
* REMOVE MISSING USING ARRAY - A VARY USEFUL TRICK FOR DATA PROCESSING;
ARRAY ITEMS DPQ010 - DPQ090; DO OVER ITEMS; IF ITEMS IN (7 9) THEN ITEMS =.; END; RUN;
* COMPUTE CRONBACH ALPHA FOR RELIABILITY ASSESSMENT AS IN CHAPTER 2;
* THE COMPUTED ALPHA=0.83;
PROC CORR ALPHA DATA=SASDATA.DPQ_J NOMISS;
VAR DPQ010 DPQ020 DPQ030 DPQ040 DPQ050 DPQ060 DPQ070 DPQ080 DPQ090; RUN;
* COMPUTE DEPRESSION SCORE AND STORE IT IN TEMP1;
DATA TEMP1; SET SASDATA.DPQ_J;
* CREATE DEPRESSON SCORE BY SUMMING UP ITEM SCORES, DO THIS AFTER ALPHA IS COMPUTED;
DEPRESS = DPQ010+DPQ020+DPQ030+DPQ040+DPQ050+DPQ060+DPQ070+DPQ080+DPQ090;
LABEL DEPRESS = 'DEPRESSIVE SYMPTOMS PHQ SCALE SCORE';
KEEP DEPRESS SEQN;
* CHECK DATA; PROC CONTENTS; RUN; PROC FREQ DATA=TEMP1; RUN;
** 3 PROCESS BMI DATA AS ANOTHER CONFOUNDER;
* READ, CONVERT AND PROCESS THE ORIGINAL WHQ_J TO GET WEIGHT AND HEIGHT, BMI AND
CREATE TEMP2;
LIBNAME XPTDATA XPORT " C:\QUANTLAB\A_DATA\ORIGINAL\WHQ_J.XPT" ACCESS=READONLY;
PROC COPY INLIB=XPTDATA OUTLIB=SASDATA; PROC CONTENTS; RUN;
* RECODE AND KEEP VARIABLES WHD010(HEIGHT INCH) WHD020(WEIGHT LB) WHQ030(SELF-
ASSESSMENT) SEQN;
DATA TEMP2; SET SASDATA.WHQ_J;
IF  WHD010 IN (7777 9999) THEN WHD010=.;  * CODE SYSTEM MISSING;
IF  WHD020 IN (7777 9999) THEN WHD020=.;
HEIGHT  = WHD010 * 0.0254;      *INCH TO METER;
WEIGHT  = WHD020 * 0.45;     *LB TO KG;
BMI = (WEIGHT/(HEIGHT * HEIGHT));
LABEL HEIGHT = 'REPORTED HEIGHT IN CM',
       WEIGHT = 'RPORTED WEIGHT IN KG',
       BMI = 'BODY MASS INDEX USING REPORTED DATA';
* USE PROC UNIVARIATE TO HEIGH WEIGHT AND BMI AFTER COMPLETE RECODING;
KEEP HEIGHT WEIGHT BMI WHQ030 SEQN;
PROC CONTENTS DATA = TEMP2; RUN;
** 4 READ DATCH5 CREATED IN SAS PROGRAM 5.2 INTO TEMP3 FOR EXPANDING;
DATA TEMP3; SET SASDATA.DATCH5; RUN;
** 5 EXPAND DATCH5: SORT TEMP1 TEMP2 TEMP3, AND MERGE BY SEQN;
PROC SORT DATA=TEMP1; BY SEQN; RUN;
PROC SORT DATA=TEMP2; BY SEQN; RUN;
PROC SORT DATA=TEMP3; BY SEQN; RUN;
DATA SASDATA.DATCH5; MERGE TEMP1 TEMP2 TEMP3; BY SEQN; RUN;
* CHECK VARIABLES;
PROC CONTENTS DATA = SASDATA.DATCH5; RUN;
*******************************************************************************;
```

SAS Program 5.3 is self-explanatory. Depression score (DEPRESS) is computed simply by summing up item scores after recoding missing data. Missing can be detected by running the **PROC FREQ**. Height and weight are converted into meter and kg respectively before they are used to compute the body mass index (BMI). With this step of data processing, a list of 20 variables plus SEQN are included in DATCH5. In addition to this chapter, many variables included in this dataset will be used in later chapters for analysis.

The selection of depression and BMI as confounders to confirm the X (tobacco smoking) and Y (blood pressure) is based on previous knowledge. Studies have already documented that BMI (CovX₁) is associated with X – tobacco smoking (Clair et al. 2011) and Y- high blood pressure (Dua et al. 2014). Meanwhile, as a mental health measure, depression (CovX₂) is consistently associated with X – tobacco smoking (Chaiton et al. 2009). Long-term depression may also increase the risk of Y – blood pressure, particularly diastolic blood pressure (Meng et al. 2012).

5.6.2   Multiple Regression to Include Confounders

As described early in this section, statistically, the multiple regression analysis with confounders will be the same as the analysis of demographic factors, only the purpose of analysis differs. Thus, the same approach used in Sect. 5.4 will be used here as seen in SAS Program 5.4. This program consists of three parts, reflecting the steps for analysis to control for confounders:

1. Create a work dataset **B** by reading the expanded DATCH5 that contains the two newly added variable BMI and DEPRESS.; and select the study participants who are not on anti-hypertensive mediation.
2. Conduct a linear correlation analysis to assess the correlations of the two confounders DEPRESS and BMI with the outcome Y (BPSYST). In addition, three demographic factors (AGE GENDER RACE2) are included. We included AGE to test the highly correlated confounder with X – years of smoking (SMKYRS) .
3. Conduct a multiple linear regression analysis to control for the confounders one at a time first and then together. No regression for SMKYRS – BPSYST relation is included since this analysis was already conducted in Sect. 5.4, the result can be used here to support the analysis for confounders.

```
***********************************************************************************
* SAS PROGRAM 5.4. ANALYSIS OF CONFOUNDERS USING DATCH52
*********************************************************************************;
** 1 CREATE WORK DATASET B FOR ANALYSIS;
*  EXCLUDE MISSING FOR SYSTBP AND OBSERVATIONS ON ANTI-HBP MEDICATION;
DATA B; SET SASDATA.DATCH5; IF SYSTBP NE .;  IF HBPMED NE 1;
IF SMKYRS EQ . THEN SMKYRS = 0; * CODE PARTICIPANTS WITH MISSING TO ZERO (NO SMOKING);
RUN;
** 2 CORRELATION ANALYSIS OF ALL RELATED VARIABLES;
PROC CORR DATA = B;
VAR BPSYST SMKYRS AGE GENDER RACE2 DEPRESS BMI; RUN;
** 3 REGRESSION TO CONTROL CONFOUNDERS, /STB FOR STANDARD REG COEFFICIENTS
      PLOTS=NONE WAS USED TO SUPRESS ALL PLOTS;
PROC REG DATA = B PLOTS=NONE;
MODEL BPSYST = SMKYRS DEPRESS BMI/STB;
RUN;
*********************************************************************************;
```

To save space, results from analysis of single confounders are not included in SAS Program 5.4. Students are encouraged to add two more models, one for DEPRESS only and another for BMI only. After completion of all analyses, results should be compared across different models.

5.6.3   Results from Correlation Analysis

SAS output from SAS Program 5.4.2 for correlation analysis is presented in Fig. 5.14. Results from the correlation analysis indicated that one selected confounder DEPRESS (no. depressive symptoms) was significantly and positively associated with SMKYRS (years of smoking, r = 0.0998, p < 0.01), but not significantly associated with the outcome SYSTBP (systolic blood pressure, r = −0.0195, p > 0.05).

Pearson Correlation Coefficients Prob > |r| under H0: Rho=0 Number of Observations							
	SYSTBP	SMKYRS	DEPRESS	BMI	AGE	GENDER	RACE2
SYSTBP MEASURED SYSTOLIC BLOOD PRESSURE, MEAN,	1.00000 3033	0.19675 <.0001 3033	-0.01945 0.2992 2851	0.16388 <.0001 2892	0.40619 <.0001 3033	-0.15376 <.0001 3033	-0.05686 0.0017 3033
SMKYRS YEARS OF SMOKING FROM ONSET TO THE SURVEY TIME,	0.19675 <.0001 3033	1.00000 3033	0.09979 <.0001 2851	-0.00240 0.8975 2892	0.44463 <.0001 3033	-0.20201 <.0001 3033	0.16808 <.0001 3033
DEPRESS DEPRESSIVE SYMPTOMS PHQ SCALE SCORE	-0.01945 0.2992 2851	0.09979 <.0001 2851	1.00000 2851	0.08800 <.0001 2724	-0.05032 0.0072 2851	0.10032 <.0001 2851	0.08405 <.0001 2851
BMI BODY MASS INDEX USING REPORTED DATA	0.16388 <.0001 2892	-0.00240 0.8975 2892	0.08800 <.0001 2724	1.00000 2892	-0.02902 0.1187 2892	0.02383 0.2002 2892	0.00825 0.6573 2892
AGE AGE IN YEAR,	0.40619 <.0001 3033	0.44463 <.0001 3033	-0.05032 0.0072 2851	-0.02902 0.1187 2892	1.00000 3033	-0.04602 0.0112 3033	0.05549 0.0022 3033
GENDER GENDER 1=MALE 2=FEMALE,	-0.15376 <.0001 3033	-0.20201 <.0001 3033	0.10032 <.0001 2851	0.02383 0.2002 2892	-0.04602 0.0112 3033	1.00000 3033	0.00164 0.9279 3033
RACE2 WHITE = 1 OTHER = 0	-0.05686 0.0017 3033	0.16808 <.0001 3033	0.08405 <.0001 2851	0.00825 0.6573 2892	0.05549 0.0022 3033	0.00164 0.9279 3033	1.00000 3033

Fig. 5.14 Correlations among influential factor X (years of smoking), outcome Y (systolic blood pressure), confounders, and demographic factors; Output of the correlation analysis from SAS Program 5.4.2

The other confounder BMI was positively associated with SYSTBP (r = 0.1639, p < 0.01), but not significantly associated with SMKYRS (r = −0.0024, p > 0.05). Strictly speaking, this variable is not qualified as a confounder since it only associated with outcome Y, not the influential factor X of interest. As a demonstration, the variable BMI is still included in the analysis as a confounder.

As expected, the variable AGE is significantly associated with X – SMKYRS (r = 0.4446, p < 0.01) and Y – BPSYST (r = 0.4062, p < 0.01). Furthermore, the AGE and SMKRRS correlation is more than two times greater than the SMKYRS-Y relation ($r = 0.1968$). Based on the discussion and Fig. 5.14, inclusion of this variable as a CovX may substantially alter the SMKYRS – BPSYST relationship, leading to a biased result.

5.6.4 Multivariate Regression Controlling for Depression and BMI

Outcome from SAS Program 5.4.3 is shown in Fig. 5.15. After controlling confounders (DEPRESS and BMI), the estimated $\beta_1 = 0.2004$ ($p < 0.01$) for X (SMKYRS, years of smoking). From previous SAS output (Fig. 5.7, bottom panel in Sect. 5.4), the estimated unadjusted $\beta'_1 = 0.2000$ ($p < 0.01$) for X (SMKYRS). There is a slight increase in the adjusted estimate of β_1 after these two confounders are controlled.

The last column in Fig. 5.15 shows the standardized regression coefficients. The absolute value of the standard regression coefficients provides a measure of relative significance of all Xs on Y. Results in the figure show that of the three factors, the impact of X (SMKYRS) was the strongest (standard $\beta = 0.2029$) and the impact of CovX (DEPRESS) was the least (absolute standard $\beta = 0.0612$), with the impact of another CovX (BMI) in between (standard $\beta = 0.1720$).

Parameter Estimates							
Variable	Label	DF	Parameter Estimate	Standard Error	t Value	Pr > |t|	Standardized Estimate
Intercept	Intercept	1	107.71089	1.35493	79.50	<.0001	0
SMKYRS	YEARS OF SMOKING FROM ONSET TO THE SURVEY TIME,	1	0.20035	0.01836	10.91	<.0001	0.20292
DEPRESS	DEPRESSIVE SYMPTOMS PHQ SCALE SCORE	1	-0.25304	0.07714	-3.28	0.0011	-0.06123
BMI	BODY MASS INDEX USING REPORTED DATA	1	0.42835	0.04622	9.27	<.0001	0.17200

Fig. 5.15 Smoking-systolic blood pressure relation after controlling for confounders of BMI and depressive symptoms: Output of multivariate regression analysis of SAS Program 5.4.3

It is worth noting that as a byproduct, results of the multivariate analysis above shows that DEPRESS was negatively and significantly associated with Y (BPSYST, $\beta = -0.2530$, $p < 0.01$); and CovX (BMI) was significantly and positively associated with Y (BPSYST, $\beta = 0.4284$, $p < 0.01$).

To demonstrate the impact of AGE on the SMKYRS – BPSYST relationship, the previous analysis was extended to include AGE (SAS program not shown). After AGE was added as another confounder, the estimated $\beta_1 = 0.0238$ for SMKYRS, about an 88% reduction from $\beta_1 = 0.2000$. Furthermore, the SMKYRS – BPSYST association became no longer statistically significant ($p = 0.2172$, >0.05) after AGE was included. This result is not consistent with the existing knowledge that smoking is a risk factor for hypertension.

Students are asked to repeat this analysis in Practice and to try to interpret the results using the concept of vector (hint: refer to Fig. 5.12).

5.7   Comprehensive Analysis and Reporting

In the previous three sections, we introduced a step by step approach on how to confirm results from bivariate analysis to include demographic factors and confounders. As a routine in epidemiological research, a comprehensive analytical strategy is often used to wrap up a project. In this section, we present the following as an example of comprehensive multivariate analysis. It can be extended to meet the requirements for different research projects with different conditions.

5.7.1   SAS Program Example for Comprehensive Analysis

SAS Program 5.5 provides a typical comprehensive analysis. It includes four regression models from Model 1 to Model 4. These models are constructed based on various analyses introduced in Sects. 5.4 through 5.6 with demographic factors and confounders carefully selected and tested.

The program is easy to follow. Model 1 is a simple linear regression to replicate the results from bivariate analysis using a Student-test or ANOVA, knowing that the estimated regression coefficient beta may be biased. Model 2 is used to adjust for demographic factors that are selected through careful analysis. We used only two variables as examples, but more demographic and socioeconomic variables can be added. Model 3 is used to adjust for confounders. As with Model 2, more confounders can be added to Model 3 if needed. Last, Model 4 is used to include both demographic and confounding variables.

```
******************************************************************************************
* SAS PROGRAM 5.5. MODELING DEMOGRAPHIC AND CONFOUNDERS TOGETHER FOR REPORTING
******************************************************************************************;
PROC REG DATA = B PLOT = NONE;
* MODEL 1: BIVARIATE ANALYSIS USING SIMPLE REGRESSION;
MODEL SYSTBP = SMKYRS;
RUN;
* MODEL 2: MULTIPLE REGRESSION TO ADJUST DEMOGRAPHIC FACTORS;
PROC REG DATA = B PLOT = NONE;
MODEL SYSTBP = SMKYRS GENDER RACE2;
RUN;
* MODEL 3: MULTIPLE REGRESSION TO CONTROL FOR CONFOUNDERS;
PROC REG DATA = B PLOT = NONE;
MODEL SYSTBP = SMKYRS DEPRESS BMI; RUN;
* MODEL 4: MULTIPLE REGRESSION INCLUDING DEMOGRAPHIC FACTORS AND CONFOUNDERS;
PROC REG DATA = B PLOT = NONE;
MODEL SYSTBP = SMKYRS GENDER RACE2 DEPRESS BMI/STB;  * /STB FOR STANDARDIZED BETA
RUN;
******************************************************************************************;
```

5.7.2   Results from Comprehensive Analysis

Results for Models 1–3 have already been presented in Sects. 5.4 through 5.6. Figure 5.16 presents the results from Model 4. The adjusted estimate of $\beta_1 = 0.1949$ ($p < 0.01$) for SMKYRS. This estimate provides a unbiased measure quantifying the smoking – blood pressure relationship after adjusting for the difference in gender and race and controlling for the confounders of depression and body mass index.

Parameter Estimates							
Variable	Label	DF	Parameter Estimate	Standard Error	t Value	Pr > |t|	Standardized Estimate
Intercept	Intercept	1	114.04270	1.66061	68.67	<.0001	0
SMKYRS	YEARS OF SMOKING FROM ONSET TO THE SURVEY TIME,	1	0.19490	0.01885	10.34	<.0001	0.19782
GENDER	GENDER 1=MALE 2=FEMALE,	1	-3.81935	0.64068	-5.96	<.0001	-0.11262
RACE2	WHITE = 1 OTHER = 0	1	-3.19186	0.67071	-4.76	<.0001	-0.08908
DEPRESS	DEPRESSIVE SYMPTOMS PHQ SCALE SCORE	1	-0.16218	0.07735	-2.10	0.0361	-0.03933
BMI	BODY MASS INDEX USING REPORTED DATA	1	0.43662	0.04608	9.48	<.0001	0.17512

Fig. 5.16 Smoking-systolic blood pressure relation after adjusting demographic factors and controlling for confounders of BMI and depressive symptoms: Output of comprehensive regression from SAS Program 5.3

In addition to the adjusted effect of smoking, the impact of other variables (covariates) on the outcome is also estimated. Using the standardized regression coefficients, the rank of impact for these factors from high to low were years of smoking, BMI, gender, race, and depression with $p < 0.01$ for all except depression with $p < 0.05$.

5.7.3   Create Table 3 with Analytical Results

With results from Models 1–4, a table, often the third table in a manuscript (Table 3), is created to report results. To facilitate research, Table 5.3 is an example or template of Table 3 with results from the four different models, each presented with a column. Model 1 shows results with no adjustment or control of any variables, Model 2 adjusts for demographic factors only, Model 3 controls for confounders only, and Model 4 adjusts and controls for both.

In Table 5.3, the "…" is a place holder reserved for inclusion of additional demographic and/or confounding variables. First, more demographic factors can be included. Demographic and socioeconomic factors provide a measure of the heterogeneity of a study sample, which could be a threat to the validity of the estimated X ~ Y relationship. In addition to gender and race, other typical demographic factors include educational attainment, employment status, annual income, migration status (if foreign born), and citizenship (US citizen, and other).

Table 5.3 Association between years of smoking and systolic blood pressure: Results from multivariate linear regression after controlling for confounders and adjusting for demographic factors

Variable	Model 1, $\hat{\beta}$ (SE)	Mode 2, $\hat{\beta}$ (SE)	Mode 3, $\hat{\beta}$ (SE)	Mode 4, $\hat{\beta}$ (SE)
Influential factor X				
Years of smoking	0.2000** (0.018)	0.1914** (0.019)	0.2004** (0.018)	0.1924** (0.019)
Demographic factors				
Gender (M = 1, F = 2)		−4.0082** (0.624)	n/a	−3.7666** (0.635)
Race(White = 1, other = 0)		−3.2856** (0.665)	n/a	−3.0966** (0.665)
...		...	...	...
Other factors				
Depression (PHQ score)		n/a	−0.2530** (0.077)	−0.1745** (0.077)
BMI (kg/m^2)		n/a	0.4284** (0.046)	0.4339** (0.046)
...		n/a	...	...
...		n/a	...	...
F-value (p)	122.06 (<.001)	64.25 (<0.01)	68.47(<.01)	53.72 (<.001)
R^2	0.039	0.060	0.070	0.090

Note: BMI: Body mass index; PHQ: Patient Health Questionnaire Scale; M for male and F for female. Model 1 for simple linear regression, Model 2 adjusting demographic factors, Model 3 controlling confounders and Model 4 control both; $\hat{\beta}$: estimated regression coefficient; *: p < .05 and **: p < .01

Second, confounders directly threaten the validity of an observed X ~ Y relationship. More confounders can be added to examine the smoking-high blood relationship in addition to gender and race. Obvious examples include levels of physical activity, stress, and alcohol use/abuse, to name a few.

Last, for studies with more than one outcome variable, one table for each outcome variable must be used. For example, when the current study is extended to investigate the diastolic blood pressure, another table must be included.

5.7.4   Results Interpretation – Conditional Interpretation Approach

Up to this point, the analysis of demographic factors and confounders is completed using multivariate linear regression to confirm the X ~ Y relation revealed from bivariate analysis. It is the time now to interpret or to understand the analytic results. Just like the selection of confounders and other covariates, interpretation of results from the multivariate analysis is also *both an art and science*. There is no so-called standard procedure to follow. In this book, the author uses a conditional approach to interpret and present the analytical findings.

To verify an X ~ Y relation in a model by adding a set of covariates, including demographic variables, socioeconomic factors, and other confounders, we eventually *set up a framework in which to examine a hypothetic X ~ Y relationship*. In our example presented above, when gender and race are included as demographic factors, and depression and BMI are included as confounders, we place the smoking-blood pressure relationship in this framework. Any estimated result would be biased without considering the impact of these factors.

Specifically, the estimate $\beta_1 = 0.1914$ from Model 2 in Table 5.3 is a quantitative measure of the association between years of smoking and systolic blood pressure given the differences in gender and racial composition, and it can be written as β (smoking | gender, race) = 0.1914, and be interpreted as the results conditioned on the inclusion of the covariates or adjusted for the impact of the heterogeneity of the study sample (population).

Likewise, the estimated $\beta_1 = 0.1924$ from Model 4 provides a quantitative measure better than that from Model 2 and Model 3 to assess the smoking – blood pressure relationship because it considered both demographic factors and confounders. This result can be written as β (smoking | gender, race, depression, BMI) = 0.1924. The increases in the estimated β from 0.1919 to 0.1924 is not because of inclusion of more variables, but rather put the X ~ Y relationship in a more comprehensive framework defined by the four covariates.

Sharp readers may have already noted that the estimated regression coefficient β for year of smoking varies with different types/numbers of covariates. It is the covariates that are used in the multivariate model that put the X ~ Y relationship in the framework; or the framework to examine the X ~ Y relationship is defined by these variables we selected. Therefore, the conclusion must be drawn within the defined conceptual framework. This presents a challenge to all researchers – how to select variables that best quantify the X ~ Y relationship with data?

Consequently, a key point of this chapter is intended to present to readers that any estimate for an X ~ Y relation from real data is relative; and the goal is to obtain a less-biased result using the multivariate models, or to find a best result from various possible models allowed by data. Understanding the point of *relativity* is very important. This is because *it is neither scientifically necessary nor philosophically possible to include all possible variables to build a perfect conceptual framework for an X-Y relationship*. A medical, behavioral, or health problem can be understood in the world that is familiar to us. Quantitative research will progress as knowledge accumulates, and *there is no end point to addressing all medical, health and behavioral problems in epidemiology*.

5.7.5   Reporting

With the understanding and interpretation of results from multivariate analysis described above, we can frame our statements to report results from the analysis. Reporting results is much more flexible than interpreting them. Although no standardized statements can be used, the following are some examples.

First, demographic and socioeconomic factors are included in almost all observational studies to examine factors associated with a health outcome. In this case, the following statement can be twisted to fit to a specific study to draft a conclusion statement:

"After adjusting for the demographic factors of gender and race, results from multiple regression confirmed the bivariate result that smoking was a significant risk factor of high blood pressure."

If both demographic variables and confounders are included, the following statement can be used to report the results presented in Table 5.3.

"Systolic blood pressure was significantly associated with years of smoking among US adults, after adjusting for differences in gender and racial composition and controlling for potential confounding effects from depression and BMI using a multivariate regression approach."

5.8   Causal Conclusion and Bradford Hill Criteria

Different from laboratory or experimental studies, it is highly challenging if not impossible to determine if a confirmed X ~ Y relationship is causal when data from observational studies are used, particularly if the data are cross-sectional in nature. Application of multivariate regression in analyzing observational studies empowers researchers to verify a hypothetic X ~ Y relationship by adjusting for the heterogeneity of the study sample and controlling for impactful confounders. Although, multivariate analysis will not guarantee an X ~ Y relationship as causal, findings from such analysis provides valuable data supporting the causal inference.

Causal inference is another evolving area of scientific research in general and in epidemiology in particular. The Bradford Hill Criteria proposed in the 1960s (Hill 1965) have experienced a lot of development to accommodate new evidence (Weed 2018). These criteria are widely used as guidance for causal inference with findings from empirical data. Let X be an influential factor, and Y be the outcome. The following are 10 Bradford Hill criteria that are often cited in research:

1. *Strength of an association*: This criterion is also known as effect size criterion, and it says that the stronger an association between X and Y, or a larger effect size of X on Y, the more likely the X ~ Y association would be causal.
2. *Consistency (reproducibility)*: A X ~ Y association is more likely to be causal if the same or similar associations are observed in many studies conducted by

different researchers using samples from different study populations residing in different geographic areas with the data analyzed using different methods.

3. *Specificity (uniqueness)*: It would be more likely to be causal if an X ~ Y association is observed only for the Y of interest, but not another Y's.

4. *Temporality (time sequence)*: For an X ~ Y association to be causal, the X must occur before the Y.

5. *Dose-response*: If changes in Y are proportionate to changes in X, the X ~ Y relation is likely to be causal. This criterion was originally stated as a "biological gradient", which failed to include non-biological factors that are more common in epidemiology today.

6. *Plausibility*: If a significant X ~ Y association is based on or supported by a solid theory or an established mechanism, it is likely to be causal.

7. *Coherence*: If findings of an X ~ Y association from a population-based study are also consistent with those from laboratory studies, the association is more likely to be causal.

8. *Experiment support*: It is likely to be causal if an observed X ~ Y relation from epidemiological studies underscore the need for an experimental test of the relation.

9. *Analogy*: The X ~ Y association is more likely to be causal if the same association is observed in studies that integrate findings from a large number of studies (i.e., meta-analysis) or from national and internal agencies such as the National Institute of Cancer and the World Health Organization.

10. *Reversibility*: The X ~ Y association is likely to be causal if removal of X results in no change in Y.

Findings from our analysis in this chapter on smoking and systolic blood pressure meet several of the Bradford Hill Criteria, including criteria 1–5, strong and consistent positive X ~ Y relationship with and without controlling for covariates, years of smoking is prior to high blood pressure (temporality), and dose-response relation (significant and positive linear regression coefficient). Lastly, if judged by criterion 9, the smoking-systolic blood pressure relation needs further investigation since strict epidemiological analysis with the powerful Mendelian randomization meta-analysis did not confirm the smoking-high blood pressure relation (Linneberg et al. 2015).

5.9 Limitations

Limitations are often discussed in reporting results with reference to the Bradford Hill criteria. In addition, unmeasured confounders must be addressed (refer Fig. 5.13). For example, the author must admit that the results could differ with more confounders being included.

5.10   Practice

5.10.1   Data Processing and Statistical Analysis

1. Further practice of data processing, including combination of datasets, methods to deal with missing data, and creation of new variables.
2. Repeat all analyses presented in the chapter, and conduct comprehensive analysis using SAS Program 5.5 by adding more demographic and socioeconomic factors and more confounders.
3. Repeat all analyses using diastolic blood pressure in the place of systolic blood pressure as the outcome Y.
4. Gain familiarity with use of the four-model approach in multiple linear regression to confirm a hypothetic X ~ Y relationship supported by theory and revealed from bivariate analysis, including Model 1 that only contains X and Y; Model 2 that contains X ~ Y, plus demographic factors; Model 3 that contains X ~ Y, plus confounders; and Model 4 that contains X ~ Y, plus both demographic factors and confounders.
5. When conducting regression analysis with X plus other factors, please add one factor at a time to see how the X ~ Y relation changes because of each factor. Use the result to assist in variable selection to finalize a model.
6. Optional: Conduct analysis to include AGE as a covariate to replicate the results presented right before Sect. 5.7 and interpret the impact of a very strong confounder on the X ~ Y relation by using the vector principles illustrated in Fig. 5.11.

5.10.2   Update Research Paper

1. If you use a continuous Y for your study project, please use the multiple regression approach to confirm the X ~ Y relationship you hypothesized for your project that is also supported by bivariate analysis.
2. Create Table 3 of your project using the template Table 5.3 to report results from the four models you constructed and used in analysis; and review your results carefully and compare the results with those in in Table 2 of your project from bivariate analysis.
3. Interpret and report your results from this analysis.
4. Revise and update your Table 2 if additional bivariate analyses are added.
5. For students with a continuous Y, it is now the time for you to finalize your research project and prepare the final paper. Please check all parts of your study, including the title, abstract (add new findings from your Table 3), materials and methods (add multivariate analysis method), and findings (add new results, and revise previous results).

6. Start to draft the last section – Discussions, conclusions and/or Implications, limitations and future research.
7. For students with other types of Y, it is the time to think of demographic factors and confounders, practice the linear regression approach, and prepare for your own project after analytical methods for different Ys will be covered in Chap. 6.

5.10.3 Study Questions

1. What is the difference between an influential factor, a covariate, a demographic factor, and a confounder? Why is an adjusted beta coefficient better than an unadjusted in measuring an X ~ Y relationship?
2. In multiple linear regression, the impact of all X's on Y are assumed to be independent. What does this mean and why it is important to understand such a relationship in etiological studies to confirm an X ~ Y relation revealed from a bivariate analysis?
3. Why can demographic factors also be used as confounders in multiple regression to verify a hypothetical X ~ Y relationship suggested by bivariate analysis?
4. If an X ~ Y relation is positive, CovX and X relation is positive, and CovX and Y relation is negative, do you think the estimated regression coefficient from a bivariate analysis for assessing the X ~ Y relation would be: (i) overestimated, (ii) underestimated, or (iii) not biased? Why and why not?
5. What are the three indicators used to assess data-model fit in linear regression analysis? What does each indicator mean? Which one will be emphasized more in etiological studies and which will be emphasized more in prediction studies?
6. What are the 10 Bradford Hill Criteria? How can these criteria be used to assist causal inference?

References

Alhawari, H.H., Al-Shelleh, S., Alhawari, H.H., Al-Saudi, A., Al-Majali, D.A., Al-Faris, L., AlRyalat, S.A.: Blood pressure and its association with gender, Body Mass Index, smoking, and family history among university students. Int. J. Hypertens. **2018**, Article ID 4186496, 5p (2018). https://doi.org/10.1155/2018/4186496

Bordacconi, M.J., Larsen, M.V.: Regression to causality: regression-style presentation influences causal attribution. Res. Politics. **2014**, 1–6 (2014). https://doi.org/10.1177/2053168014548092

Chaiton, M.O., Cohen, J.E., O'Loughlin, J., et al.: A systematic review of longitudinal studies on the association between depression and smoking in adolescents. BMC Public Health. **9**, 356 (2009). https://doi.org/10.1186/1471-2458-9-356

Clair, C., Chiolero, A., Faeh, D., et al.: Dose-dependent positive association between cigarette smoking, abdominal obesity and body fat: cross-sectional data from a population-based survey. BMC Public Health. **11**, 23 (2011). https://doi.org/10.1186/1471-2458-11-23

Dua, S., Bhuker, M., Sharma, P., Dhall, M., Kapoor, S.: Body mass index relates to blood pressure among adults. N. Am. J. Med. Sci. **6**(2), 89–95 (2014). https://doi.org/10.4103/1947-2714.127751

Hill, A.B.: The Environment and Disease: Association or Causation?. Proceedings of the Royal Society of Medicine. **58**(5), 295–300 (1965)

Linneberg, A., Jacobsen, R.K., Skaaby, T., et al.: Effect of smoking on blood pressure and resting heart rate: a Mendelian randomization meta-analysis in the CART Consortium. Circ. Cardiovasc. Genet. **8**(6), 832–841 (2015)

Meng, L., Chen, D., Yang, Y., Zheng, Y., Hui, R.: Depression increases the risk of hypertension incidence: a meta-analysis of prospective cohort studies. J. Hypertens. **30**(5), 842–851 (2012)

Ramirez, L.A., Sullivan, J.C.: Sex differences in hypertension: where we have been and where we are going. Am. J. Hypertens. **31**(12), 1247–1254 (2018)

Seeley, R., Sandoval, D.: Weight loss through smoking. Nature. **475**, 176–177 (2011)

VenderWell, T.: Principles of confounder selection. Eur. J. Epidemiol. **34**, 211–219 (2019)

Weed, D.L.: Analogy in cause inference: rethinking Austin Bradford Hill's neglected consideration. Ann. Epidemiol. **28**(2018), 343–346 (2018)

Chapter 6
Multiple Regression for Categorical and Counting Data

Using the right tools to do the right job

In Chap. 5, we introduced multiple linear regression and its application in quantitative analysis to verify a potential X ~ Y relationship by controlling for impactful confounders and adjusting for key socioeconomic and demographic factors. Controlling for confounders can enhance internal validity of a study while adjusting demographic and socioeconomic factors can improve external validity.

As described in Chap. 5, linear regression can be used in research to analyze continuous outcome variables, such as height, weight, BMI, measured blood pressure, and scores from CESD-10 for depression, etc. As detailed in Chap. 2, in addition to continuous variables, quantitative methods are needed to analyze discrete variables. For example, the following questions are often confronted in research: "What factors can cause a person to have high blood pressure?" "Why do some people die at a younger age than others?" "Why are some people more likely than others to become obese?" To answer such questions, a binary (yes/no) outcome variable must be used.

In addition to binary, variables with three or more categories are common, such as stage of a disease (none, earlier/light, moderate, later/severe), high blood pressure (normal, marginal, and hypertensive), consequences from treatment (cured, improved, and no response), frequency of depressive symptoms and cigarette smoking (none, occasionally, sometimes, often, daily), and attitudes/belief measures (strongly disagree to strongly agree). There are also variables that look like continuous but are in fact not, such as number of days stayed in hospital after admission, number of days missed medication by a patient, and number of drinks of a study participant had on a typical day.

When the outcome variable Y is no longer continuous, statistical methods other than linear regression are needed to verify a potential X ~ Y relationship. If the outcome Y is binary, *(binomial)* logistic regression is indicated. If the outcome Y has multiple categories, multinomial logistic regression is used; furthermore, if the

© The Author(s), under exclusive license to Springer Nature Switzerland AG 2021   163
X. Chen, *Quantitative Epidemiology*, Emerging Topics in Statistics and
Biostatistics, https://doi.org/10.1007/978-3-030-83852-2_6

multi-categories of Y are ordered, *ordinal logistic regression* provides a choice in addition to the multinomial logistic regression. If the outcome Y is a counting variable (i.e., days of alcohol use), Poisson regression will be a choice. Lastly, to analyze data from a matched case-control study, conditional logistic regression is ideal.

In this chapter, we will introduce the four logistic regression methods and Poisson regression, and demonstrate their applications in research to confirm a hypothetic X ~ Y relationship. Like in Chap. 5, all methods will be demonstrated with SAS Program and real data. The emphasis will be placed on the modeling procedure and result interpretation.

6.1 Introduction to Logistic Regression

Different from the linear regression described in Chap. 5, logistic regression is developed to quantify an X ~ Y relationship with Y being categorical, including binary and multi-categories. Different from a continuous variable, a categorical variable does not follow the normal distribution. In this section, we will introduce binary outcome variable, binomial distribution, and binomial logistic regression. Other types of categorical outcome variables will follow.

6.1.1 Binary Outcome Y and Binomial Distribution

Like the normal distribution for a continuous variable, in probability theory, an event with two exclusive outcomes follows a binomial distribution. Binary outcomes are used very often in epidemiology. Outcomes to address the questions described in the second paragraph at the beginning of this chapter can be measured using binary variables. Binary outcomes are also used in epidemiology to design case-control and cohort studies.

In quantitative analysis, binomial distribution can be understood as a probability distribution to estimate the chance to have a disease in a study. Given the sample size n, there is a relationship between k, the number of subjects having the disease and n-k, the number of subjects not having the disease, and the incidence rate of p of the disease. For example, if the incidence rate for a cancer $p = 3/1000$ in a population. In a study that followed 235 participants who smoked tobacco (n = 235) for 10 years, and 3 developed lung cancer (k = 3) during the period. A research question: Can smoking increase the risk for developing lung cancer?

To answer this question, we can estimate the probability for two persons to develop lung cancer assuming the cancer risk is, on average, the same for everyone in the study population. With the population incidence rate $p = 0.003$, study sample n = 235, and incidence k = 3, the probability to develop the cancer can be estimated using the formula for binomial distribution:

$$\Pr\left(k;,n;,p\right)=\Pr\left(Y=k\right)=\binom{n}{k}p^{k}\left(1-p\right)^{n-k}=\binom{235}{3}0.003^{3}\left(1-0.003\right)^{235-3}=0.028.$$

Based on this result, the estimated probability = 0.028 to have 3 lung cancer patients with a sample of 235 participants if no smoking. Cleary this probability is 9.3 (0.028/0.003) times higher than the population incidence rate p = 0.003. Epidemiologically, we may conclude that exposure to tobacco smoking is likely a risk factor for lung cancer.

Binomial distribution is determined by three parameters, p, n, and k. It consists of the foundation for logistic regression analysis. Figure 6.1 plots the binomial probability on y-axis against the number of events k on x-axis (range: 0 to 80) with sample size n = 100. The three curves are p values for three different incidence rates, respectively with p_1 = 0.028 (red), p_2 = 0.250 (green), and p_3 = 0.450 (blue). The three probabilities are selected simply for a better visual presentation to illustrate the characteristics of a binomial distribution.

From Fig. 6.1, it can be seen that as p increases from 0.028 (red line) to 0.250 (green line), the binomial distribution moves from right-skewed with a long tail toward the middle. As p increases to approach 0.500 (blue line), the binomial distribution is approaching a normal distribution with the probability peaked at around k = 50, the middle of n).

Fig. 6.1 Binomial distribution for probability p = 0.028 (red line), 0.250 (green line) and 0.450 (blue line) respectively

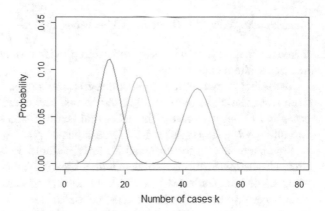

6.1.2   From Binary Outcome to Logistic Regression

Many books and papers have introduced logistic regression (Hoffmann 2016; Wright 1995). The binary distribution described in the previous section provides a knowledge base to understand logistic regression. Assuming a binomial distribution and letting $\Pr(Y = 1 | X = x)$ be the probability $p(x)$ to develop a positive outcome of Y with exposure to an influential factor $X = x$, the probability $p(x)$ be expressed as:

$$p(X) = \Pr(Y = 1 \mid X = x) = \frac{e^{\alpha + \beta x}}{1 + e^{\alpha + \beta x}} = \frac{1}{1 + e^{-\beta x}}, \tag{6.1}$$

where x is the influential factor to be examined, and parameters α and β are model coefficients to be estimated with observed data. With some rearrangement, model 6.1 can be expressed as *odds* for exposure to influential factor X as commonly used in epidemiology:

$$\text{odds} = \frac{p(X)}{1 - p(X)} = e^{\alpha + \beta x}. \tag{6.2}$$

A logistic regression *model* is thus established simply by taking a logarithm of model 6.2:

$$\log\left(\frac{p(X)}{1 - p(X)}\right) = \alpha + \beta X. \tag{6.3}$$

In the logistic regression expressed with model 6.3, $\log\left(\frac{p(X)}{1 - p(X)}\right)$, or log-odds is statistically termed as logit and modeled as Y as in a linear regression. Thus, in a logistic regression, the β coefficient quantifies the X ~ Y relationship *within the log-linear space*. When X = 0, model 6.3 becomes $\log\left(\frac{p(X)}{1 - p(X)}\right) = \alpha$. Thus, the estimated intercept α from a logistic regression provides *a measure of the baseline risk*, i.e., risk without exposure to X.

To further demonstrate the logistic regression model, Table 6.1 presents results from a simulation study with 20 observations. The outcome Y contains 9 positive cases and 11 negative cases. The influential factor X was simulated as a continuous variable ~ N (mean = 0, SD = 1.2). For simplicity, $\beta = 1$ was used in simulation.

Simulated data for the observed X and Y in Table 6.1 are plotted in Fig. 6.2. As shown in the figure, this type of data with a binary Y cannot be effectively analyzed using a linear regression with Y as a continuous variable as introduced in Chap. 5. This is because no matter how the influential factor X varies in any range, Y can only take two values: either 1 (for positive) or 0 (for negative).

To solve this problem, we can further process the data to compute the probability to have a positive outcome (i.e., Y = 1) for individual participants with different X using model 6.1. The computing is easy since $\beta = 1$ by design. For example, for the third observations with x = 1.3013, the estimated probability

$$p(X) = \frac{1}{\left[1 + \exp(-1.3013)\right]} = 0.7861.$$

The estimated $p(X)$ for all subjects are presented in column 3, Table 6.1. With these estimated probabilities, the 20 participants can be classified into "positive" or "negative" with $p(X) = 0.50$ as the cutoff. A participant will be classified as positive

Table 6.1 Simulated Data Demonstrating the Principle of Logistic Regression as a Log Linear model

Obs	Observed Y	Observed X	p(X)	Predicted Y	Odds	Log (odds)
1	0	−1.4485	0.1902	0	0.234927	−1.44848
2	0	0.3329	0.5825	1	1.395029	0.332915
3	1	1.3013	0.7861	1	3.674178	1.301329
4	0	−2.8148	0.0565	0	0.059914	−2.81484
5	1	0.5149	0.6260	1	1.673554	0.51495
6	1	0.6075	0.6473	1	1.835409	0.607267
7	1	−0.6899	0.3341	0	0.501733	−0.68969
8	0	−0.6560	0.3416	0	0.518945	−0.65596
9	0	−0.6773	0.3369	0	0.507965	−0.67734
10	1	−1.0681	0.2558	0	0.34368	−1.06805
11	0	−0.5726	0.3606	0	0.564039	−0.57263
12	0	−1.1981	0.2318	0	0.301778	−1.19806
13	0	−0.9315	0.2826	0	0.39396	−0.9315
14	1	0.0774	0.5193	1	1.080421	0.077351
15	1	1.1514	0.7598	1	3.162595	1.151393
16	0	−0.1323	0.4670	0	0.876041	−0.13234
17	0	−0.6132	0.3513	0	0.541609	−0.61321
18	1	−1.0934	0.2510	0	0.335064	−1.09343
19	0	−1.0046	0.2680	0	0.366189	−1.00461
20	1	2.8990	0.9478	1	18.15602	2.899002

Note: See Figs. 6.1 and 6.2 for visual presentation of the simulated data

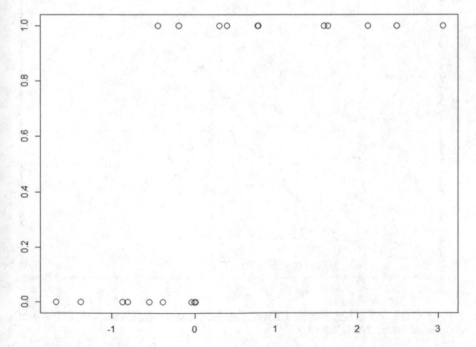

Fig. 6.2 Plot of binary outcome Y (vertical axis) with continuous X (horizonal axis) with data from Table 6.1 (1 = positive and 0 = negative)

if the estimated $p(X) > 0.50$, otherwise, be classified as negative. These results are also presented in Table 6.1 as predicted Y (column 4). Data in the table indicate that 6 of the 9 positives, and 9 of the 11 negatives are correctly predicted with the model with an accuracy of 75% [(6 + 9)/20].

Figure 6.3 plots the observed Y (open circles), estimated probability for Y (solid dots) at different X's on a smooth curve along with the exposure of X (horizontal axis). Although the observed Y is binary, the estimated probability $p(X)$ (black line) is continuous forming an S-shaped curve. In the figure, the correctly and incorrectly predicted observations are also visualized. The red dots on the S-curve above the dashed line (p=0.50) and the black dots on the S-curve below the dashed line are those that are correctly predicted; otherwise, they are incorrectly predicted.

To demonstrate logistic regression model 6.3 as a linear logit model, odds and log odds for the 20 individual participants are computed using the computed $p(X)$ in Table 6.1. For example, the estimated $p(X)= 0.234927$ for observation number 1, the odds for this subject =0.19024/(1–1.9024) = 0.234927, and log odds = ln(0.234927) = −1.44848. The estimated odds and log (odds) are presented in the last two columns of Table 6.1. When the $p(X)$ in Fig. 6.3 is replaced with log odds and plot the same data in Fig. 6.4, a totally different picture appears.

In Fig. 6.4, the observed Y (0, 1) remain binary, however, the log odds or logit (range: −3 to 3) reflecting the outcome and the influential factor X form *a straight line*. This linear relationship clearly demonstrate that a logistic regression is simply

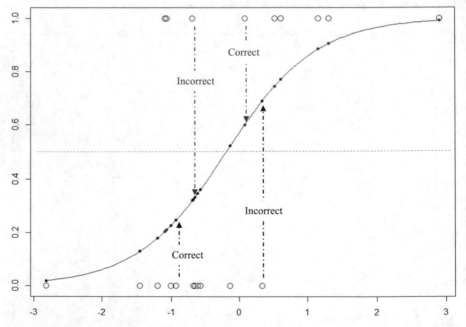

Fig. 6.3 Observed Y (binary, vertical axis) and probability (continuous, vertical axis) of Y against X (horizontal axis), data in Table 6.1

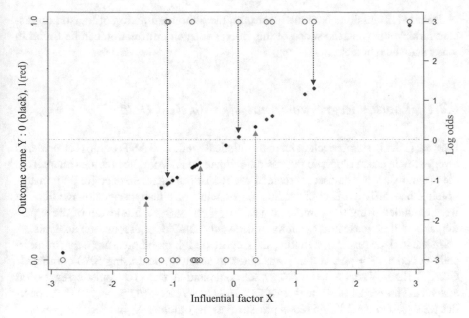

Fig. 6.4 Logistic regression as a log linear model with data in Table 6.1 and Eq. 6.3

a log linear regression, and this model is statistically expressed using model 6.3. Furthermore, correctly and incorrectly classified participants are identified in the figure. Similar to those in Fig. 6.3, all red dots above the dashed greyline with log odds = 0, and all black dots below the same line are classified correctly; and all black dots above the dashed greyline and all red dots below the same line are classified incorrectly.

6.2   Logistic Regression Solution and Risk Measurement

From Figs. 6.3 and 6.4 it can tell that the OLS method for solving a linear regression model cannot be used to solve a logistic regression model because for a logistic regression model, all the data points (the estimated probability from binomial distribution and the corresponding log odds) for individual participants are located on the regression line. However, the binomially distributed Y makes it possible to estimate the logistic regression coefficients α and β using the maximum likelihood estimator (Albert and Anderson 1984). Instead of minimizing the difference between the observed Y and model predicted Y as in the OLS for linear regression, maximum likelihood estimation attempts to find the best estimates of α and β such that the probability to obtain the observed sample is maximized.

Detailed discussion about the maximum likelihood estimation of logistic regression model is beyond the scope of this book and such information can be found in many statistical books.

6.2.1 Logistic Regression Analysis with Real Data

Practice is the best approach to learn a statistical method. SAS Program 6.1 presents a very simple case of logistic regression using the data from the previous chapter. In the program, a work dataset is created first by reading DATCH5 used for demonstration in Chap. 5. To avoid confounding, participants on anti-hypertension medication were excluded using the command: IF HBPMED NE 1. Exclusion of these participants will increase homogeneity of the study sample for association analysis.

In the logistic regression model, self-reported high blood pressure HBP (numerically coded as: 1 = yes, 0 = no) was claimed as categorical using SAS command: CLASS HBP. The **PROC LOGISTIC** command is used for logistic regression analysis. The model statement: MODEL HBP (EVENT="1") = SMKYR specifies HBP (self-reported high blood pressure) as the outcome Y, and SMKYR (years of smoking) as the influential factor X. Lastly, the option (EVENT="1") tells the computer to model the impact of X on high blood pressure (Y = 1) with reference to those without high blood pressure (Y = 0).

Based on model 6.3, the logistic regression used in SAS Program 6.1 can be expressed as:

$$\log\left(\frac{p(HBP)}{1-p(HBP)}\right) = \alpha + \beta\,(SMKYRS)$$

(6.4)

```
********************************************************************************
* SAS PROGRAM 6.1. DEMONSTRATION OF SIMPLE LOGISTIC REGRESSION ANALYSIS
********************************************************************************;
** DATA PROCESSING;
* 1 READ DATA USED IN CHAPTER 5 AND STORE IN DATASET A;
LIBNAME SASDATA "C:\QUANTLAB\A_DATA\"
DATA A; SET SASDATA.DATCH5;
* EXCLUDE PARTICIPANTS WHO ARE ON ANTI-HYPERTENSIVE MEDICATION;
IF HBPMED NE 1;
* 2 CHECK DATA AND VARIABLES;
PROC CONTENTS; RUN;

** LOGISTIC REGRESSION ASSOCIATING SMKYRS WITH HIGH BLOOD PRESSURE;
* 1 ACTIVATE SAS PROCEDURE PROC LOGISTIC;
PROC LOGISTIC DATA = A;
* 2 CLAIM THE VARIABLES THAT ARE CATEGORICAL;
CLASS HBP;
* 3 SPECIFY THE LOGISTIC REGRESSION MODEL TO ASSOCAITED X (SMKYRS) WITH Y(HBP);
MODEL HBP (EVENT="1") = SMKYRS;
RUN;
********************************************************************************;
```

6.2.2 Results from Logistic Regression

Figure 6.5 displays the main output by executing SAS Program 6.1. The first two parts of the output provide information on data-model fit. AIC (Akaike Information Criterion) and SC (Schwarz Criterion) are two statistics often used to assess if the data fit the logistic regression model well (smaller values indicating better fit). Of the three chi-square tests, likelihood ratio test in the second part of the output is the one used most often to indicate if the estimated logistic regression coefficient is significantly different from zero with $p < 0.05$ as the criteria. In this example, the likelihood ratio test with chi-square = 35.4593, $p < 0.0001$, suggests a very good data-model fit. In other words, the model results support a statistically significant smoking-high blood pressure relationship.

Consistent with the data-model fit tests, the third part of the output in Fig. 6.5 contains the key results that are reported as findings in a research study. It contains (1) the estimated intercept, $\alpha = -2.2065$; this is a measure of the baseline risk without exposure to X; and (2) the estimated slope for X (SMKYRS), $\beta = 0.0162$ and it measures the change in risk of high blood pressure along with years of

Model Fit Statistics		
Criterion	Intercept Only	Intercept and Covariates
AIC	2694.401	2660.942
SC	2700.610	2673.359
-2 Log L	2692.401	2656.942

Testing Global Null Hypothesis: BETA=0			
Test	Chi-Square	DF	Pr > ChiSq
Likelihood Ratio	35.4593	1	<.0001
Score	38.6750	1	<.0001
Wald	37.6757	1	<.0001

Analysis of Maximum Likelihood Estimates					
Parameter	DF	Estimate	Standard Error	Wald Chi-Square	Pr > ChiSq
Intercept	1	-2.2065	0.0648	1160.5461	<.0001
SMKYRS	1	0.0162	0.00264	37.6757	<.0001

Fig. 6.5 Main output of a simple logistic regression, output from SAS Program 6.1

smoking (in a log linear scale, see Fig. 6.4). The Chi-sq test indicated that $p < 0.0001$ for both the estimated α and β. The extremely significant result for the estimated β coefficient suggests a strong and positive relationship between years of smoking and high blood pressure among adults in the US.

6.2.3   Odds Ratio from Logistic Regression

A logistic regression model is built on the log-odds (or logit) as previously described in this chapter. Therefore, *results from a logistic regression provide useful data to derive odds and odds ratios (OR), the two most commonly used risk measures in* epidemiology.

By definition, odds ratio from exposure to an influential factor $X = x$ can be described as below:

$$\text{Odds ratio}(OR) = \frac{\text{odds}(Y \mid X = x)}{\text{odds}(Y \mid X = 0)} = \frac{\exp(\alpha + \beta)}{\exp(\alpha)} = \exp\left[(\alpha + \beta) - \alpha\right] = \exp(\beta).$$

(6.5)

With the β coefficient for $X = x$ estimated from the logistic regression with reference to $X = 0$ (no exposure), the OR can thus be calculated using formula 6.5. With the result from our analysis, the estimated $\beta = 0.0162$, thus,

$$\text{The estimated } OR = \exp(\beta) = \exp(0.0162) = 1.0163$$

With this result, we can conclude that for every 10 years of smoking, there would be 16.3% increase in the risk of high blood pressure. The relationship is statistically extremely significant as $p < 0.01$ level. Be advised, OR = 1.0163 means 1.63% increase in risk for one year of smoking; translate this into 10 years of smoking, the risk becomes 16.3%.

It is worth noting that caution is needed in interpreting the estimated OR. An OR is a good approximation of the relative risk RR *only if* the incidence (cohort study) or the prevalence (cross-sectional study) of the outcome variable Y is low, often below 5%. This would not be a big issue for studies addressing many acute and chronic diseases with relatively lower morbidity and mortality rates; however, it would be somewhat problematic for studies to examine many health-related behaviors that are highly prevalent, such as physical activity, condom use, tobacco smoking, and alcohol abuse.

6.3   Multiple Logistic Regression for Verification of a Bivariate Analysis

Following the introduction in Sect. 6.2, the difference between a linear and a logistic regression becomes clear. A logistic regression is simply a log-linear model. It first converts the binary Y into a continuous probability based on the binomial distribution. After converting, a log-linear model is constructed to associate X with Y. The constructed log-linear regression model makes it possible to estimate the regression coefficients using the maximum likelihood method. With the estimated model coefficients, risk measures (i.e., OR) can be derived to quantify the X ~ Y relationship. Similar to the linear regression in Chap. 5, a simple logistic regression can be extended to a multiple regression for analysis to verify a potential X ~ Y relation by including impactful covariates.

6.3.1   Multiple Logistic Regression Model

By extending the simple logistic regression Model 6.3 to include more than one influential factor X, a multiple logistic regression model can be derived:

$$\ln \frac{P}{1-p} = \alpha + \beta_1 X_1 + \beta_2 CovX_2 + \beta_3 CovX_3 + \ldots + \beta_p CovX_p \qquad (6.6)$$

In Model 6.6, X_1 is the variable that was detected through bivariate analysis as a potential influential factor to be associated with the outcome Y. $CovX_2$ to $CovX_p$ are covariates for demographic factors and confounders. If the estimated β_1 remains statistically significant at $p < 0.05$ or $p < 0.01$ level after inclusion of all $CovXs$, it provides evidence supporting the X ~ Y relationship detected from the bivariate analysis; otherwise, the X ~ Y relationship would not be supported.

Different from linear regression, odds ratio (OR) is estimated based on the results from a logistic regression to measure the level of risk on the outcome Y from exposing to an influential factor X.

6.3.2   Application of the Multiple Logistic Regression to Real Data

In this section, we will demonstrate the application of a multiple logistic regression model to verify an X ~ Y relationship suggested by a bivariate analysis. In Chap. 4, we showed that the reported years of smoking was significantly associated with reported high blood pressure (Table 4.3). Here we will use a multiple logistic regression model to verify this bivariate result. Since high blood pressure (0 = no, 1 = yes) is binomial, it presents a good example for logistic regression.

As a demonstration, the same demographic variables and confounders used in Chap. 5 will be used here. The two demographic factors are gender (male vs. female) and race (White vs. other); and the two confounders are depression (scores from the 9-item PHQ scale), and BMI (kg/meter²).

6.3.3 SAS Program for Multiple Logistic Regression

SAS Program 6.2 is an example of using various multiple logistic regression models to verify a potential X ~ Y relationship by adjusting demographic factors and controlling for confounders. The program consists of two parts: Part 1 for data processing and Part 2 for logistic regression analysis.

Capitalizing on the data used in Chap. 5 for continuous variables, Part 1 of SAS Program 6.2 shows how to derive data from another dataset to create a new dataset DATCH6 for analysis. During the process, a new variable SMKYR10 is created. This variable is rescaled using 10 years as unit, based on the result from SAS Program 6.1 in Fig. 6.5. In the result, the estimated $\beta = 0.0162$ and $OR = 1.0163$ for SMKYRS, both of which are rather small for result interpretation.

To support all the analyses planned for this section, a set of 12 variables are included in DATCH6. As a side interest, a cross-table is used to check the consistency between the reported (HBP) and measured (HBPX) high blood pressure. In addition, two variables (SMKNOW SMKDAYS) were included for use later, the variable SMKNOW will be used for ordered logistic regression and SMKDAYS will be used for Poisson regression. Several demographic and anthropologic variables (EDUCATION MARRIAGE HEIGHT WEIGHT) were included but not used. These variables are included for students who may be interested in using them for practice.

Last, a work dataset **B** is created for analysis. Participants who were on anti-hypertensive medication, or with missing data on high blood pressure were excluded from the data to avoid confounding. A different dataset name **B** is used to avoid confusion with dataset **A** in the previous part of analysis in SAS Program 6.1.

```
*******************************************************************************
* SAS PROGRAM 6.2. MULTIPLE LOGISTIC REGRESSION TO VERIFY AN X-Y RELATIONSHIP
*******************************************************************************;
** PART 1: CREATE DATCH6 FOR ANALYSIS BASED ON THE DATCH5 USED IN CHAPTER 5;
LIBNAME SASDATA "C:\QUANTLAB\A_DATA\"
* CREATED DATASET DATCH6 BY READING DATCH5 USED IN CHAPTER 5;
DATA SASDATA.DATCH6; SET SASDATA.DATCH5;
* RESCALE THE INDEPENDENT VARIABLE SMKYRS FOR BETTER RESULT INTERPRETATION;
SMKYR10 = SMKYRS/10;
LABEL SMKYR10 = 'YEARS OF SMOKING MEASURED USING 10 YEARS AS UNIT';
* SELECT VARIABLES FOR USE CHECK THE SELECTED VARIABLES;
KEEP AGE GENDER RACE2 EDUCATION MARRIAGE HEIGHT WEIGHT BMI DEPRESS SMKYR10 SMKNOW
SMKDAYS HBP HBPX HBPMED; PROC CONTENTS; RUN;
* CHECK CONSISTENCY BETWEEN HBP AND HBPX;
PROC FREQ DATA=LIB.DATCH6; TABLES HBP*HBPX/MISSING; RUN;
* CREATE WORK DATASET B FOR USED IN ANALYSIS;
DATA B; SET SASDATA.DATCH6;
* EXCLUDE PARTICIPANTS WHO ARE ON ANTI-HYPERENSIVE MEDICATION;
IF HBPMED NE 1;
* EXCLUDE PARTICIPANTS WITH NO DATA ON HIGH BLOOD PRESSURE;
IF HBPX NE .; RUN;

** Part 2: LOGISTIC REGRESSION FOR COVARIATE JUSTIFICATION AND CONTROL;
* LINAER CORRELATION OF ALL RELATED VARIABLES;
PROC CORR DATA = B;
VAR HBPX HBP SMKYR10 GENDER RACE2 BMI DEPRESS; RUN;
* MODEL 1 - SIMPLE LOGISTIC REGRESSION TO QUANTIFY HBPX SMOKING RELATION;
PROC LOGISTIC DATA = B;
CLASS HBPX;  *SPECIFY THIS VARIABLE AS CATEGORICAL;
* SPECIFY LOGISTIC REGRESSION MODEL AMD THE EVENT TO BE MODELED;
MODEL HBPX (EVENT="1") = SMKYR10 / EXPB; *EXPB ASKS FOR ODDS RATIO;

RUN;
* MODEL 2- LOGISTIC REGRESSION TO ADJUST THE TWO DEMOGRAPHIC FACTORS;
PROC LOGISTIC DATA = B;
CLASS HBPX GENDER RACE2;
MODEL HBPX (EVENT="1") = SMKYR10 GENDER RACE2 / EXPB;
RUN;
* MODEL 3 - LOGISTIC REGRESSION TO CONTROL THE TWO CONFOUNDERS;
PROC LOGISTIC DATA = B;
CLASS HBPX GENDER RACE2;
MODEL HBPX (EVENT="1") = SMKYR10 BMI DEPRESS / EXPB;
RUN;
* MODEL 4 - LOGISTIC REGRESSION INCLUDING BOTH DEMOGRAPHIC AND CONFOUNDERS;
PROC LOGISTIC DATA = B;
CLASS HBPX GENDER RACE2;
MODEL HBPX (EVENT="1") = SMKYR10 GENDER RACE2 BMI DEPRESS/ EXPB;
RUN;
*******************************************************************************;
```

Part 2 of SAS Program 6.2 demonstrates the use of multiple logistic regression in verifying a hypothetic X ~ Y relationship with a binary or dichotomous Y. Like the multiple linear regression models in Chap. 5, the logistic regression starts with a linear correlation to explore the relationships among all the related variables. Data derived in this step can be used for variable selection for further analysis. For example, in the analysis, the two alternative measures for high blood pressure (HBP and HBPX) are included. Results from this analysis can be used to help select one from the two for further analysis. After correlation, a set of four logistic regression models, as in Chap. 5 are used to progressively confirm the X ~ Y relationship suggested by the bivariate analysis, with Model 1 for simple logistic regression, Model 2 to adjust for demographic factors, Model 3 to control confounders and Model 4 to include both demographic factors and impactful confounders.

In these models, the selection of demographic factors is based on the literature, in addition to results from the correlation analysis. Published studies often report significant differences in smoking and depression by gender (Weinberger et al. 2012) and racial groups (Berg et al. 2012). These two variables are thus used to demonstrate the application of logistic regression to adjust for demographic factors. Likewise, potential confounding effect of the BMI and depression on the smoking-high blood pressure relationship has been documented in literature (Widome et al. 2009); these two variables are included to demonstrate the application of logistic regression to control for confounders.

6.4   Analytical Results and Interpretation

In this section, we will present and discuss the analytical results from part 2 of SAS Program 6.2, including the simple correlation analysis and the four logistic regression models: Model 1 for simple logistic regression, Model 2 adjusting for demographic factors, Model 3 controlling for confounders, and Model 4 simultaneously adjusting demographic factors and controlling for confounders.

6.4.1   Results from Linear Correlation Analysis

Simple linear correlation analysis in SAS Program 6.2 contains all 7 variables for the demonstration, including the two alternative measures of the outcome Y (HBPX and HBP), the influential factor X_1 (SMKYR10), the two demographic factors X_2 (**GENDER**) and X3 (RACE2), and the two confounders X_4 (BMI) and X_5 (DEPRESS). Figure 6.6 contains the main output – correlation matrix.

First, results in the figure indicate that the correlation between the measured high blood pressure HBPX and SMKYR10 was r = 0.1342 ($p < 0.01$); this value was greater than r = 0.1026, the same relation if the high blood pressure was measured using self-reported HBP. This result is used as evidence supporting the use of HBPX rather than HBP for verification analyses in the four models that follow.

With HBPX being selected as Y, results in Fig. 6.6 further show that HBPX was significantly associated with all covariates except DEPRESS. These include **GENDER** ($r = -0.0481, p < 0.01$), RACE2 ($r = -0.0377, p < 0.05$), and BMI ($r = 0.0603, p < 0.01$)). Furthermore, GENDER ($r = -0.1953$, $p < 0.01$), RACE2 ($r = 0.1811$, $p < 0.01$), and DEPRESS (r = 0.0930, $p < 0.01$) were each positively associated with X_1 (SMKYR10).

These results suggest that (1) the smoking - hypertension relationship may differ by gender and racial groups, and; (2) the smoking-high blood pressure relationship may also be confounded by BMI and DEPRESS. To generalize the study findings to a homogenous population with regard to gender and race, potential impact of the demographic factors must be adjusted; and to ensure high internal validity, influence of the two confounders must be controlled.

It is worth noting that although three of the four variables used in this part of analysis are not continuous (not suitable for linear correlation), we used correlation analysis here simply for exploration purposes.

Pearson Correlation Coefficients Prob > |r| under H0: Rho=0 Number of Observations							
	HBPX	HBP	SMKYR10	GENDER	RACE2	BMI	DEPRESS
HBPX HIGH BLOOD PRESSURE BASED EXAMINATION	1.00000 3721	0.18081 <.0001 3721	0.13422 <.0001 3673	-0.04814 0.0033 3721	-0.03766 0.0216 3721	0.06025 0.0003 3540	-0.00047 0.9784 3269
HBP HIGH BLOOD PRESSURE 1=YES 0 = NO,	0.18081 <.0001 3721	1.00000 3721	0.10261 <.0001 3673	-0.05104 0.0018 3721	0.03426 0.0366 3721	0.13581 <.0001 3540	0.10562 <.0001 3269
SMKYR10 YEARS OF SMOKING MEASURED USING 10 YEARS AS UNIT	0.13422 <.0001 3673	0.10261 <.0001 3673	1.00000 3673	-0.19535 <.0001 3673	0.18109 <.0001 3673	-0.01115 0.5100 3493	0.09300 <.0001 3226
GENDER GENDER 1=MALE 2=FEMALE,	-0.04814 0.0033 3721	-0.05104 0.0018 3721	-0.19535 <.0001 3673	1.00000 3721	-0.00372 0.8204 3721	0.02796 0.0962 3540	0.10110 <.0001 3269
RACE2 WHITE = 1 OTHER = 0	-0.03766 0.0216 3721	0.03426 0.0366 3721	0.18109 <.0001 3673	-0.00372 0.8204 3721	1.00000 3721	0.00867 0.6063 3540	0.07132 <.0001 3269
BMI BODY MASS INDEX USING REPORTED DATA	0.06025 0.0003 3540	0.13581 <.0001 3540	-0.01115 0.5100 3493	0.02796 0.0962 3540	0.00867 0.6063 3540	1.00000 3540	0.08561 <.0001 3126
DEPRESS DEPRESSIVE SYMPTOMS PHQ SCALE SCORE	-0.00047 0.9784 3269	0.10562 <.0001 3269	0.09300 <.0001 3226	0.10110 <.0001 3269	0.07132 <.0001 3269	0.08561 <.0001 3126	1.00000 3269

Fig. 6.6   Results from simple linear correlation analysis: Output from SAS Program 6.2

6.4.2   Results from Model 1: Simple Logistic Regression

Figure 6.7 presents the main output from Model 1 – Simple Logistic Regression in the SAS Program 6.2. Like in Fig. 6.5 for the introductory analysis, since maximum likelihood estimation was used to solve for logistic regression, three tests are used to assess the global hypothesis with all beta = 0, including log likelihood test, Score test and Wald test. Results from the three tests all indicated a good data-mode fit with chi-square greater than 106 and $p < 0.001$.

The estimated $\beta = 0.1620$ ($p < 0.0001$) for X_1 (SMKYR10). This result means, *with a one-unit (10 years here) increase in X_1, the logit of high blood pressure increases by 0.1620 units*. The bottom part of Fig. 6.7 presents the estimated odds ratio (OR) and [95% CI] = exp.(β) = 1.176 [1.117, 1.238]. These results were automatically computed by adding "/EXPB" to the logistic regression model in the SAS program. Since 95% CI of the OR does not include 1.00, the estimated OR is statistically significant at $p < 0.05$ level. Based on the estimated OR, it can be concluded that for every 10-years of smoking, the risk of hypertension will increase 17.6% after adjusting the significant demographic factors and control for impactful confounders.

Model Fit Statistics		
Criterion	Intercept Only	Intercept and Covariates
AIC	2694.401	2660.942
SC	2700.610	2673.359
-2 Log L	2692.401	2656.942

Testing Global Null Hypothesis: BETA=0			
Test	Chi-Square	DF	Pr > ChiSq
Likelihood Ratio	35.4593	1	<.0001
Score	38.6750	1	<.0001
Wald	37.6757	1	<.0001

Analysis of Maximum Likelihood Estimates						
Parameter	DF	Estimate	Standard Error	Wald Chi-Square	Pr > ChiSq	Exp(Est)
Intercept	1	-2.2065	0.0648	1160.5461	<.0001	0.110
SMKYR10	1	0.1620	0.0264	37.6757	<.0001	1.176

Odds Ratio Estimates		
Effect	Point Estimate	95% Wald Confidence Limits
SMKYR10	1.176	1.117 1.238

Fig. 6.7 Results from Model 1 for simple logistic regression: Ooutput of SAS Program 6.2

6.4.3   Computing R^2 for Logistic Regression

The statistic R^2 is often used in epidemiology to assess the importance of an influential factor X in interpreting an X ~ Y relationship because it tells the amount of variation in Y as explained by the X included in the model. However, R^2 cannot be directly calculated for logistic regression (no variance measure of Y) as in linear regression. To solve this challenge, a measure named as pseudo R^2 can be estimated using the McFadden methods (Freese and Long 2006):

$$R^2 = 1 - \left[\log \text{likelihood} \left(\text{intercept with covariate} \right) / \log \text{likelihood} \left(\text{intercept only} \right) \right]$$

(6.7)

Although conceptually different from the R^2 for linear regression, this pseudo R^2 can be interpreted like in the linear regression. The pseudo R^2 also varies between 0 and 1; a larger R^2 indicates a greater amount of variation in Y being explained by the influential factor X; and a small R^2 indicates the need to consider additional influential factors.

As an illustration, the top part of the SAS output in Fig. 6.7 shows that the -log likelihood = 2692.401 for the *intercept only*, (similar to the total variance in linear regression) and the log likelihood = 2656.942 for the *intercept + covariate* (variations in Y explained by X). Thus, the pseudo or McFadden's R^2 = 1–2656.942/269 2.401 = 1–0.9868 = 0.0132 (or 1.32%).

This result indicates that only small part of Y is explained by X (years of smoking). This result thus suggests the existence of many other influential factors for high blood pressure in addition to tobacco use if the smoking - high blood pressure relation follows the logistic regression model. Additional studies should be conducted to include other potential influential factors to better understand the etiology of high blood pressure and provide more adequate evidence supporting prevention interventions.

6.4.4 Results from Model 2: Multiple Logistic Regression Considering Demographic Factors

The main results of Model 2 in SAS Program 6.2 are presented in Fig. 6.8. The estimated β_1 = 0.2234 for X_1 (SMKYR10) after the two demographic factors X_2 (**GENDER**) and X_3 (RACE2) were included. The estimated β_1 for X_1 is greater than the β_1 = 0.1620 for the same variable X_1 (SMKYR10) without considering the two demographic factors from Model 1 (result in Fig. 6.7).

Analysis of Maximum Likelihood Estimates							
Parameter		DF	Estimate	Standard Error	Wald Chi-Square	Pr > ChiSq	Exp(Est)
Intercept		1	-2.4546	0.0778	994.3447	<.0001	0.086
SMKYR10		1	0.2234	0.0278	64.6415	<.0001	1.250
GENDER	1	1	0.0728	0.0541	1.8108	0.1784	1.076
RACE2	0	1	0.2259	0.0605	13.9302	0.0002	1.253

Odds Ratio Estimates		
Effect	Point Estimate	95% Wald Confidence Limits
SMKYR10	1.250	1.184 1.320
GENDER 1 vs 2	1.157	0.936 1.430
RACE2 0 vs 1	1.571	1.239 1.992

Fig. 6.8 Main results from Model 2 adjusting for demographic factors: Output of SAS Program 6.2

Differences in the estimated β_1 in the results discussed above suggest that the effect of X_1 (SMKYR10) was under-estimated from the bivariate analysis if the impact of the two demographic factors are not considered.

Likewise, as a byproduct, the covariate X_3 (RACE2) was significant associated with Y (HBPX). The result suggests that being White was associated with increased risk of high blood pressure. The association between **GENDER** and HBPX was not statistically significant ($p > 0.05$).

6.4.5   Results from Model 3: Multiple Logistic Regression Controlling for Confounders

Likewise, Fig. 6.9 displays the main output of Model 3 in SAS Program 6.2. After controlling for the two confounders X_4 (BMI) and X_5 (DEPRESS), the estimated $\beta_1 = 0.2208$, the effect of X_1 (SMKYR10) on high blood pressure. This adjusted estimate is also greater than the unadjusted estimate of $\beta_1 = 0.1620$ for the same X_1 in Model 1.

Similar to the two demographic factors, the results presented in Fig. 6.9 suggest that the impact of X_1 on the risk of high blood pressure Y would be underestimated if the two confounders were not considered.

Analysis of Maximum Likelihood Estimates						
Parameter	DF	Estimate	Standard Error	Wald Chi-Square	Pr > ChiSq	Exp(Est)
Intercept	1	-3.0750	0.2345	171.8841	<.0001	0.046
SMKYR10	1	0.2208	0.0285	59.8029	<.0001	1.247
BMI	1	0.0285	0.00755	14.2636	0.0002	1.029
DEPRESS	1	-0.0182	0.0141	1.6640	0.1971	0.982

Odds Ratio Estimates		
Effect	Point Estimate	95% Wald Confidence Limits
SMKYR10	1.247	1.179 1.319
BMI	1.029	1.014 1.044
DEPRESS	0.982	0.955 1.009

Fig. 6.9   Main results from Model 3 controlling for confounders: Output of SAS Program 6.2

6.4.6   Results from Model 4: Considering Both Demographic Factors And Confounders

Last, Fig. 6.10 displays the main results from Model 4 in SAS Program 6.2 that simultaneously considered both the two demographic factors and the two confounding factors. The adjusted $\beta_1 = 0.2307$, $p < 0.01$ for X_1 (SMKYR10). Of the four logistic regression models, this adjusted β_1 was the highest. The result suggests the need to consider both demographic factors and confounders; otherwise, the results will be biased (under-estimated) if only bivariate analysis is used.

The result of a largest adjusted β_1 from Model 4 is also expected. This is because the analysis from Model 2 and Model 3 both indicated an underestimation of the effect of X_1 (SMKYR10) using Model 1. When all the covariates were included in Model 4, the underestimates were all corrected, resulting in the largest increase in the estimated beta coefficient for the effect of smoking years on the risk of high blood pressure.

Analysis of Maximum Likelihood Estimates							
Parameter		DF	Estimate	Standard Error	Wald Chi-Square	Pr > ChiSq	Exp(Est)
Intercept		1	-3.2067	0.2405	177.8509	<.0001	0.040
SMKYR10		1	0.2307	0.0299	59.7007	<.0001	1.259
GENDER	1	1	0.0743	0.0585	1.6148	0.2038	1.077
RACE2	0	1	0.2097	0.0631	11.0296	0.0009	1.233
BMI		1	0.0293	0.00765	14.6863	0.0001	1.030
DEPRESS		1	-0.0133	0.0142	0.8750	0.3496	0.987

Odds Ratio Estimates		
Effect	Point Estimate	95% Wald Confidence Limits
SMKYR10	1.259	1.188 1.335
GENDER 1 vs 2	1.160	0.923 1.459
RACE2 0 vs 1	1.521	1.188 1.948
BMI	1.030	1.014 1.045
DEPRESS	0.987	0.960 1.015

Fig. 6.10 Main results from Model 4 considering impact of all covariates: Output of SAS Program 6.2

Based on the adjusted beta coefficient for X_l from Model 4, the adjusted *OR* [95% CI] = 1.259 [1.188,1.335] for the smoking measure after both demographic factors and confounders are considered.

6.4.7   Result Interpretation and Conclusions

In conclusion, findings from the multiple logistic regression analysis verified the result from bivariate analysis that smoking is a risk factor for hypertension among US adults. The effect of smoking on hypertension has increased after the main demographic factors and impactful confounding variables are considered using various logistic regression models. Based on the finding from this study, smoking for every 10 years is associated with a 25.9% (ranging from 18.8 to 33.5%) increase in the risk of hypertension. This result is not affected by gender and race and is independent of body weight and poor mental health status.

It is worth noting that in this demonstration, only two demographic factors and two confounders were used. In practice, more demographic factors and more confounders should be considered given the multifactual nature of the disease of high blood pressure.

6.4.8   Exploration with HPB as Outcome Y

As a further exploration, we run Model 4 (not shown in SAS Program 6.2) by replacing HBPX (measured high blood pressure) with HBP (self-reported high blood pressure). With the substitution, the adjusted $\beta_1 = 0.1305$, $p < 0.001$, and *OR* [95% CI] = 1.139 [1.073,1.210].

For practice purposes to further the understanding of the analytical method, students are asked to repeat the analyses in SAS Program 6.2 using different measures of Xs and Ys, then compare the results between the two (see practice question 3 presented at the end of this chapter).

6.5   Conditional Logistic Regression for Matched Case-Control Study

In epidemiology, matched case-control design is often used to enhance internal validity of a study to examine the association between an influential factor X and an outcome Y. In this case, the conventional logistic regression described above will be less efficient to obtain accurate estimates of the relationship between X and Y, as well as the type I error for statistical inference. In such case, the *conditional logistic regression* can be used instead to appreciate the value of the case-control design (Connolly and Liang 1988).

Although conditional logistic regression differs from the logistic regression in principle and computing methods, the same SAS procedure **PROC LOGISTIC** is still used for modeling analysis. Furthermore, the analytical results, including data-model fit, estimated β coefficients, *OR* and 95% CI are the same. Two things that differentiate the two methods are (1) data arrangement and (2) model specification.

6.5.1   Data Format for Conditional Logistic Regression

To conduct conditional logistic regression analysis, data must be arranged in the format shown in Table 6.2. The data format is similar to that introduced in Chap. 2 except one column: PAIRID. One ID number is assigned to each matched case and control pair as PAIRID, in addition to the ID for individual participants in the sample. For example, the first two cases in Table 6.2 are a matched pair with first participant suffering from hypertension (HBPX =1) and the second did not (HBPX = 0). The PAIRID can be extended to include 1: n matches with n varying from 1 to 3, occasional upto 10 or more matches for rare conditions.

The columns for other variables are the same as in linear and logistic regression in general, including demographic factors and confounders.

Table 6.2 Data format of matched case-control studies for conditional logistic regression analysis

ID	PAIRID	HBPX	AGE	SEX	RACE2	DEPRESS	BMI	SMK10	...
1	1	0							
2	1	1							
3	2	0							
4	2	1							
5	3	0							
6	3	1							
...	...	...							

6.5.2   SAS Program for Conditional Logistic Regression Analysis of Matched Case-Control Data

All the steps described in Sects. 6.3 and 6.4 are applied here for conditional logistic regression except for the part for model specification. SAS Program 6.3 presents a simple example for conditional logistic regression. The program is similar to all the logistic regression models covered in previous sections except one program line:

```
STRATA PAIRID;
```

This SAS statement indicates that conditional logistic regression treats individually matched pairs as the independent units for analysis, rather than individual participants. In this way the type I error can be estimated correctly.

```
***********************************************************************************
* SAS PROGRAM 6.3. CONDITIONAL LOGISTIC REGRESSION FOR MATCHED CASE-CONTROL STUDY;
***********************************************************************************;
PROC LOGISTIC DATA = YOUR DATA;
* MODEL SPECIFICATION;
MODEL Y = X1 COVX2 COVX3 ...;
STRATA PAIRID;   * CONSIDERING MATCHED PAIRS AS STRATA INDICATED BY ID IN THE DATASET;
RUN;
***********************************************************************************;
```

6.6   Multinomial and Ordinal Logistic Regression

As described at the beginning of this chapter, for an outcome variable Y that contains more than two categories, the binomial logistic regression cannot be used. For a multi-category outcome Y, it can be divided into two broad groups: nominal (naming) and ordered (ranking). *These two types of Y can both be modeled using the multinomial logistic regression method.* For an ordered multi-level Y, relative to multinomial logistic regression, ordinal logistic regression can provide additional information about the X ~ Y relationship (Bender and Grouven 1997). In this section, we will introduce these two logistic regression methods, including demonstrations with real data.

6.6.1   Multinomial Logistic Regression

Multinomial outcomes Y are often used in etiological studies. For example, a study can be conducted to determine if smoking X is associated with Y - suffering from any of the six diseases labeled as 1 (lung cancer), 2 (*chronic and obstructive pulmonary diseases*), 3 (*coronary heart disease*), 4 (*breast cancer*), 5 (prostate cancer), and 6 (*diabetes*). In this case, Y is measured using 6 categories. A study can also be conducted to quantify the relationship between an influential factor X (i.e., depression) and an outcome Y (i.e., smoking), in which the Y can be measured using ranks as 1 (*no smoking*), 2 (*smoked sometimes*), and 3 (*smoked daily*). In a study to assess the satisfaction with care from patients as outcome, a 5-level Likert scale can be used with 1 (*extremely unsatisfactory*) to 5 (*extremely satisfactory*); this represents another case of a ranked Y. Multinomial logistic regression is devised to analyze these multicategorical Ys.

Multinomial logistic regression is an extension of the binomial logistic regression with Y being measured using k levels. In the three examples above, k = 6 for the first one, k = 3 for the second one, and k = 5 for the last one. Let us start with the example in which Y is measured with 3 levels: Y = 1 for no smoking, Y = 2 for smoked someday, and $Y = 3$ for smoked every day. Using $Y = 1$ as the reference, modeling the association between X and $Y = 2$ (smoked somedays) becomes a binomial logistic regression as Model 6.3:

$$\ln \frac{\Pr(Y = 2)}{\Pr(Y = 1)} = \beta_1 X \tag{6.7}$$

In this model, the regression coefficient β_1 quantifies the relationship between X and $Y = 2$ with $Y = 1$ as the reference.

Likewise, modeling the relationship between X and the $Y = 3$ relative to $Y = 1$ becomes another binary logistic regression as Model 6.3:

$$\ln \frac{\Pr(Y = 3)}{\Pr(Y = 1)} = \beta_2 X \tag{6.8}$$

In this model, the regression coefficient β_2 quantified the X and Y ($Y = 3$) relative to the reference group ($Y = 1$).

A three-level multinomial logistic regression is simply a combination of these two binary logistic regression models 6.7 and 6.8. With Y measured using three levels, two β coefficients will be estimated to describe the X ~ Y relationship with one level selected as the reference. Statistically, a multinomial logistic regression quantifies the X ~ Y relationship using k-1 β coefficents if Y is measured with k levels. Relative to binomial, multinomial logistic regression will provide more detailed information about the X ~ Y relationship.

6.6.2   Empirical Test with Real Data

The relationship between smoking and depression among US population has been reported in the literature (McClave et al. 2009). To demonstrate the multinomial logistic regression method, the same data from Sect. 6.2 are used. A 3-level outcome Y (*current smoking*) was used. The variable was measured based on self-reported data from the 2017–2018 NHANES. In the original data, daily smoking was coded as 1, smoked somedays as 2, and not smoked as 3. A new variable SMK3L was created as Y for analysis by recoding the original data such that 0 = not smoked, 1 = smoked in some days, and 2 = smoked daily. The independent variable X(DEPRESS) and covariates such as BMI were previously defined in Sect. 5.6 and SAS Program 5.2. In the demonstration analysis, the variables **AGE**, **GENDER**, and RACE2 are used as demographic factors given the obvious difference in smoking and depression by these factors; and BMI is used as confounder since overweight and obese has been documented to affect smoking behavior as well as depression.

With these data, two β coefficients will be estimated using the multinomial logistic regression to measure the association of the influential factor X (DEPRESS) with

the outcome Y (SMK3L) with the *Y* being measured using three levels. To verify the
X ~ Y relationship suggested by the bivariate analysis, the same modeling approach
introduced in Chap. 5 for linear regression and the binomial logistic regression in
Sect. 6.3 of this chapter can be used, including (i) a simple linear correction to
assess relationships among all the variables, (ii) model 1 - a simply multinomial
logistic regression containing only the independent variable X, (iii) model 2 adjusting for demographic factors only, (iv) model 3 controlling for confounders only, and
(v) model 4 considering both demographic and confounding factors. To avoid dupli-
cation, only two of the five models, (ii) and (v) are included in the demonstration.

6.6.3   Data Processing for Multinomial Logistic Regression

Data processing for the demonstration of multinomial logistic regress is included in
SAS Program 6.4 part 1. The program starts by reading dataset DATCH5 to create a
work dataset C. Several program lines are thus used to show how to process the data
for analysis. The three-level Y (SMK3L) is created based on the variable SMKNOW in
the NHANES data. In the original survey, for participants who responded positively
(yes) to a question on cigarette smoking in the past 30 days, they were further asked
the frequency of smoking with 1 = smoking daily and 2 = smoking sometimes;
while for participants who responded negatively to the smoking question, system
missing was assigned to avoid asking the smoke frequency question. To create a
new *outcome Y*, we first recoded the system missing as 3 (*not smoked*) for the original variable SMKNOW. After the recoding, the new outcome *Y* (SMK3L) was created
by reversely coding the recoded SMKNOW (i.e., subtracting 3 from the original values) such that 0 (*not smoked*), 1 (*smoked sometimes*), and 2 (*smoked daily*). This
recoding will also facilitate result interpretation.

In the demonstration analysis, DEPRESS, a variable used as a confounder in
previous examples is now used as the *influential factor X*. As usually, demographic
factors (i.e., **AGE**, **GENDER**, and RACE2) and confounder BMI are included as
covariate CovXs.

In addition to SMK3L, other variables in the same dataset can be used for practice. As an example, we created a 3-level variable and labeled it as WEIGHT3L,
based on the original variable body weight (WHQ030) from the NHANES data. This
variable can be used as *Y* for practice to test relevant X ~ Y relationships.

As usual, after data processing, **PROC CONTENTS** is used check the variables in
the processed dataset C. For more detailed information about the data, other SAS
procedures   previously   introduced   can   be   used   too,   such   as
PROC FREQ and **PROC UNIVARIATE**.

6.6.4   SAS Program for Multinomial Logistic Regression

As an example, the second part of SAS Program 6.4, Part 2 presents two multinomial logistic regression models showing the program codes for multinomial logistic regression. The first one is a simple multinomial logistic regression for a bivariate analysis; and the second one is a multiple multinomial logistic regression to confirm the X (DEPRESS) –Y(SMK3L) relationship by adjusting the three demographic factors and one confounder.

```
*****************************************************************************
SAS PROGRAM 6.4. MULTINOMIAL LOGISTIC REGRESSION FOR MULTI-CATEGORICAL DATA
*****************************************************************************;
** PART 1. DATA PROCESSING;
LIBNAME SASDATA "C:\QUANTLAB\A_DATA";
* READ DATASET DATCH5 USED IN CHAPTER 5 INTO DATA C AND CREATE NEW VARIABLES;
DATA C; SET SASDATA.DATCH5;
* CODE THE SYSTEM MISSING AS NOT SMOKED;
IF SMKNOW EQ . THEN SMKNOW = 3;
* REVERSE CODING SUCH THAT 0=NOT SMOKE, 1=SMOKED SOMETIMES, 2=SMOKED DAILY;
SMK3L = 3-SMKNOW;
* INCLUDE A SELF-REPORTED BODY WEIGTH FOR STUDENTS TO PRACTICE;
IF WHQ030 ^IN (1 2 3) THEN WHQ030 = .;   * RECODE MISSING;
* REVERSE CODE SUCH THAT 0=OK, 1=UNDERWEIGTH AND 2 = OVERWEIGHT;
WEIGHT3L = 1-WHQ030;
LABEL SMK3L    = '0 = NOT SMOKED 1 = SMOKED SOMETIMES 2 = SMOKED DAILY',
      WEIGHT3L = '0 = OK 1 = UNDERWEIGTH 2 = OVERWEIGHT';
PROC CONTENTS; RUN;
** PART 2: MODELING ANALYSIS
* MODEL 1: SIMPLE LOGISTIC REGRESSION;
PROC LOGISTIC DATA = C;
CLASS SMK3L(REF = '0')/PARAM=REF;
MODEL SMK3L = DEPRESS /LINK=GLOGIT;
RUN;
* MODEL 2: ADJUST DEMOGRAPHIC FACTORS AND CONTROL FOR CONFOUNDERS;
PROC LOGISTIC DATA = C;
CLASS SMK3L(REF = '0') GENDER (REF='1') RACE2 (REF='0')/PARAM=REF;
MODEL SMK3L = DEPRESS AGE GENDER RACE2 BMI/LINK=GLOGIT;
RUN;
*****************************************************************************;
```

SAS program for multinomial logistic regression differs from the (binomial) logistic regression in the following two program lines:

```
CLASS SMK3L(REF = '0')/PARAM=REF;
MODEL SMK3L = DEPRESS /LINK=GLOGIT;
```

In the program line started with the SAS key word CLASS, reference group must be specified using (REF = 'ref of your selection'), followed by PARAM=REF to specify the method for parameter estimation using the reference. In the line to specify the model, the "LINK=GLOGIT" must be specified such that a multinomial logistic regression model will be used with logit (P) of Y rather than the values of Y (0, 1, 2) as continuous outcome.

6.6.5 Results from Model 1: Simple Multinomial Logistic Regression

The main output of Model 1 in SAS Program 6.4 is similar to that from the logistic regression (see Fig. 6.7). First, it includes a model fit statistics section. The -2Log L in this section can be used to compute pseudo R^2. It also has a section on testing the global null hypothesis that BETA = 0, reporting the likelihood ratio test, score test, and Wald test using chi-square with $p < 0.05$ as an indication of good data-model fit. The output unique for the multinomial logistic regression is presented in Fig. 6.11.

Testing Global Null Hypothesis: BETA=0			
Test	Chi-Square	DF	Pr > ChiSq
Likelihood Ratio	113.3473	2	<.0001
Score	131.5468	2	<.0001
Wald	121.8004	2	<.0001

Type 3 Analysis of Effects			
Effect	DF	Wald Chi-Square	Pr > ChiSq
DEPRESS	2	121.8004	<.0001

Analysis of Maximum Likelihood Estimates						
Parameter	SMK3L	DF	Estimate	Standard Error	Wald Chi-Square	Pr > ChiSq
Intercept	1	1	-2.1508	0.0551	1523.7584	<.0001
Intercept	2	1	-3.2528	0.0965	1135.2968	<.0001
DEPRESS	1	1	0.0899	0.00817	121.1092	<.0001
DEPRESS	2	1	0.0370	0.0169	4.8077	0.0283

Odds Ratio Estimates				
Effect	SMK3L	Point Estimate	95% Wald Confidence Limits	
DEPRESS	1	1.094	1.077	1.112
DEPRESS	2	1.038	1.004	1.073

Fig. 6.11 Main results from Multinomial Logistic Regression Model 1: Output from SAS Program 6.4

Second, the SAS output contains a section named as "Type 3 Analysis of Effects". Type 3 analysis is the test to assess the effect of X on Y, overall and not by category. In our example, type 3 analysis for DEPRESS is extremely significant with chi-square = 95.48 (DF = 2), $p < 0.0001$. This suggests that the association between the number of depressive symptoms and frequency of smoking is statistically extremely significant.

Third, in the section "Analysis of Maximum Likelihood Estimates", multinomial logistic regression provided two α intercepts and two β slopes for X (DEPRESS) on two levels of Y (SMK3L) with no smoking as the reference. The estimated model coefficients $\alpha's$ and $\beta's$ as well as the odds ratios (ORs) can be interpreted as in general logistic regression.

The two estimated slopes were β_1=0.0899 ($p < 0.001$) and β_2=0.0370 ($p < 0.05$) for the influential factor X (DEPRESS) on the outcome Y (SMK3L) measured using 3 levels. The estimated β_1 indicatef that for each point score increase in DEPRESS, the risk from no smoking to smoking someday (i.e., from 0 to 1) would increase by 0.0899 units in log-odds; likewise, the estimated β_2 shows for a one unit increase in DEPRESS score, the risk from no smoking to daily smoking (0 to 2) would increase by 0.0370 units in log-odds.

Corresponding to the two estimated β slopes, the estimated odds ratio (OR) and 95% CI are presented in the last part of Fig. 6.11.

6.6.6   Results from Model 2: Multiple Multinomial Logistic Regression

The main results from Model 2, the multiple multinomial logistic regression are presented in Fig. 6.12. The left part of the figure contains the estimated $\alpha's$ and $\beta's$ for X_1 (DEPRESS), the influential factor, three demographic factors, X_2 (AGE), X_3 (GENDER), and X_4 (RACE2) and one confounder X_5 (BMI); the right part of the figure contains the estimated ORs and 95% CIs.

First, comparing to the result in Fig. 6.11, the estimated β_1= 0.0987 ($p < 0.001$), greater than 0.0899 ($p < 0.001$), the estimate from Model 1 for the simple logistic regression; and the estimated β_2= 0.0470 ($p < 0.0001$), also greater than 0.0370 ($p < 0.05$), the estimate also from Model 1.

With the estimated β coefficients, odds ratio (OR) for X_1 (not shown in Fig. 6.12 to save space) the estimated OR [95% CI] = 1.104 [1.085, 1.123] for nonsmokers progressing to smoking someday; and the OR [95% CI] = 1.048 [1.013, 1.084] for non-smokers directly progressing to daily smokers.

Based on results from Model 2 and estimated OR, depressive symptoms were statistically significantly associated with frequency of smoking. Relative to non-smokers, increases in one depressive symptom would result in a 10.4% increase in the risk for a nonsmoker to progress to an occasional smoker; and 4.8% increase in the risk for a non-smoker directly jumping to smoke daily, adjusting the main demographic factors and impactful confounders were considered. Students can calculate the ORs to confirm the results.

Analysis of Maximum Likelihood Estimates						
Parameter	SMK3L	DF	Estimate	Standard Error	Wald Chi-Square	Pr > ChiSq
Intercept	1	1	-0.5790	0.2298	6.3486	0.0117
Intercept	2	1	-2.0673	0.3923	27.7723	<.0001
DEPRESS	1	1	0.0987	0.00882	125.0186	<.0001
DEPRESS	2	1	0.0470	0.0174	7.3220	0.0068
AGE	1	1	-0.0107	0.00263	16.5850	<.0001
AGE	2	1	-0.0154	0.00473	10.6525	0.0011
GENDER 2	1	1	-0.5432	0.0883	37.8630	<.0001
GENDER 2	2	1	-0.5826	0.1577	13.6442	0.0002
RACE2 1	1	1	0.5669	0.0882	41.2909	<.0001
RACE2 1	2	1	-0.00632	0.1665	0.0014	0.9697
BMI	1	1	-0.0307	0.00672	20.8415	<.0001
BMI	2	1	-0.00139	0.0111	0.0158	0.9000

Fig. 6.12 Main results from multinomial logistic regression that adjusted demographic factors and controlled confounder: Output of SAS Program 6.4

Lastly, as in other multivariate analyses, a byproduct of the multiple logistic regression as in Model 2 is the data on potential associations of the demographic and confounding factors (i.e., AGE, GENDER, RACE2, and BMI) on the outcome Y (DEPRESS). Although supportive to the current study, these byproducts are useful for proposing new studies. Likewise, students can manually calculate the ORs.

6.6.7   Conclusion Remarks

The analytical method of multinomial logistic regression not only enhances our ability to analyze data with Y being measured as multiple categorical, but it also provides more detailed information regarding an X ~ Y relationship (a dose-response relation in the example) we want to examine. The concept is easy, and the SAS programs in this section can be used as a template to analyze the data of your own and obtain the results to address a study question.

6.7   Ordinal Logistic Regression for Ordered Outcomes

In Sect. 6.6 for multinomial logistic regression, each level of the outcome Y was modeled separately in the analysis to assess the X ~ Y relationship. In such analyses, the multi-category Y can be both nominal and ordinal, providing certain flexibility to quantify a hypothetic X ~ Y relationship.

Despite detailed results, multinomial logistic regression ignores the cumulative effect of X on Y if the multi-levels of Y are ordered (Bender and Grouven 1997). For example, in our example with a 3-level smoking measure (SAS Program 6.3), although the two estimated β coefficients measured the impact of X on the two levels of Y with reference to no smoking, cumulative risk has not estimated for the effect from level 0 (no smoking as the reference) to level 1(smoked sometimes) and further to level 2(smoked daily). Ordinal logistic regression is a method devised to obtain this missed information (Bender and Grouven 1997).

6.7.1   A Brief Introduction to the Ordinal Logistic Regression

In ordinal logistic regression for a Y with k ordered levels, the cumulative distribution of Y up to level j, i.e., $Y \leq j$ is contrasted to the level of $>j$:

$$\ln \frac{\Pr(Y \leq j)}{\Pr(Y > j)} = logit(P(Y \leq j) = \beta X. \tag{6.9}$$

Clearly, an ordinal logistic regression associates the influential factor X with a cumulative proportion of Y over the ordered levels. In this case, although Y contains multiple levels, only one β coefficient will be used to quantify the overall X ~ Y relationship, rather than k-1 β coefficients each quantifying the impact of X on one-level change in Y. SAS Program 6.5 below shows an *ordinal* logistic regression using the data to examine the smoking – depression relationship.

6.7.2   SAS Program for Ordinary Logistic Regression

SAS Program 6.5 is an example of ordinal logistic regression. The program codes are similar to the multinomial logistic regression with two exceptions. (1) The key word DECENDENG is used behind the outcome Y to specify the order of the variable; (2) no link function is specified at the end of the MODEL statement.

Like in SAS Program 6.4, in this program, Model 1 is a simple ordinal logistic regression without considering any covariates; and Model 2 is a multiple ordinal logistic regression with AGE, GENDER, RACE2 and BMI included as covariates.

As a demonstration, we will provide SAS output in detail from Model 1 only. Results from Model 2 analysis will be left for practice.

```
**************************************************************************************
* SAS Program 6.5. ORDINAL LOGISTIC REGRESSION
**************************************************************************************;
** MODEL 1: SIMPLE ORDINAL LOGIST REGRSSION;
PROC LOGISTIC DATA = C;
CLASS SMK3L (DECENDENG) /PARAM=REF;
MODEL SMK3L = DEPRESS;
RUN;
** MODEL 2: ORDINAL MULTIPLE LOGISTIC REG TO INCLUDE COVARIATES;
PROC LOGISTIC DATA = C;
CLASS SMK3L (REF = '0') GENDER (REF='1') RACE2 (REF='0')/PARAM=REF;
MODEL SMK3L = DEPRESS AGE GENDER RACE2 BMI/ LINK=GLOGIT;
RUN;
**************************************************************************************;
```

6.7.3   Results from Model 1 and Interpretation

Many of the ordinal logistic regression results are similar to those of the multinomial logistic regression. These results include (i) data-model fit, -2log likelihood (for computing pseudo-R^2), (ii) three chi-square tests for the global hypothesis beta $= 0$, (iii) maximum likelihood estimate of α and β, and (iv) odds ratio (OR).

Figure 6.13 displays the main part of SAS output from Model 1 in SAS Program 6.5. From the figure it can be seen that estimated slope $\beta = 0.0758$ ($p < 0.01$) for DEPRESS. Different from the multinomial logistic regression, this β coefficient provides a measure of effect cumulative of depressive symptoms on smoking that was measured using a three-level variable with reference to no smoking. Corresponding to the β coefficient, estimated OR [95% CI] $= 1.079$ [1.063. 1.095]. This result suggests that depression is associated with about a 7.9% increase in risk of every one-step up in smoking frequency along with the 3 levels for each

Analysis of Maximum Likelihood Estimates					
Parameter	DF	Estimate	Standard Error	Wald Chi-Square	Pr > ChiSq
Intercept	2	1	-3.5919	0.0833	1859.9007	<.0001
Intercept	1	1	-1.8556	0.0490	1433.3184	<.0001
DEPRESS		1	0.0758	0.00758	100.1304	<.0001

Odds Ratio Estimates			
Effect	Point Estimate	95% Wald Confidence Limits	
DEPRESS	1.079	1.063	1.095

Fig. 6.13 Results from ordinal logistic regression: Output of Model 1, SAS Program 6.5

depressive symptom – a cumulative effect that cannot be obtained from the multi-nomial logistic regression.

The significance of an ordinal logistic regression can be revealed by comparing the results in Fig. 6.13 with those in Fig. 6.11 for multinomial logistic regression using Model 1 in SAS Program 6.4. When levels of smoking were analyzed as mul-tinomial variable with k levels, β coefficients are estimated for k-1 levels with one level as the reference. Since smoking was measured using three levels, two β coef-ficients β_1 and β_2 are estimated using multinomial logistic regression (i.e., Model 1 in SAS Program 6.4), each measuring the risk of one level of Y comparing to the reference level. However, when the same data are analyzed using the ordinal logistic regression, only one β coefficient is estimated to measure risk of X on Y as Y varies upward alone the ranked/leveled measure relative to the reference.

6.7.4   Application in Verifying Hypothetic X ~ Y Relationships

Like in other logistic regression models previously introduced in this section, Model 2 in SAS Program 6.5 is an example of ordinal multiple logistic regression to verify the X_1 (DEPRESS) – Y(SMK3L) relationship by including four covariates AGE, GENDER, RACE2, and BMI. Among the four covariates, three are demographic factors (AGE, **GENDER**, and RACE2) and one is a confounder (BMI).

This part of the program will be kept for practice, and no results are displayed and none of the result will be discussed here. As a reference, the estimated $\beta = 0.1018$ ($p < 0.001$) for DEPRESS, and this estimated β is greater than 0.094 ($p < 0.01$) esti-mated from Model 1 without controlling for covariate. If you do everything cor-rectly, you should get the same result.

6.8   Poisson Regression for Y as a Counting Variable

As discussed in Chap. 2, counting data are another type of outcome Y that are also used in medical, health, and behavioral research studies. Typical examples include blood cell count, copies of viruses, DNA adducts, hospital days, number of smoking days, and number of drinking days. Numerically, these data look like continuous variables, such as age, body height and weight; but statistically they are not continu-ous and do not follow the normal distribution.

Let us use days of hospital stay as an example. If the data on days of hospital stay for patients in a hospital are considered, it is not uncommon that a few patients may have stayed in hospital for a very long time, for weeks or even months after admis-sion; while most patients stay less than a whole day or only 1 or 2 days. This type of data cannot be analyzed efficiently using the linear regression introduced in Chap. 5 since the data do not follow the normal distribution. This type of data also cannot be analyzed using the logistic regression previously introduced in this chap-ter because they do not follow the binomial or multinomial distribution.

One unique characteristic of the counting data is that their distribution is skewed to the right with a lot of participants having zero or very smaller counts and a few participants with very large counts. Statistically, this type of data often follows the *Poisson distribution*. Typical examples include but are not limited to the following: copies of viruses, gene mutations, rare diseases such as cancer, car accidents by day, the number of births per hour during a day, the number of calls received for emergent events, and days of hospital stay. If the observed data follow Poisson distribution, such data can be effectively analyzed using a Poisson regression model.

6.8.1 A Brief Introduction to the Poisson Regression

Although not as popular as logistic regression, the Poisson regression method has been well-established (Hoffmann 2016). As the name suggests, Poisson regression is based on the Poisson distribution with λ_i represents the count of an outcome variable Y for i[th] participant in a study sample. The sample is selected from a population with λ = mean count of the population. In this setting, the probability distribution of $Y = \lambda_i$ ($\lambda_i > 0$) follows Poisson distribution: $\Pr\{Y = y| \lambda\} = [e^{-\lambda} \lambda^y]/y!$. A unique feature of the Poisson distribution is that its sample mean equals the standard deviation (SD) and equals the population mean λ. In practice to check if data follow Poisson distribution, we can compute the mean and SD of the outcome Y with sample data and compare if the two are close to each other.

Like in the logistic regression, a Poisson regression model links the Poisson distribution of an outcome variable Y to an influential factor X through an exponential model: $\lambda_i = e^{\alpha + \beta x}$. Taking a logarithm of the model, the log-linear Poisson regression is generated:

$$\log(\lambda_i) = \alpha + \beta x \tag{6.10}$$

Like logistic regression, the maximum likelihood method is used to solve for a Poisson regression model, to estimate regression coefficients of the model, and to conduct significant tests. More detailed description of the Poisson regression can be found in many classic statistical books (Hoffmann 2016).

6.8.2 Preparation for Poisson Regression Analysis

Different from the linear and logistic regression, before Poisson regression analysis, the distribution of Y must be examined to check: (i) if the distribution is skewed, (ii) if it is skewed to the right (i.e., a few subjects with large counts and many subjects with small counts), and (iii) if the mean and SD are close to each other.

If the analytical results indicate that the distribution of Y is skewed but skewed toward a wrong direction - the left (many subjects with large counts and few subjects with small counts), action must be taken to convert the left-skewed data into right-skewed before modeling analysis.

In the SAS Program 6.6 next, we will show how to check if a variable follows the Poisson distribution. If not, how to convert a left-skewed distribution to a right-skewed distribution.

6.8.3   SAS Program for Poisson Regression with Real Data

SAS Program 6.6 demonstrates the Poisson regression analysis method with dataset DATCH6 created for this chapter. In the data processing step, a work dataset D is created by access the created dataset DATCH6. In this demonstration, the number of days smoked in the past 30 days (SMKDAYS) was used as Y, DEPRESS was used as X_1, and **AGE, GENDER,** and RACE2 as covariates X_2, X_3 and X_4, respectively.

Since the analysis focuses on the variable measuring days of smoking as Y, in the data processing step, the first task is to select participants who were smokers and exclude participants who were not. This inclusion and exclusion operation are achieved using one line of SAS program in the data step: IF 1 <= SMKDAYS <= 30. With this criterion any participants who smoked on any day during the past 30 days were included.

```
*******************************************************************************
* SAS PROGRAM 6.6 DEMONSTRATION OF DATA PREPARATION AND POISSON REGRESSION
*******************************************************************************;
** PART 1: PROCESS DATA USING DATCH6 THAT WAS CREATED IN SAS PROGRAM 6.2;
LIBNAME SASDATA "C:\QUANTLAB\A_DATA";
* 1. CREATE A NEW DATASET D, SELECT PARTICIPANTS AND PROCESS THE SELECTED DATA;
DATA D; SET SASDATA.DATCH6;
* 2. SELECT ONLY THOSE WHO SMOKED IN THE PAST 30 DAYS;
IF 1 <= SMKDAYS <= 30;
* 3. CONVERT THE Y TO POISSON DISTRIBUTION;
Y = 31 - SMKDAYS; RUN;
* 4. CHECK THE DISTRIBUTION OF Y AND COMPUTE MEAN AND SD USING PROC UNIVARIATE;
PROC UNIVARIATE DATA=D;    * THIS ANALYSIS CAN BE USSED BEFORE STEP 3 AND AFTER STEP 2;
HISTOGRAM Y; RUN;
** PART 2. POISSON REGRESSION USING PROC GENMOD AND POISSON DISTRIBUTION;
* ACTIVATE THE PROC GENMOD IN SAS FOR POISSON REGRESSION;
PROC GENMOD DATA = D;
* SPECIFY ALL VARIABLES THAT ARE CATEGORICAL, INCLUDING Y;
CLASS Y GENDER RACE2 / PARAM=GLM;
* SPECIFY THE POISSON REGRESSION MODEL;
MODEL Y = DEPRESS AGE GENDER RACE2 /DIST=POISSON TYPE3;
RUN;
*******************************************************************************;
```

6.8.4   Check the Distribution of Outcome Y

As an important step of Poisson regression, the distribution of Y is checked first. This step is completed using the **PROC UNIVARIATE** in SAS previously learned Chap. 3, Sect. 3.3. Putting the variable SMKDAYS in the place of Y in the program

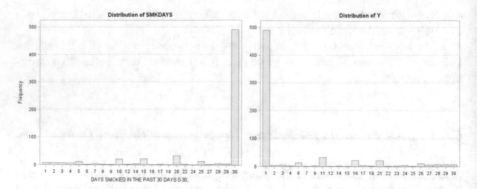

Fig. 6.14 Distribution of Y (days of smoking) before and after conversion: Output from SAS Program 6.6

and executing the program code by highlighting it first and then click "run", two types of results will be generated.

The first part is the estimated mean of smoking days = 5 and SD = 8. Although not equal, they are close to each other, and the difference could be due to sampling errors.

The second part is presented in the left side of Fig. 6.14. This is the distribution of Y generated using from the program code `HISTOGRAM` with the Y being measured using the variable `SMKDAYS`. It is clear that the distribution is highly skewed with few participants having small counts and many having large counts. Unfortunately, the distribution is skewed to the left, opposite to the Poisson distribution. To analyze the data using Poisson regression, the data must be converted so that the distribution is skewed to the right.

To convert the left-skewed distribution to the right, a new Y was created using the formula `Y = 31 - SMKDAYS`. Since the highest number of smoking days in a month is 30, subtracting the reported smoking days from 31 will convert the distribution from skewed left to the right. The right panel of Fig. 6.14 display the output from the same **PROC UNIVARIATE** with the converted Y. When the converted variable Y is used, the distribution looks like following the Poisson distribution with a large number of participants having very small counts and a small number of participants having very large counts. Therefore, such data can be analyzed using a Poisson regression model.

Remember, the Y is numerically reversed now. With the revision, Y = 1 means "smoked every day for 30 days in the past month" and Y = 30 means "smoked only on one day in the past month". As a result, findings *from the* analysis *must be interpreted reversely with a negative relation as positive and a positive relation as negative*. We will see this next in the real data analysis.

6.8.5 Poisson Regression Analysis Using SAS

As shown in the last part of SAS Program 6.6, different from linear and logistic regression, SAS did not provide a procedure for Poisson regression. Poisson regression is thus completed using the **PROC GENMOD**. The syntax for Poisson regression looks very similar to the logistic regression introduced early in this chapter. The following options make the **PROC GENMOD** a Poisson regression.

First, the outcome variable Y is modeled as categorical by adding Y to the variable list after the SAS key word: CLASS. Remember, in our data, Y is numerical. If this variable is not claimed as categorical, Poisson regression analysis cannot be conducted. In addition, all other non-continuous influential factors are added; here GENDER and RACE2 are used as two examples. At the end of this program line, "PARAM=GLM"" is specified for model parameter estimation using the general linear model (GLM).

Second, in the line for model statement, the following must be added "DIST=POISSON TYPE3". This option instructs the computer to estimate model parameters assuming a Poisson distribution. This is a key option for Poisson regression modeling analysis.

Last, the option TYPE3 in the same line asks the computer to do a type 3 test. What is type 3 test? Remember the outcome Y (counted data) is now modeled as categorical (CLASS) in Poisson regression. However, only one regression coefficient β rather than multiple βs for each count will be used to quantify the X ~ Y relationship although the Y is not continuous. Type 3 asks the computer to conduct such analysis to test the significance of the estimated β. This is similar to type 3 test in multinomial logistic regression.

6.8.6 Results About Data-Model Fit

Poisson regression model is solved using the maximum likelihood estimation method as in logistic regression analysis. Therefore, the first output of a Poisson regression is a list of nine criteria for assessing goodness of data-model fit, including deviance, chi-square, log likelihood, AIC, BIC, etc. The left part of Fig. 6.15 presents these criteria for the Poisson regression using SAS Program 6.6. Although

Criteria For Assessing Goodness Of Fit			
Criterion	DF	Value	Value/DF
Deviance	855	7583.3175	8.8694
Scaled Deviance	855	7583.3175	8.8694
Pearson Chi-Square	855	10756.5293	12.5807
Scaled Pearson X2	855	10756.5293	12.5807
Log Likelihood		2835.7237	
Full Log Likelihood		-4925.9241	
AIC (smaller is better)		9861.8483	
AICC (smaller is better)		9861.9185	
BIC (smaller is better)		9885.6329	

Analysis Of Maximum Likelihood Parameter Estimates								
Parameter		DF	Estimate	Standard Error	Wald 95% Confidence Limits		Wald Chi-Square	Pr > ChiSq
Intercept		1	1.7984	0.0575	1.6856	1.9111	977.10	<.0001
DEPRESS		1	-0.0267	0.0033	-0.0331	-0.0202	66.01	<.0001
AGE		1	-0.0065	0.0010	-0.0085	-0.0044	39.24	<.0001
GENDER	1	1	-0.0263	0.0318	-0.0886	0.0360	0.68	0.4083
GENDER	2	0	0.0000	0.0000	0.0000	0.0000		
RACE2	0	1	0.4059	0.0327	0.3419	0.4699	154.39	<.0001
RACE2	1	0	0.0000	0.0000	0.0000	0.0000		
Scale		0	1.0000	0.0000	1.0000	1.0000		

Fig. 6.15 Main results from Poisson regression analysis: Output from SAS Program 6.6

p-values are not computed, the large chi-square values and degreed of freedom (DF) suggest good data-model fit.

6.8.7 Poisson Regression Results and Interpretation

The right part of Fig. 6.15 presents the estimated regression coefficients. The estimated $\beta = -0.0267$ ($p < 0.01$) for the X_1 on the outcome Y. This is a measure of the association of influential factor X_1 (DEPRESS, the number of depressive symptoms in the past two weeks) with the reverse-coded outcome Y (SMKDAYS) while adjusting for the three demographic factors **AGE**, **GENDER**, and RACE2.

As mentioned early, since Y was reverse-coded before it was used for regression analysis, the negative sign of the estimated β must be reversed to correctly reflect direction of the X ~ Y relationship. Therefore, the real regression coefficient for DEPRESS should be: $\beta = 0.0267$ rather than -0.0267, namely, experiencing more depressive symptoms was associated with increased days of smoking in the past month.

We have already learned that Poisson regression is solved using a log linear model (Model 6.10) like in logistic regression. Therefore, odds ratios (OR) can be computed directly using the estimated β: $OR = \exp(\beta) = \exp(0.0267) = 1.027$. This result suggests that having one depressive symptom is associated with a 2.7% increase in the number of days of smoking in the past 30 days. This result was statistically extremely significant at $p < 0.001$ level after controlling for significant covariates.

6.9   Chapter Summary: Non-continuous Y to Verify X ~ Y Relationship

In this chapter, we introduced five methods to verify an X ~ Y relationship for non-continuous outcome variable Y. These methods include (binary) logistic regression, multinomial logistic regression, ordinal logistic regression, conditional logistic regression, and Poisson regression. We have demonstrated the application of these methods in practical use with real data. These methods, plus the linear regression introduced in Chap. 5 consist of the six most widely used multivariate analytical tools in epidemiology to advance etiological research studies.

In epidemiology, categorical outcome variables are used more often than continuous variables to assess an X ~ Y relationship suggested by a bivariate analysis. In cohort studies, categorical outcome Y is often used. In case-control studies, the outcome Y is always categorical, including binary (case, vs. control) or multicategory (i.e., dividing outcome measure into 3 or more levels); and further, a multi-category variable can be either simply nominal or ordered. The last case is the counting variables as Y. These variables look like continuous but are in fact not; this type of variables cannot be efficiently analyzed using any other methods except Poisson regression.

6.10 Practice

6.10.1 Statistical Analysis and Computing

1. Practice the simple logistic regression analysis by running SAS Program 6.1 yourself first. After gaining a mastery of the method, use the same approach to analyze data of your choice with a binary outcome Y and an influential factor X.
2. Practice the use of logistic regression to verify an X ~ Y relation using SAS Program 6.2 by including demographic factors and confounders. Spend time to review the results, particularly changes in the regression coefficients and ORs after inclusion of covariates.
3. Replace **HBPX** (hypertension determined by measured blood pressure) with **HBP** (self-reported hypertension) in all steps of analysis in SAS Program 6.2. Make comparisons of results between the two analytical approaches with different Y and think of the importance to select the right variable for quantitative analysis.
4. Practice the multinomial logistic regression analysis by re-running SAS Program 6.4. Spend time to review the results to gain an understanding of the method and its application.
5. Try to analyze some variables of your own choice using different variables and different logistic regression models.
6. Practice the Poisson regression analysis method using SAS Program 6.6 and dataset **DATCH6**.

6.10.2 Study Project Update

1. For students who used a binary, a multi-categorical, or a counting outcome variable to test an X ~ Y relationship in your own projects, please select an appropriate analytic method to verify your results by inclusion of demographic factors and confounders in four steps with four models, with model 1 to quantify the relation from bivariate analysis, model 2 to adjust demographic factors, model 3 to control for confounders, and model 4 to adjust/control for both.
2. Create Table 3 following the template in sect. 5.7.3, Chap. 5 and use the table to summarize the results from your own analysis.
3. Write up your interpretations of the analytical results.
4. Update all other parts of your paper to reflect the findings from the multivariate analysis, starting from the title to, Introduction, Materials and Methods, Findings, Discussion and Conclusions.
5. For students who use a continuous outcome Y, please refine your analysis after learning the methods for categorical outcomes. If you would like to switch to using a binary or multi-categorical Y, it is the time to do so now.

6.10.3 Study Questions

1. In a study project, a student wants to examine the relationship between internet usage and being overweighted. Which method should this student use to verify this relationship by considering demographic factors and controlling for confounders? Please consider all possible outcome measures (i.e., continuous, binary, and categorical).
2. When a log-linear model is used in multiple regression analysis, ORs can be calculated using the estimated beta regression coefficients for all influential factors. Please compute OR for the following beta coefficients:

Estimated beta	1.25	0.36	0.01	−0.25	−0.45	−1.58
OR =?						

3. In answering Question 2, do you see any trend by inspecting the relationship between the beta coefficients and ORs from question 2?
4. What is Type 3 test? When and why is type 3 test is needed?

References

Albert, A., Anderson, J.A.: On the existence of maximum likelihood estimates in logistic regression models. Biometrika. **71**(1), 1–10 (1984)

Bender, R., Grouven, U.: Ordinal logistic regression in medical research. J. R. Coll. Physicians Lond. **31**(5), 546–551 (1997)

Berg, C.J., Kirch, M., Hooper, M.W., McAlpine, D., An, L.C., Boudreaux, M., Ahluwalia, J.S.: Ethnic group differences in the relationship between depressive symptoms and smoking. Ethn. Health. **17**(1–2), 55–69 (2012)

Connolly, M.A., Liang, K.Y.: Conditional logistic regression models for correlated binary data. Biometrika. **75**(3), 501–506 (1988)

Freese, J., Long, J.S.: Regression Models for Categorical Dependent Variables Using Stata. Stata Press, College Station (2006)

Hoffmann, J.P.: Regression Models for Categorical, Count, and Related Variables: An Applied Approach. University of California Press, CA, USA (2016)

McClave, A.K., Dube, S.R., Strine, T.W., Kroenke, K., Caraballo, R.S., Mokdad, A.H.: Associations between smoking cessaion and anxiety and depression among U.S. adults. Addictive Behavior. **34**(6–7), 491–497 (2009)

Weinberger, A.H., Pilver, C.E., Desai, R.A., Mazure, C.M., McKee, S.A.: The relationship of major depressive disorder and gender to changes in smoking for current and former smokers: longitudinal evaluation in the US population. Addiction. **107**(10), 1847–1856 (2012)

Widome, R., Linde, J.A., Rohde, P., Ludman, E.J., Jeffery, R.W., Simon, G.E.: Does the association between depression and smoking vary by body mass index (BMI) category? Prev. Med. **49**(5), 380–383 (2009)

Wright, R.E.: Logistic regression. In: Grimm, L.G., Yarnold, P.K. (eds.) Reading and Understanding Multivariate Statistics, pp. 217–244. American Psychological Association (1995)

Chapter 7
Survival Analysis and Cox Regression for Time-to-Event Data

The process is more important than the outcome.

In Chap. 5, we learned the methods to confirm a potential X~Y relationship with multiple linear regression to address questions with the outcome Y being measured as a continuous variable, such as blood pressure, body height, and weight as well as BMI derived using height and weight, and scale scores for depression using the PHQ-9. In Chap. 6, we extended the analytical methods to include methods for various non-continuously measured Ys, including the binomial logistic regression for a dichotomous Y (i.e., having a disease or not, used drugs or not), multinomial logistic regression for a multi-categorical Y (i.e., frequency of drinking, severity of a diseases, levels of response to an intervention), ordinal logistic regression for a ranked Y, conditional logistic regression for case-control studies with Y being assessed through a matched design, and Poisson regression for a counting Y (i.e., count of cells, bacteria and viruses, rare diseases, car accidents, the number of emergency calls, and days of hospital stay).

In this chapter, we will learn methods to analyze another type of Y: Time-to-event (TTE). An outcome Y measured using the TTE data differs from both the continuous Y as described in Chap. 5 and the non-continuous Y as described in Chap. 6. As the name suggests, TTE data measures the time duration from the beginning till the time point when an event of interest occurred. TTE data are common in medicine and public health; but they cannot be efficiently analyzed using the methods we described in the previous two chapters, including linear, logistic, and Poisson regression. All these methods are useful to analyze the ultimate results, not the process or time course by which the outcome (event) develops. Therefore, evidence extracted from TTE data will be more informative than other types of data to advance the etiology and to evaluate therapies for disease treatment and interventions for disease prevention and health promotion.

To learn this method, we will first introduce the concept and various types of TTE data, research questions that can best be addressed with TTE data, and the methods to analyze TTE data. We will focus on the multivariate methods and their applications in verifying a potential X~Y relationship with TTE data. Likewise, all

X. Chen, *Quantitative Epidemiology*, Emerging Topics in Statistics and
Biostatistics, https://doi.org/10.1007/978-3-030-83852-2_7

the data and analytical methods will be demonstrated using SAS programs and the 2017–18 NHANES data.

7.1 Introduction to Studies with Time-To-Event Data

7.1.1 The Concept of Time-To-Event Data

In medical, health, and behavioral studies with longitudinal data to examine a hypothetic X~Y relationship, changes in the outcome Y are used as data to examine if the Y is associated with the exposure X. For example, to examine if the lack of physical activity (X) is associated with increases in bodyweight (Y), two groups of participants are observed, one practicing regular physical activity (X = 0) and another not (X = 1). These participants will be followed for a period of time (say for 24 months) to assess their body weight in kilograms (Y). Since the body weight Y is a continuous variable, such data can be analyzed using linear regression methods.

In addition to bodyweights, participants can be divided into different groups using the BMI calculated based on the weight and height. Following the published criteria for BMI, participants can be divided into: (a) normal weight (BMI<25) and (b) overweight (BMI>25). By dividing participants into two groups, a dichotomous Y is created, and such data can be efficiently analyzed using logistic regression to assess the physical activity - bodyweight relationship. If more than two levels are used, such as normal weight, overweight, and obesity (BMI>30), multinomial logistic regression can be used to examine the physical activity and bodyweight relationship.

In research practice, however, the outcome Y, either measured as the weight at the end of the study for linear regression, or the body weight status (i.e., normal, overweight, obese) as in the logistic regression measured at the end of a study, did not occur all at the same time when the study ends but during the whole study period. Changes in body weight and/or the status of body weights for all participants occur over time. With a longitudinal design, bodyweight of individual participants can be measured repeatedly. With such longitudinally measured data, the time to observe changes in Y can be derived for individual participants. The measured *time duration* for an observed change in Y is the so-called time-to-event (TTE) data.

TTE data consist of three basic components: the beginning date, the date when the expected event occurred, and the time duration from the beginning date to the date when the expected event occurred. With the beginning date and the ending date, time-to-event is simply a subtraction of later from the former. The methods introduced in this chapter are developed to analyze this type of data for outcome Y.

Three types of TTE data are often used in epidemiological studies: TTE from longitudinal studies, TTE constructed from cross-sectional studies, and TTS constructed with clinical recorded data. We will introduce these types of data next.

7.1.2   Time-To-Event Data with Longitudinal/Cohort Design

One source of TTE data is longitudinal studies, including studies with a cohort design (Fig. 7.1). In these studies, the beginning date t_0 is recorded for individual participants. Follow-up assessments are thus arranged on a pre-determined time interval (say, every week, every month, every 3 months…) to monitor the occurrence of the expected event as the outcome Y (i.e., disease occurrence, recovery from treatment, death, etc.). If an expected event occurred, the date or time when the event occurred is recorded as t. If no event occurred at one follow-up assessment, the observation is continued till the next assessment. Repeat the process until the study ends.

Fig. 7.1 Time to event data – Cohort (longitudinal) design

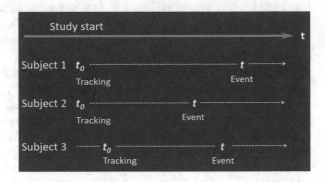

It would be ideal if all participants entered the study exactly on the same day when a study is launched. In this case, the starting date t_0 would be the same for all – the beginning date of the study. In this case, researchers only need to record t at which the expected event occurred. However, in practice, individual participants often enter a study sequentially after the study is launched. In this case, efforts must be devoted to recording the beginning date t_0 for individual participants, in addition to the t for timing of onset of the event.

With the recorded t and t_0 for individual participants, *TTE* is thus computed by subtracting t_0 from t:

$$TTE = t - t_0 \tag{7.1}$$

When collecting data to measure the time to event, different time scales can be used as the unit of *TTE* for different outcome measures. The unit of a time scale can vary from the shortest to the longest of minutes, hours, days, months, or years. For events in infants and young children, very short units are often used, including hours, minutes, and even seconds. For acute infectious diseases such as pneumonia and digestive system infections, day and hour are typical units used for measuring TTE; while for chronic conditions, such as heart diseases, cancers, dependence of substance use, and mental health problems, weeks, months, and years are typical units used for mearing TTE. It is worth noting that TTE data from longitudinal/cohort design are confounded by participants' age since participants of a longitudinal studies were often not born in one year. This issue has often been ignored in many reported studies.

7.1.3　Time-To-Event Data from Cross-Sectional Surveys

In the field of public health and preventive medicine, more data are available from cross-sectional studies than from cohort or longitudinal studies. In many cross-sectional studies, participants are also asked to report (1) important health-related events that happened in the recent past, and (2) the age when an event first occurred in life. For example, in the 2017–18 NHANES, adult participants were asked if they ever had high blood pressure; if yes, they were further asked the age when they were first told by their doctors about it (see Chap. 4). In the National Survey on Drug Use and Health (NSDUH), adolescent participants were asked if they "ever smoked cigarettes in life, including a few puffs"; for those who responded positively to the question, they were further asked "How old were you when you smoked a cigarette, including a few puffs the first time in life (age in year)?"

As shown in Fig. 7.2, with retrospectively reported data on a health-related event as the two examples described above, the reported age when an event first occurred in life can be used as the *TTE*. When participants recalled the age when they experienced an event for the first time, the reported age is eventually a measure of the time duration from birth to the year when the event occurred – a special type of *TTE* data.

Fig. 7.2 Time to event data – Cross-sectional design with survey data

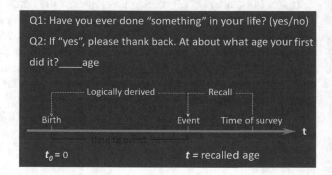

Different from the data derived from longitudinal studies, the reported chronological age from cross-sectional data is used as a measure of the TTE. A unique and also very important feature of such data is that they allow researchers to quantitatively characterize the age pattern of onset of a medical, health, or behavior-related event. Typical events include the onset of many diseases, developmental stages, menarche, sexual debut, onset of condom use, initiation of alcohol and tobacco, onset of suicidal ideation, etc. Knowledge on the age pattern of onset for any of these outcomes is of great significance in supporting the evidence-based planning and strategic decision-making for research to understand the epidemiology and for practice in public health and medicine for targeted prevention and treatment at the earliest time possible.

With cross-sectional data, different time units can also be used for different purposes. For example, for issues related to young children, TTE can be measured using smaller time units (i.e., days, weeks, or months) for higher time-resolution; while for adults, TTE can be measured using larger time units, say by a single year of age or multi-year age intervals (i.e., every 5 years or every 10 years) to reveal the overall pattern by age.

One concern with the TTE data derived from cross-sectional studies is the errors from self-reporting due to memory loss and/or recall bias. Statistically, such errors are often normally distributed with a zero mean. Therefore, the impact of such errors would be a minimal when the recalled data are used to obtain point estimates for the time duration, here the age of onset.

TTE data derived from cross-sectional studies have been used quite often in published studies to examine the age pattern of onset of disease, health status and behavior, including heart disease (Ahmad et al., 2017), cancer (Lim et al. 2018), smoking (Chen et al., 2006; Kendler et al., 2013), and drinking (Donovan and Molina 2011; Hingson et al. 2006). Findings from these studies provide data essential to understand the epidemiology of the problem and to make decisions and form policies for timely treatment and early prevention.

Capitalizing on the 2017–18 NHANES data, in this chapter, we will use self-reported age when a participant was first diagnosed with high blood pressure to demonstrate the methods for analyzing TTE data.

7.1.4   Time-To-Event Data from Clinical Records of Patient Data

Clinical records for individual patients provide a third source of *TTE* data. Clinical records for patients are originally gathered by healthcare professionals in patient care as part of the standard clinical practice procedure. The data are often prepared and stored in the format of electronic medical records (EMR) or electronic health records (EHR) to promote big data and data sciences (Ross et al. 2014). There is an increasing trend in using the EMR and HER data for research in medicine and public health.

Figure 7.3 shows how the clinical records-based *TTE* data are derived from the EMR or HER data. After the diagnosis of a disease is made, the formally recorded date of the diagnosis provide an accurate measure of t, the time an event occurred. In clinical practice, patients are often asked to recall the time when they first experienced anything that was related to the disease. For example, after being diagnosed with COVID-19, the patients will often be asked when (i.e., t_0) they first experienced a related symptom such as a fever, headache, and/or sore throat. This retrospective generated t_0 makes it possible to obtain data for TTE, the time from the

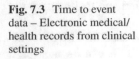

Fig. 7.3 Time to event data – Electronic medical/health records from clinical settings

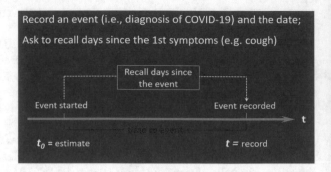

appearance of first symptoms to the time when a clinical diagnosis of COVID-19 was made.

TTE data derived from EMR/HER data are very useful for research and practice. Evidence can be derived from such data to advance our understanding of the development process of various diseases. In addition, patients may also be asked to report age of onset, age when they got married, age when first exposed to a risk factor in the past, time when having been in contact with other persons with the same diseases (for infectious diseases), year when moving to a different location in a country, and year when migrating from other countries to the United States, etc. These data can be used to assess influential factors on the onset of a medical or health-related problem.

The TTE data derived from the EMR/HER differ in principle from the TTE data derived from longitudinal and cohort studies. With patient data collected in healthcare settings, data for t are recorded in real time by medical professionals following the standard protocols. The recorded date is thus more accurate than the recalled date from longitudinal survey studies.

TTE data derived from EMR/HER also differ from those derived from cross-sectional survey studies. With patient data, data for t_0 are obtained through recall; while in cross-sectional survey studies, data for t are collected through recall. Knowledge of the differences described above is of certain importance for epidemiologists to selectively use data, taking advantages and avoiding limitations of the TTE data derived from different sources.

7.2   Survival Function and Weibull Distribution for Time-To-Event Data

As discussed at the beginning of this chapter, research data covered in Chaps. 5 and 6 are used to measure the outcome Y itself directly, such as current health status (sick or not sick), satisfaction with personal life (satisfied, neutral, not satisfied), marijuana use (times of use recently), engagement in risky sexual behavior (never, a few times, often), etc. Different from these data, the TTE data discussed in this chapter measures *the time course* by which a medical, health, or behavior-related outcome developed as an event. The TTE data make it possible to statistically quantify the time course using well-established statistical tools. One such tool is survival analysis (Lee and Go 1997).

7.2.1   Quantify the Time Course with Survival Function

As the name suggests, survival analysis is a method that was first developed to examine the age pattern of mortality after birth for demography and for life insurance computing (Keyfitz and Caswell 2005). Let T be a continuous variable measuring time, t as the observed duration of survival (non-negative), $f(t)$ as the probability density function, and $F(t)$ as the cumulative distribution of t, thus: $F(t) = P(T \leq t)$. With $F(t)$, the function to characterize the time course of survivorship, by definition can be written as:

$$S(t) = 1 - F(t). \tag{7.2}$$

Model 7.2 is the well-known survival function. This function describes the time course from birth at time zero to death at time t for all t when $t \leq T$. With mortality data by age, $F(t)$ measures the cumulative probability of death by age up to age t (range: 0–1). When $F(t = age)$ is known, the probability of survival up to age t: $S(t = age)$ is simply computed as $1-F(t)$.

When generalizing to all events in addition to death, model *7.2 can be used to characterize the time-to-event for any event of interest.* Typical examples include from the first symptom to the first diagnosis of a disease, from the first diagnosis to the start of treatment, from the beginning of treatment to the time of a significant effect, age of menarche and sexual debut (implicitly measured from birth), from birth to the age when first smoked a cigarette, from the start of physical activity to the time when a significant decline in body weight was observed; the list is endless. Survival analysis has also been used in industry to assess the life of a merchant for quality control and in the market research to assess the influential factors associated with the duration of credit card holders (Dirick et al. 2017).

7.2.2   Hazards Function and Instantaneous Risk of Event Occurrence

With the survival model described using Eq. 7.2, another function is defined: *the probability of the occurrence of an event in a population that has not yet occurred but will occur in a very short moment, Δt:*

$$h(t) = \lim_{\Delta t \to 0} \frac{\Pr(t \leq T < t + \Delta t)}{\Delta t S(t)} = \frac{F'(t)}{S(t)}$$

(7.3)

Model 7.3 is the well-known **hazard function**. It is a conditional probability that measures the likelihood of occurrence of an event of interest at any time immediately after time t for a person who has not yet developed the event up to time t. In demography and actuarial science, the hazard is known as the *force of* mortality; in medicine and public health, it is termed more generally as the *hazard rate*.

In this book for epidemiology, the name hazard or hazard rate is used. Technically, the hazard rate provides a measurement of the *instantaneous risk* for an event to occur. The event will include, in addition to death, all outcomes of interest that are relevant for medicine, health, and behaviors, including the normal developmental stages, occurrence of any diseases, changes in a health status, and initiation of any health-related behaviors.

The cumulative distribution function $F(t)$ increases monotonically with time t because it quantifies the probability of all persons in population who developed the outcome up to time t; the survival function $S(t)$ declines monotonically with time t since it quantifies the probability for a person in a population who has not developed the event yet up to time t; while the hazards function $h(t)$ can increase and decline with time. For example, from birth to young adulthood, the risk of death declines with age; while the same risk increases with age after adulthood until the end of life (Keyfitz and Wescall 2005). Therefore, the hazards function is often used in epidemiology to measure risk.

With survival analysis, the following three types of research questions can be addressed:

1. With $S(t)$, the proportion of individuals who remain free of the event of interest (but remaining at-risk) after a certain period of time of t can be estimated;
2. With $F(t)$ or $1 - S(t)$, the proportion of individuals who have already had developed the event of interest (cumulative prevalence rate) after a certain period of time t can be estimated; and
3. With $h(t)$, questions regarding the risk of developing the event of interest at a particular point in time t among those who remained event-free (at-risk) from the beginning until the time point can be estimated.

7.2.3   Survival Function and Weibull Distribution

Like the binomial distribution for logistic regression and polynomial distribution for multinomial logistic regression, to conduct survival analysis, the quality of TTE data must be checked to assess if they follow the Weibull distribution. Let λ be a constant, the cumulative distribution $F(t)$ can be expressed as an exponential function:

$$F(t) = 1 - \exp(-\lambda t). \tag{7.4}$$

With model 7.4, the survival function can be derived as $S(t) = \exp(-\lambda t)$. Let the cumulative hazard function $H(t) = \lambda t$ and the hazard function $h(t) = p\lambda^p t^{p-1}$, the distribution of survival time t, $F(t)$ can be described using a generalized exponential distribution model:

$$F(t) = 1 - \exp(-\lambda t)^p, \tag{7.5}$$

Model 7.5 is a form of Weibull distribution in which the value of p determines the direction of $h(t)$ - the hazard function. Figure 7.4 displays the Weibull density distributions of $h(t)$ for three different conditions.

In a hazard function, the $h(t)$ will increase with time to form a peak when $p > 1$ (the blue and red lines in Fig. 7.4); and $h(t)$ will progressively decline when $p \leq 1$ (the black line in Fig. 7.4). The Weibull distribution *consists of the statistical foundation to test if the observed TTE data can be analyzed using survival models*. If observed TTE data follow the Weibull distribution, the plots of log time (t) against log $(-\log(S(t)))$ will fall roughly on a straight line (Mudholkar et al. 1996). This property makes it possible to check the quality of any TTE data for survival analysis.

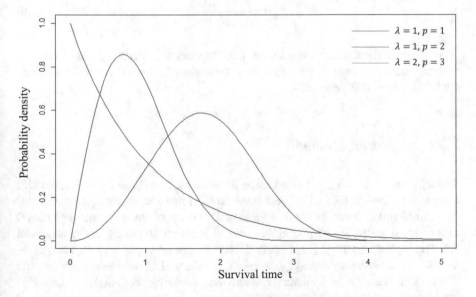

Fig. 7.4 Weibull density distribution for three different λ and p combinations

7.3   Estimation of Survival Functions

Various methods are developed and used to model time-to-event data using the survival functions described in Sect. 7.2. Two methods often reported in literature are the Kaplan-Meier (K-M) product-limit method and the actuarial method. The K-M method is often used to analyze TTE data with a small sample size (e.g., clinical based studies with patient data) while the actuarial method is often used to analyze TTE data with a large sample size (e.g., data derived from national survey studies). We will introduce these two methods.

7.3.1   Kaplan-Meier Method

The Kaplan-Meier method is statistically known as the product-limit estimation method (Kaplan and Meier 1958). As a non-parametric method, the K-M method is directly based on the definition of survival function $S(t)$ with discrete time. Let $n(t)$ = the number of participants who remain alive at time t, and $d(t)$ = number of participants that have died up to time t, the probability of survival at any time t, or $S(t)$ can be calculated as:

$$S(t) = \frac{n(t) - d(t)}{n(t)} \tag{7.6}$$

With the $S(t)$ estimated using model 7.6, other related survival functions can be derived, including cumulative probability function $F(t)$, hazard function $h(t)$, and cumulative hazard function $H(t)$.

7.3.2   Actuarial Method

The actuarial method is also known as the lifetable method (Cutler and Ederer 1958; Keyfitz and Caswell 2005). Different from the K-M method, this method uses a predetermined time interval rather than the actually observed survival time (age range) of individual participants to build the survival function $S(t)$ using the same model 7.6. The typical age range (commonly dabbed as age group) is 5 years, such as 0-, 5-. 10-, 15-... With the defined age intervals, a table will be used to present $n(t)$ and $d(t)$ as data. With the data, all survival functions, including $F(t)$, $S(t)$, $h(t)$, and $H(t)$ are then calculated using a spread sheet.

Different from the K-M method, the estimated survival curve is not affected by the random variation in survival time for individual subjects. As a result, the estimated survival functions F(t) and S(t) and the curves for these functions are smooth and visually attractive. While the same results using the K-M methods are step-like since the observed time is directly used in parameter estimation while the observed survival time often contains random variations.

7.3.3   Censoring in Survival Time

An important feature of the methods for survival analysis is that these methods can deal with a special type of missing data, known as censored.

As Fig. 7.5 shows, in conducting a study to assess the time course of an outcome event, a study must be completed during a certain time period with a starting and an ending date. There would be no missing data if all participants developed the event of interest by the time when a study ends. However, in many cases, a large number of participants have not yet developed the event (e.g., cancer, heart disease, drug dependence, etc.) by the time a study ends (t_0 is known, but not t). In this case, it is uncertain whether and when the study event will occur for the participants who have not yet developed the event by the end of a study. These participants will thus end up with no data for their outcome Y. In survival analysis, we term these participants as having a *right* censored or right-truncated data.

Fig. 7.5 Two types of censoring in collecting and analyzing survival data

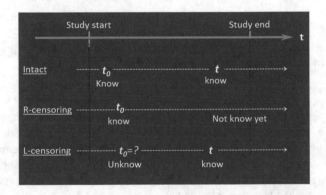

Studies with right censored data cannot be analyzed using all the methods described in Chaps. 5 and 6. This is because those methods focus on the outcome event itself, not the time course to the event. Since it is unknow if the event will occur for the participants, they must be excluded from the data in traditional analysis. However, survival analysis methods are devised to handle such missing data. Instead of the event of interest, a *survival analysis method focuses on the time course to the event*; thus, data from participants with complete data are used to predict the survivorship after time T when the study ends for the participants with right-censored data: $S(t) = Prob (t > T)$.

In addition to the right censoring, *left censoring* may exist (bottom panel of Fig. 7.5). Left censoring is common in data that are collected in clinical settings. For example, researchers can determine the exact time t when a disease of interest is diagnosed; however, they may not be able to determine t_0, the time when the symptoms of a disease first occurred. In addition to the appearance of symptoms, it is also not uncommon to experience difficulties in determining t_0 of first exposure to an influential factor for any health outcome, such as the time when first exposed to an environment pollutant, and the time when first experienced depression, the time when first noted as being overweighted.

7.4   Survival Modeling Analysis with Real Data

The best approach to learn a new method is to apply it to the real data. To demonstrate the methods for survival analysis, data from the same source, the 2017–18 NHANES are used. Instead of death, high blood pressure will be used as the outcome; and the age when participants were first aware that they had high blood pressure will be used as TTE. This TTE data serves as an example of the time-course data that are not associated with death but the occurrence of a disease. Survival analysis will be used to characterize the age pattern of high blood pressure onset. SAS program codes for data processing, statistical analysis, and interpretation of typical results are provided for learning and practice.

7.4.1   Data Source and Variables

The data for survival analysis will be derived from the datasets used in previous chapters, including those from DATCH2 used in Chap. 2 to obtain demographic factors and DATCH3 used in Chap. 3 to obtain variables to measure high blood pressure and age when first diagnosed with high blood pressure as TTE. Four demographic variables are age, gender, race, and education; and two high blood pressure variables are: (1) if they have high blood pressure (variable name: HBP, 1 = yes, 0 = no) and (2) age when they were first aware of having high blood pressure (variable name: AGEHYPR).

With these variables, survival analysis is conducted to assess the risk (hazard) of high blood pressure onset from the time at birth age t_0 to any age t up to $T = 80+$ years, the highest age group included in the NHANES data. With the inclusion of gender, race, and education, the survival analysis can be conducted, stratified by subgroups measured using these variables, and to assess cross-group differences.

7.4.2   SAS Programs for Survival Analysis

SAS Program 7.1 is prepared as an example for survival analysis. The program consists of three parts: Part 1 is for data preparation, showing how to read data used in Chapter 2 and Chap. 3 to select the variables. First, two temporary datasets,

TMP1and TMP2 are recreated to store the data obtained from the datasets DATCH2 (dataset for Chap. 2) and DATCH3 (dataset for Chap. 3), respectively. As usual, the **PROC CONTENTS** is used to make sure that the obtained data are the data needed. Before combining two datasets to create DATCH7 for analysis, the two datasets, TMP1and TMP2, must be sorted by the universal id number SEQN common for the two temporary datasets.

```
***************************************************************************************
SAS PROGRAM 7.1 SURVIVAL ANALYSIS
***************************************************************************************;
** PART 1, DATA PREPARATION, SEQN IS USED FOR DATA MERGING;
*  OBTAIN DEMOGRAPHIC FACTORS FROM DATA USED IN CHAPTER 2;
LIBNAME SASDATA "C:\QUANTLAB\A_DATA";
DATA TMP1; SET SASDATA.DATCH2;
KEEP AGE GENDER RACE5 EDUCATION SEQN; RUN;
*  OBTAIN HIGH BLOOD PRESSURE MEASURES FROM DATA USED IN CHAPTER 3;
DATA TMP2; SET SASDATA.DATCH3;
KEEP HBP AGEHYPR SEQN;
PROC CONTENTS; RUN;
* CREATE DATCH7 BY COMBINING TMP1 WITH TMP2 FOR SURVIVAL ANALYSIS;
PROC SORT DATA=TMP1; BY SEQU; RUN;
PROC SORT DATA=TMP2; BY SEQN; RUN;
DATA TMP; MERGE TMP1 TMP2; BY SEQN; RUN;
PROC CONTENTS DATA=TMP; RUN;

** PART 2 DATA PROCESSING: CENSORING AND RECODING;
*  CHECK DATA FOR CENSORING USING PROC FREQ PLUS OPTION: /MISSING, RESULTS SHOW 8
SUBJECTS WITH MISSING ON HBP (EXCLUDED) and 3273 WITH MISSING DATA ON AGEHYPR --
SUBJECTS WITH RIGHT CENSORING;
PROC FREQ DATA = TMP;
TABLES AGEHYPR * HBP/MISSING;
RUN;
* RECODE VARIABLE FOR SURVIVAL ANALYSIS;
DATA SASDATA.DATCH7; SET TMP;
IF HBP NE .; * EXCLUDE PARTICIPANTS WITH MISSING DATA ON HBP;
* DEFINE A NEW VARIABLE CENSORED TO MEASURE CENSORING;
CENSORED = 0;   * SET IT TO ZERO FIRST;
* CODE THOSE WITH MISSING AGEHYPR AS CENSORED;
IF HBP    EQ 0 AND AGEHYPR EQ . THEN CENSORED = 1;
* USE THE AGE AT SURVEY TO REPLACE MISSING ON AGEHYPR;
IF CENSORED EQ 1 AND AGEHYPR EQ . THEN AGEHYPR = AGE;
RUN;
* CHECK IF THE VARIALE CENSORED IS CORRECTLY CODED;
PROC FREQ DATA= SASDATA.DATCH7; TABLES CENSORED *HBP; RUN;

** PART 3 SURVIVAL ANALYSIS;
DATA A; SET SASDATA.DATCH7
* MODEL 1, KAPLAN-MEIER PRODUCT LIMIT METHOD;
PROC LIFETEST DATA = A METHOD=KM;
TIME AGEHYPR * CENSORED (1);
RUN;
* MODEL 2 ACTUARIAL METHOD WITH SPECIFIED TIME INTERVAL AND PLOT OPTIONS;
* PLOT OPTIONS - S FOR SURVIVAL H FOR HAZARD AND LLS FOR WEIBULL TEST
PROC LIFETEST DATA = A INTERVALS=0 TO 80 BY 5 PLOTS=(S, H, LLS) METHOD=ACT;
TIME AGEHYPR * CENSORED (1);
RUN;
* MODEL 3 BY GENDER AS STRATA, WILCOXON TEST FOR GENDER DIFFERENCE;
PROC LIFETEST DATA = A INTERVALS=0 TO 80 BY 5 PLOTS=(S, H, LLS) METHOD=ACT;
TIME AGEHYPR * CENSORED (1);
STRATA GENDER / TEST=(WILCOXON);
RUN;
* MODEL 4 BY RACE (5 LEVELS). THE VARIABLE EDUCATION IS LEFT FOR PRACTICE;
PROC LIFETEST DATA = A INTERVALS=0 TO 80 BY 5 PLOTS=(S, H, LLS) METHOD=ACT;
TIME AGEHYPR * CENSORED (1);
STRATA RACE5 / TEST=(WILCOXON);
RUN;
***************************************************************************************;
```

Part 2 of the program represents a key step in data processing for survival analysis – checking for participants who reported not having high blood pressure at the time when the 2017–18 NHANES was conducted. This step is completed using the SAS program codes: TABLES AGEHYPR * HBP/MISSING under the **PROC FREQ**. This step can help (1) identify all participants with missing data for HBP and (2) detect participants with HBP = 0 (no high blood pressure) and missing data for the variable AGEHYPR. Participants with missing data on key variables are often excluded, such as missing data on HBP and AGEHYPR.

Based on our discussion in Sect. 7.3, participants who did not have high blood pressure at the time of the study had missing data for AGEHYPR. They consist of a subsample of participants with *right-censored data*. If analyzed using the methods in Chaps. 5 and 6, these participants with missing data for AGEHYPR must be excluded. However, in survival analysis, data for these subjects can be used. What needs to be done is to code these participants as censored. A new variable **CENSORED** (0, 1) is created such that **CENSORED** = 1 for participants with HBP = 0 and missing data for AGEHYPR. The newly coded variable **CENSORED** is thus used as a condition to recode the AGEHYPR by set AGEHYPR = **AGE** (age of the participant at the time of study). In other words, the reported age of the participants at the time of the survey was used to replace the missing data, or the time course for the participants who have not yet developed the outcome at the time when the study is completed. When used together with **CENSORED** (0, 1), the SAS program knows how to handle the AGEHYPR for participants with and without missing data in constructing the survival functions.

Part 3 of the program presents four survival analysis models, Model 1 shows survival analysis using the K-M method, and Models 2–4 show survival analysis using the actuarial method. Of the three models, Model 2 is a duplicate of Model 1 with the actuarial method; models 3 and 4 are for stratified analysis using the actuarial method, including cross-strata comparisons using Wilcoxon test. Wilcoxon is a non-parametric method to assess whether the cross-strata difference in survival pattern is true or due to random sampling errors.

In all the four models, The SAS procedure **PROC LIFETEST** for survival analysis is used. This procedure is designated for use to analyze TTE data. Different from the regression models in the previous two chapters that start with the key word MODEL, then the dependent variable Y, the survival model starts with the key word TIME, followed by the time-to-event variable, here AGEHYPR, multiplied by the variable **CENSORED** (0, 1) newly created with 0=no censoring and 1=censored.

It is worth noting that in Models 2–4 when the actuarial method is used for survival analysis, the age range and age-intervals are specified. In our example, the age range is set from 0 to 80, the range allowed by data; a 5-year interval was used as routine. These specifications can be modified in practice. For example, even for the practice data, the analysis can be limited to the age range of 0–65; different age-intervals can also be used such as 2-year or 10-year age intervals.

7.4.3 Results from Model 1 and Model 2 and Interpretation

Figure 7.6 presents two survival curves $S(t) = 1 - F(t)$ estimated using processed data. The left part of the figure shows the results estimated using the K-M method and the right part shows the results estimated using the actuarial method. Consistent with the introduction to the methods in the previous section, when the observed time is directly used to construct the survival functions with the K-M method, the estimated survival curve $S(t)$ will not be smooth but decline by steps. The steps are eventually the time to event of individual participants. This phenomenon would be more obvious in small-scale longitudinal studies, including randomized controlled trials. It is worth noting that the NHANES data are technically not suitable for the K-M method because of the large sample size; K-M method is used here only for illustration purposes.

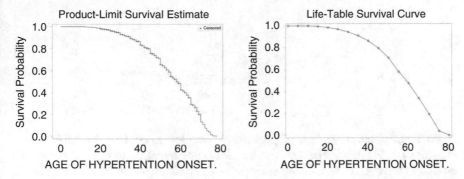

Fig. 7.6 Survival Curves of age pattern of high blood pressure from Models 1 and 2, SAS Program 7.1

The right part of Fig. 7.6 shows that different from K-M method, the survival curve $S(t)$ estimated using the actuarial method is relative smoother. The plotted data points are 5 years apart as specified in Model 2, SAS Program 7.1. This curve describes the age pattern of survival (here age pattern high blood pressure onset). As age increases, the estimated curve $S(t)$ declined progressively. There is a twist interpreting the results since the $S(t)$ in this analysis is not for death but for having high blood pressure for the first time in life (onset). Instead of survival, the curve tells us the age pattern of the probability for not having high blood pressure (free from high blood pressure) from birth up to age t after birth, all the way to 80 years of age.

As an epidemiologist, we would also like to know the probability of having high blood pressure for the first time by age. Unfortunately, the **PROC LIFETEST** from SAS does not provide such a plot. This is because this SAS procedure was developed for analyzing survival data. The results we need can be derived by subtracting the estimated $S(t)$ from 1.00 across all age groups. Detailed values of $S(t)$ by age for the $S(t)$ plot in Fig. 7.6 can be found in the SAS output using the **PROC LIFETEST** (see Fig. 7.8 later in this section).

Figure 7.7 presents the estimated hazard $h(t)$, or risk of having high blood pressure by age at any time from birth up to 80 years of age for the US population. This result can be interpreted as the risk of developing high blood pressure at any moment in time as age increases. Following this result, the risk to develop high blood pressure was rather low before 20, and it increases gradually throughout adulthood, followed by a rapid increase after age 65.

Fig. 7.7 Hazard or instantaneous risk of having high blood pressure by age: Output from SAS Program 7.1, Model 2

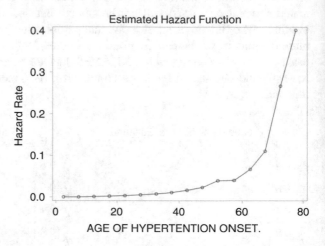

For learning purposes, Fig. 7.8 presents the detailed output from Model 2 in SAS Program 7.1. While viewing this figure, please pay attention to the following columns: (1) Interval for age, (2) Number failed (here reported having had high blood pressure), (3) Number censored, (4) Survival, (5) Failure, and (6) Hazard. In addition to describing the findings, these results can help improve our understanding of the survival analysis methods.

Interval						Conditional						Evaluated at the Midpoint of the Interval			
[Lower,	Upper)	Number Failed	Number Censored	Effective Sample Size	Conditional Probability of Failure	Conditional Probability Standard Error	Survival	Failure	Survival Standard Error	Median Residual Lifetime	Median Standard Error	PDF	PDF Standard Error	Hazard	Hazard Standard Error
0	5	0	0	4876.0	0	0	1.0000	0	0	58.8578	0.3377	0		0	
5	10	0	0	4876.0	0	0	1.0000	0	0	53.8578	0.3377	0		0	
10	15	23	0	4876.0	0.00472	0.000981	1.0000	0	0	48.8578	0.3377	0.000943	0.000196	0.000946	0.000197
15	20	50	0	4853.0	0.0103	0.00145	0.9953	0.00472	0.000981	43.9691	0.3369	0.00205	0.000289	0.002071	0.000293
20	25	74	386	4610.0	0.0161	0.00185	0.9850	0.0150	0.00174	39.2109	0.3421	0.00316	0.000365	0.003236	0.000376
25	30	107	376	4155.0	0.0258	0.00246	0.9692	0.0308	0.00250	34.5837	0.3546	0.00499	0.000477	0.005218	0.000504
30	35	133	371	3674.5	0.0362	0.00308	0.9443	0.0557	0.00341	30.1338	0.2853	0.00684	0.000582	0.007373	0.000639
35	40	166	345	3183.5	0.0521	0.00394	0.9101	0.0899	0.00439	25.7599	0.2955	0.00949	0.000719	0.010708	0.000831
40	45	209	321	2684.5	0.0779	0.00517	0.8626	0.1374	0.00549	21.6292	0.3050	0.0134	0.000896	0.016202	0.00112
45	50	238	271	2179.5	0.1092	0.00668	0.7955	0.2045	0.00675	17.8594	0.3121	0.0174	0.00107	0.023101	0.001495
50	55	300	259	1676.5	0.1789	0.00936	0.7086	0.2914	0.00802	14.4505	0.3170	0.0254	0.00136	0.039306	0.002258
55	60	203	266	1114.0	0.1822	0.0116	0.5818	0.4182	0.00935	11.6489	0.2969	0.0212	0.00139	0.040099	0.0028
60	65	180	301	627.5	0.2869	0.0181	0.4758	0.5242	0.0102	8.4548	0.3235	0.0273	0.00181	0.066977	0.004922
65	70	93	164	215.0	0.4326	0.0338	0.3393	0.6607	0.0112	5.7428	0.3756	0.0294	0.00249	0.110386	0.011002
70	75	32	0	40.0	0.8000	0.0632	0.1925	0.8075	0.0131	3.1250	0.4941	0.0308	0.00322	0.266667	0.035136
75	80	8	0	8.0	1.0000	0	0.0385	0.9615	0.0125	2.5000	0.8839	0.00770	0.00249	0.4	0
80	.	0	0	0.0	0	0	0	1.0000	0						

Fig. 7.8 Detailed Results from Model 2: Output from SAS Program 7.1

It is worth noting that results presented under the column "Survival" are the estimated $S(t)$ by age that has been used to produce the plot in Fig. 7.6, the right panel.
The column "Failure" is computed by $1- S(t)$, and it measures the probability of
having high blood pressure for the first time by age (age of onset). Values in this
column can thus be plotted to provide information for epidemiology. This part will
be left for students. Please spend time to plot the data and compare it with Figs. 7.6
and 7.7 to gain more understanding of the results from survival analysis.

As the last part of the survival analysis, Fig. 7.9 presents the analytical results for
statistical testing to examine whether the TTE data used in the demonstration analysis (i.e., the data regarding the reported age when having had high blood pressure
for the first time in life) follows the Weibull distribution. If the data follows the
Weibull distribution, the plot of log ($-\log(S(t))$) over the log (age of high blood pressure onset) should fall more or less on a straight line. Findings from Fig. 7.9 appears
to say that our data roughly follows the Weibull distribution: Overall all the data
points are more or less on a straight line with some variations at the beginning and
the ending part of the line. Technically, the TTE data from participants' self-reporting about the age when they had high blood pressure for the first time in life from
the 2017 to 18 NHANES are suitable for survival analysis.

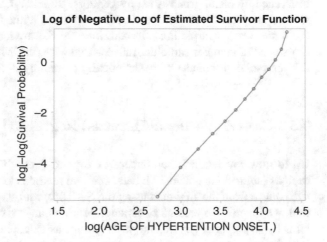

Fig. 7.9 Test if the time-to-event data follow Weibull distribution

7.4.4   Results from Model 3 and Model 4

Figure 7.10 displays the $S(t)$ curves estimated using Model 3 and Model 4, respectively. The left part of the figure is for the results from Model 3 that compared the
male-female difference in survival curves for high blood pressure. According to the
estimated survival function, US females (orange line) were less likely than males
(blue line) to develop high blood pressure from age 25 to 60 years old and were
more likely to after age 70; the risk for both genders was similar in other age ranges.
Wilcoxon test indicated that gender difference was statistically significant ($p < 0.05$).

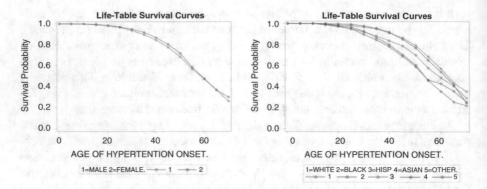

Fig. 7.10 Gender and racial difference in survival curves that measure risk of high blood pressure onset by age in the US population. 2017–18 NHANES data (Wilcoxon test p < 0.05 for gender differences and p<0.01 for racial group differences)

The right part of Figure 7.10 shows the result from Model 4 that compared the racial differences in the estimated survival curves across the defined 5 racial groups of White, Black, Hispanic, Asian, and Other. The results suggest a much greater difference by racial groups than by genders. In general, the risk from low to high was for Hispanic (green line), Asian (brown line), White (blue line), Black (orange line), and Other (purple line). In addition, the risk by racial groups showed some crossovers at younger and older ranges. Likewise, the Wilcoxon test indicated that that the racial differences were statistically extremely significant (p < 0.01).

7.5 Cox (Proportional Hazards) Regression Model

Up to now, we learned the concept of time-to-event (TTE) data, three different designs (sources) to obtain TTE data, and two methods to extract information about age pattern from the TTE data using the SAS program **PROC LIFETEST**. In addition, we learned the method to conduct stratified analysis to compare the time patterns by strata using gender and racial groups as examples. In this section, we will introduce the well-known Cox or proportional hazards regression model to assess factors related to TTE like other regression methods in the previous two chapters.

Cox or proportional hazard regression model is based on the survival model. However, it moves one step further to assess multiple influential factor Xs on the survival time Y. This is very much similar to the other multiple regression models. However, the proportional hazards regression will be more efficient than the other regression methods. Although stratified survival analysis can be used to assess influential factors like the examples used in Sect. 7.4, the proportional hazards regression will make the analysis much more efficient.

Similar to other multiple regression models described in Chaps. 5 and 6, the Cox or proportional hazard regression model can be used to examine multiple influential factors Xs. However, different from the other regression methods is that the Cox or proportional hazards regression uses the time to an outcome event Y, not the Y itself. In addition, the Cox or proportional hazard regression method can deal with data in which the outcome variable Y has missing values, which none of the other regression methods can.

7.5.1 Introduction to the Cox Regression Model

Cox regression model is also known as proportional hazards regression model; these two terms are often used interchangeably in the literature. After it was established in the 1970s (Cox 1972), the method has been increasingly used in research studies, particularly studies conducted in the field of medicine and public health (Spruance et al. 2004; Moolgavkar et al. 2018). In some cases, the word "hazard" is used in the place of "hazards" to describe the model.

The Cox regression model is constructed using the hazard function $h(t)$ from survival analysis to quantify the risk of an influential factor X associated with the outcome Y, the time t to the event of interest. Starting as an exponential model, $h(t)$, the risk or hazard for an event to occur at any time t can be expressed as:

$$h(t) = h_0(t) \times \exp\left(\beta_1 X_1 + \beta_2 X_2 + \ldots + \beta_p X_p\right). \tag{7.7}$$

In this regression model, the risk for an event to occur at any time t is expressed as (1) a baseline risk $h_0(t)$, multiplied by (2) an exponential of the effect from p influential factors Xs, measured using a set of β coefficients. This is quite similar to the other regression models in the exponential family such as the logistic regression and Poisson regression.

It is worth noting that it is the multiplicative relationship between the baseline hazard $h_0(t)$ and the hazards that are attributed to the p influential factors that gives the Cox regression model the name: Proportional hazards regression *model*. The name implies that changes in hazard $h(t)$ is proportional to the effect of individual influential factors Xs. It is worth noting that the multiplicative nature makes the Cox regression model different from the additive nature in a linear regression model as described in Chap. 5. In a linear regression model, each X contributes to the Y independently and additively; while in a Cox regression model, individual Xs affect the Y not independently but multiplicatively.

Based on the discussion above, the baseline hazard $h_0(t)$ in Eq. 7.7 can be interpreted as the risk when none of the estimated β coefficients for all p factors X_1, $X_2 \ldots X_p$ is significantly different from zero since $\exp(0) = 1$. The term $\exp(\beta_i X_i)$ is termed as the *hazard ratio* (*HR*), and it measures the influence or hazard of the i_{th} factor X_i on the Y (time to event). Hazard ratio or HR is a commonly used risk measure; this measure is very similar to many other risk ratios, such as odds ratio (OR) or relative risk (RR). Different from other measures, the HR measures the risk of time course for an event to occur the first time in life, rather than whether an event will occur or not as in other regression methods.

With the Cox regression model, the HR can be estimated for multiple influential factors Xs. Like in a logistic regression model, with an estimated HR, the impact of an influential factor can be assessed quantitatively as follows:

If $HR = 1$ or not significantly different from 1 for a factor X_i, this factor has no effect on the hazard $h(t)$;

If $HR < 1$ at least at p<0.05 level for a factor X_i, this factor reduces the hazard $h(t)$; and

If $HR > 1$ at least at p<0.05 level for a factor X_i, this factor increases the hazard $h(t)$.

Cox regression model is **semi-parametric** since the model does not assume the shape of the baseline hazard $h_0(t)$. However, to correctly use a Cox regression method, the following conditions must be satisfied:

1. Independence: The survival time of individual participants in the study sample must be independent from each other;
2. Changes in an influential factor X result in proportional changes in $h(t)$, since there is a multiplicative relationship between the independent variables Xs and the dependent variable$h(t)$; and
3. The hazard ratios for individual influential factor Xs does not change over time (constant hazard assumption), although they can differ from each other.

7.5.2   Multiple Cox Regression Model and Parameter Estimation

Like other multiple regression models, the multiple Cox regression model 7.7 can be used to confirm a hypothetic X~Y relationship suggested by bivariate analysis in the case when the outcome Y is measured using the time to event data. Instead of examining multiple Xs on $h(t)$ all at once, we use the multiple Cox regression analysis to verify a proportional hazard X~Y relationship with Y being the time to an event of interest.

Multiple Cox regression model is created by taking a logarithm transformation of Eq. 7.7: $Y = \alpha + \beta_1 X_1 + \beta_2 X_2 + \ldots + \beta_p X_p$, where $y = \ln(h(t))$ and $\alpha = \ln(h_0(t))$. Let X_1 be the factor of interest to confirm its relationship with Y (expressed as log hazard), and the remaining $p - 1$ Xs as the $CovX_i$ ($i = 2, 3, \ldots p$), the Cox regression model becomes:

$$Y = \alpha + \beta_1 X_1 + \beta_2 covX_2 + \ldots + \beta_p covX_p. \tag{7.8}$$

Model 7.8 is exactly like Model 5.6 described in Chap. 5 where the multiple linear regression was first introduced as a confirmatory model to verify a hypothetic and bivariate analysis-suggested X~Y relationship while controlling for covariates.

In statistics, the parameters α and β of a Cox regression model are estimated using the *maximum* likelihood estimation *method*. This method is similar to that used for other exponential and logarithm-transformed linear regression models (i.e., logistic regression and Poison regression) described in Chap. 6. Likewise, the statistics such as -2 LOG L (likelihood), AIC, and BIC are used to assess data – model fit; likelihood ratio, Score, and Wald tests (chi-square) are used to test the overall null hypothesis that $\beta = 0$. With the estimated -2 LOG L, pseudo-R^2 can be computed manually to assess the contribution of individual Xs on the outcome variable Y, expressed as the log hazards $h(t)$.

7.5.3   Steps for Cox Regression Analysis to Verify an X~Y Relationship

When the dependent variable Y is measured using the time to event, the following steps are recommended for Cox regression analysis:

Step 1: Conduct survival analysis to quantitatively characterize the outcome Y, i.e., the time to event. By conducting this step of analysis, knowledge will be obtained on whether (1) the variable Y and the variable for censoring are correctly coded, (2) a survival curve is generated correctly reflecting the Y, and (3) all analytical results are meaningful, including the test for Weibull distribution. Step 1 analysis will be completed using the methods, including the SAS programs described in Sect. 7.4.

Step 2: Like in Chaps. 5 and 6, fit the processed data to Model 1, a Cox regression model that contains only the influential factor X of interest that is to be confirmed. If results from this step of modeling indicate no significant relationship between the X and the Y, stop and start over again to revise your hypothesis and conduct exploratory analysis as described in Chap. 4.

Most times you may find a significant X~Y relationship if the bivariate exploratory analysis is carefully planned and correctly conducted. This is because Model 1 is essentially a bivariate analysis, and the result should be consistent with that from the bivariate analyses as described in Chap. 4. A significant X~Y association from Step 2 analysis will bring you to the next step of analysis.

Step 3: Fit the data to the remaining three multiple Cox regression models: Model 2 to adjust for demographic factors only; Model 3 to control for confounders only; Model 4 to adjust for demographic factors and to control confounders all together. As described in previous chapters, in each of the three models, particularly Models 2 and 3, please add only one variable at a time to examine its impact; and drop the variables that do not show much impact.

7.6   Application of a Multiple Cox Regression with Real Data

As a demonstration for Cox regression analysis, results from the bivariate analysis in Chap. 4 will be used here. In that chapter, we found that smoking (X) could be positively associated with high blood pressure (Y) among US adults. To verify the X~Y relationship, we can use the age when a participant was diagnosed with high blood pressure for the first time in life as Y. As shown in Fig. 7.2, this is a typical TTE data from survey studies. With this outcome, the smoking - high blood pressure relationship can be verified using Cox regression.

Following the steps described in the previous section, Step 1 analysis was completed in Sect. 7.4. Results from the analysis indicated that the two key variables are coded correctly, including the outcome Y (age onset of high blood pressure) and the variable for censoring (0, 1) with 1 for those who have not yet had high blood pressure at the time when data collection was completed; and 0, otherwise. The derived TTE data follow the Weibull distribution, and are successfully expressed by a survival model.

In this section, we will conduct the remaining steps of analyses to confirm if X (cigarette smoking) is a true risk factor for the onset of high blood pressure.

7.6.1   Variables for Analysis

Outcome variable Y (AGEHYPR): Years to the onset of high blood pressure. This variable was already described in detail in Sect. 7.4.

Influential factor X (LIFESMK): Lifetime smoking (yes/no). This variable is preferred over other smoking measures (i.e., if smoking now, number of cigarettes smoked per day, and biomarkers of tobacco exposure) because the goal is to examine the impact of smoking on the onset of high blood pressure that occurred in the past. In this case, lifetime smoking, i.e., ever smoked in life, includes past and present smoking. It might have occurred during the time course the high blood pressure was diagnosed for individual participants.

Demographic variables as CovX's: As a demonstration, two are included: $CovX_2$ (GENDER), male and female and $CovX_3$ (RACE5), five racial groups of White, Black, Hispanic, Asian, and Other. By including these two factors, the analytical results can be generalized to a genderless and raceless population.

Confounders as CovX's: To demonstrate the method, one confounder included: $CovX_4$ (EDUCATION), less than high school, high school, college or more. Levels of education can affect both smoking behavior and high blood pressure. Education has been reported to be negatively associated with high blood pressure (Dyer et al. 1976) as well as tobacco smoking (Tomioka et al. 2020).

7.6.2   Data Source and SAS Program

Data for this demonstration analysis are derived from those used in this and a previous chapter. The data for high blood pressure, the two demographic factors, and the one confounder were included in DATCH7 for the survival analysis in Sect. 7.4. Data for the smoking measures will be derived from DATCH4, the dataset used for exploratory bivariate analyses in Chap. 4. Instead of going back to the original NHANES data, the dataset DATCH7 will be expanded by adding the smoking variables from DATCH4.

SAS Program 7.2 details the steps for data processing (Part 1) and Cox regression analysis to confirm an X~Y relationship (Part 2). In Part 1, the dataset DATCH7 created for survival analysis in Sect. 7.4 is updated to include smoking measures derived from dataset DATCH4 that was used in Chap. 4. This step was completed using two temporary datasets TMP3 and TMP4, sorting them by SEQN first and then merging by SEQN. Since the dataset DATCH4 contains both child and adult participants of the 2017–18 NHANES and DATCH7 contains only the adult participants, to merge the two datasets, a special method in SAS was used to merge only adult data from the two datasets. The following program line shows the trick:

```
MERGE TMP3(IN=A) TMP4(IN=B); IF A AND B; BY SEQN;
```

In this line of SAS code, data will be merged for participants who present in both TMP3 (DATCH7) and TMP4 (DATCH4). This is achieved by assigning a value of 1 to a new variable A, for a participant in TMP3 and a value of 1 to another variable B, for the same participant in TMP4. The merging operation will be executed *only* when a participant is presented in both datasets as controlled by the logic statement: IF A AND B.

For comparison purposes, a variable that measures the number of cigarettes smoked per day (SMKNUMS) is included for interested students to practice.

```
******************************************************************************
SAS PROGRAM 7.2 PROPORTIONAL HAZARD (COX) REGRESSION ANALYSIS
CONTINUE FROM SAS PROGRAM 7.1
******************************************************************************;
** PART 1 DATA PREPARATION
*  READ DATCH7 USED IN SURIVAL ANALYSIS INTO TMP3 FOR FURTHER PROCESSING;
LIBNAME SASDATA "C:\QUANTLAB\A_DATA";
DATA TMP3; SET SASDATA.DATCH7; PROC CONTENTS; RUN; * N=5134 IN THIS DATASET;
*  OBTAIN DATA ON SMOKING FROM DATCH4 USED IN CHAPTER 4 KEEP LIFESMK AND SMKNUMS;
DATA TMP4; SET SASDATA.DATCH4;
* CODE SYSTEM MISSING IN THE VARIABLE SMKNUMS - NO CIGARETTES PER DAY;
IF SMKNUMS GT 60 THEN SMKNUMS =. ;
IF LIFESMK EQ 2 AND SMKNUMS EQ . THEN SMKNUMS=0;
KEEP LIFESMK SMKNUMS SEQN; PROC CONTENTS; RUN;        * N=9027 TOTAL PARTICIPANTS;
* CHECK IF THE MISSING CODED CORRECTLY;
PROC FREQ DATA=TMP4; TABLES SMKNUMS*LIFESMK/MISSING; RUN;
* SORT DATA FOR MERGING;
PROC SORT DATA = TMP3; BY SEQN; RUN;
PROC SORT DATA = TMP4; BY SEQN; RUN;
* CREATE A NEW DATASET BY REPLACING THE OLD DATCH7 WITH NEWLY ADDED VARIABLES;
* VARIABLE A AND B ARE USED TO EXCLUDE SUBJECTION IN B BUT NOT IN A;
DATA SASDATA.DATCH7;
MERGE TMP3(IN=A) TMP4(IN=B); IF A AND B; BY SEQN;
PROC CONTENTS; RUN;  * N=5134 PARTICIPANTS IN THE MERGED DATASET;

** PART 2 PROPORTIONAL (COX) REGRESSION MODEL ANALYSIS WITH DATA;
* CREATE A WORK DATASET B FOR ANALYSIS AND CHECK MISSING;
DATA B; SET LIB.DATCH7; PROC FREQ; RUN;
* MODEL 1 ASSESS LIFETIME SMOKING AND AGE OF HIGH BLOOD PRESSURE ONSET;
PROC PHREG DATA = B;
CLASS LIFESMK;
MODEL AGEHYPR * CENSORED(1) = LIFESMK/RL;
RUN;
* MODEL 2 ADJUSTING MALE FEMALE GENDER AND RACIAL GROUPS;
PROC PHREG DATA = B;
CLASS LIFESMK GENDER RACE5;
MODEL AGESVIVAL * CENSORED(1) = LIFESMK GENDER RACE5/RL;
RUN;
* MODEL 3 CONTROLLING FOR EDUCATION AS CONFOUNDER;
PROC PHREG DATA = B;
CLASS LIFESMK EDUCATION;
MODEL AGEHYPR * CENSORED(1)= LIFESMK EDUCATION/RL;
RUN;
* MODEL 4 ADJUST DEMOGRAPHIC FACTORS AND CONTROL FOR CONFOUNDER;
PROC PHREG DATA = B;
CLASS LIFESMK GENDER RACE5 EDUCATION;
MODEL AGEHYPR * CENSORED(1) = LIFESMK GENDER RACE5 EDUCATION/RL;
RUN;
******************************************************************************;
```

Part 2 of the SAS Program presents the four Cox regression models to confirm the X (lifetime smoking) and Y (time to high blood pressure onset) relationship. The SAS procedure **PROC PHREG** is used for the proportional hazard or Cox regression analysis. Non-continuous variables are specified using the key word CLASS. Like in linear and logistic regressions, the Cox regression model is specified using the key word MODEL with the outcome Y * the variable measuring censoring, here **CENSORED** (1). This specification tells the computer not to drop the participants with censored data but use the age at the study time if the value = 1 in the parenthesis, since this is what we defined as censored. Last point, the option RL is used to the end of the MODEL statement, asking the computer to estimate the HR and the corresponding 95% confidence interval.

As usual, of the four models specified in the SAS Program, Model 1 is a simple bivariate regression with the smoking measure LIFESMK as X_1; in Model 2, the two demographic factors GENDER and RACE5 are used as $CovX_2$ and $CovX_3$; in Model

3, the confounder EDUCATION is analyzed as $CovX_4$; and in Model 4, all three CovXs are modeled, including the two demographic factors, $CovX_2$ and $CovX_3$, and the confounder $CovX_4$ (with reference to Eq. 7.8).

The Cox regression models in SAS Program 7.2 are used simply as an illustrative analysis. In real studies, more CovXs can be added to meet the needs of individual studies, including more demographic factors, such as income, marital status, number of children; and more confounding factors as suggested by literature and simple bivariate analysis.

7.7 Results and Interpretation

To illustrate the methods for Cox regression analysis and result interpretation, several pieces of results from the SAS output are selectively presented and discussed in detail. Although brief and selective, the purpose is to try to generate a template for you to use in interpreting and reporting findings from your own research studies.

7.7.1 Results from the Simple Cox Regression Model 1

Figure 7.11 presents several pieces of selected results from executing Model 1 in SAS Program 7.2. This is the simplest part of the modeling analysis to quantify the relationship between lifetime smoking and age onset of high blood pressure. The first part shows the influential factor X_1 (LIFESMK) and how it was coded. In the original data, LIFESMK was coded as 1 = yes and 2 = no. However, in the analysis, the original code of 1 was modeled as 1 (yes) and 2 was modeled as 0 (no). In other words, the model provides information about the impact of lifetime smoking on the hazard (risk) of onset of high blood pressure by age with reference to those who did not smoke in lifetime. *It is very important to check this part before seeing other results from the analysis.*

The second part contains the three statistics for data-model fit, including the -2 LOG L (negative 2 log likelihood estimate), AIC, and BIC. Likewise, there is no cutoff for these criteria measures, the rule is: *the smaller the value, the better.* Similarly, the global hypothesis test indicates that chi-square = 6.54 (keep two decimals) from likelihood ratio test, and p = 0.01 (two decimals). This result suggests that Model 1 is valid.

The last part of the output displays results from the significance test for the influential factor X_1(LIFESMK). Type 3 test shows that the Wald chi-square = 6.61, p = 0.01. The estimated $\beta_1 = 0.1210$ for LIFESMK, and the chi-square = 6.61, $p < 0.05$. Correspondingly, the estimated HR = exp (0.1210) = 1.129, and the 95% CI = 1.029, 1.238. These results suggest that lifetime smoking is *likely* a factor that *may* increase the risk of early onset of high blood pressure at younger ages among adults in the United States.

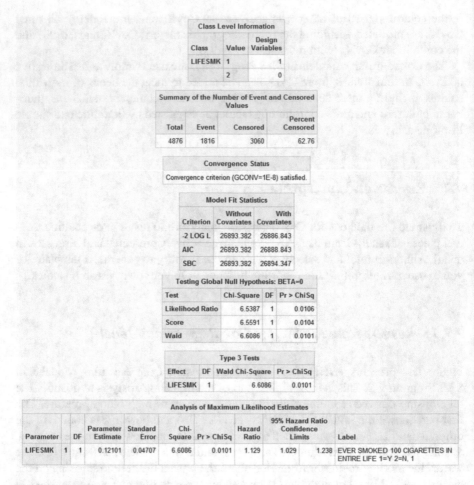

Fig. 7.11 Results from simple Cox Regression Model 1: Output of SAS Program 7.2.2

7.7.2   Estimate R^2 for Proportional Hazard Regression

As described in Chap. 6 for logistic regression, R^2 or the amount of variance explained by an influential factor X_1 from a Cox regression cannot be estimated as in the linear regression in Chap. 5. However, with the estimated -2LOG L, the pseudo-R^2 can be calculated using the McFauden formula (Eq. 6.7).

In our case, results in Fig. 7.11 show that the -2LOG L = 26893.38 for the condition without a covariate (equivalent to intercept only in logistic regression), and 2LOG L =26886.84 for the condition with a covariate (equivalent to the intercept plus covariates in logistic regression). Using the McFauden formula, the pseudo-R^2 can be computed as follows:

$$R^2 = 1 - (26893.38 / 26888.84) = 1 - 0.9998 = 0.02\%.$$

Here we can see that although the variable LIFESMK is statistically significant, it can only explain a tiny part of the variations in the hazards of high blood pressure onset by age. In other words, although this factor may be important, many other factors are to be considered as covariates to obtain valid measures to assess the impact of lifetime smoking on the onset of high blood pressure in younger ages.

7.7.3   Temporary Conclusion from Model 1

Based on the results from the Cox regression Model 1 analysis as presented in Fig. 7.11, we can conclude that the processed data fit the Cox regression model well as indicated by the data model fit statistics and the global null hypothesis testing statistics. Furthermore, smoking in lifetime, the influential factor X derived from the bivariate analysis, remained to be significantly associated with the risk of early onset of high blood pressure among the adult population in the US. However, the observed results may not be valid since the US population in 2017–18 was not homogenous, and so was the sample for the 2017–18 NHANES. Thus, the lifetime cigarette smoking and the prevalence of high blood pressure by age may also differ by gender and race. Further analysis is needed to adjust for these differences.

7.7.4   Results from Cox Regression Model 2 Adjusting Demographic Factors

The Cox regression Model 2 in SAS Program 7.2 is designed to verify the results from Model 1 by including gender and racial groups as demographic factors. As indicated in the stratified survival analysis in Sect. 7.4 (Fig. 7.10), the hazards for the onset of high blood pressure by age differed significantly by the male-female gender and the five racial groups. By inclusion of these two demographic factors in Model 2, the impact of each variable on the Y is reflected by the estimated beta coefficient. As such, the estimated regression coefficient β_1 for X_1 (lifetime smoking) will be an adjusted measure of the independent effect of X_1 on the hazards for high blood pressure. If the estimated regression coefficient for X_1 remains statistically significant after inclusion of the demographic factors, the hypothetic X~Y relation could be valid; otherwise, not.

Figure 7.12 presents some selected findings from the Cox regression Model 2. To save space, we did not include the part on data-model fit. The estimated statistic -2 LOG L = 21445.888, much smaller than 26893.382, the same statistic for Model 1 (Fig. 7.11). Other important findings from the Model 2 analysis are summarized below:

Testing Global Null Hypothesis: BETA=0			
Test	Chi-Square	DF	Pr > ChiSq
Likelihood Ratio	100.1663	6	<.0001
Score	102.8096	6	<.0001
Wald	100.3824	6	<.0001

Type 3 Tests			
Effect	DF	Wald Chi-Square	Pr > ChiSq
LIFESMK	1	1.8832	0.1700
GENDER	1	0.5413	0.4619
RACE5	4	90.7086	<.0001

Analysis of Maximum Likelihood Estimates									
Parameter		DF	Parameter Estimate	Standard Error	Chi-Square	Pr > ChiSq	Hazard Ratio	95% Hazard Ratio Confidence Limits	Label
LIFESMK	1	1	0.07692	0.05605	1.8832	0.1700	1.080	0.968 1.205	EVER SMOKED 100 CIGARETTES IN ENTIRE LIFE 1=Y 2=N, 1
GENDER	1	1	0.04008	0.05447	0.5413	0.4619	1.041	0.935 1.158	1=MALE 2=FEMALE, 1
RACE5	1	1	-0.30096	0.12160	6.1254	0.0133	0.740	0.583 0.939	1=WHITE 2=BLAKC 3=HISP 4=ASIAN 5=OTHER, 1
RACE5	2	1	0.03305	0.12068	0.0750	0.7842	1.034	0.816 1.309	1=WHITE 2=BLAKC 3=HISP 4=ASIAN 5=OTHER, 2
RACE5	3	1	-0.60464	0.12742	22.5163	<.0001	0.546	0.426 0.701	1=WHITE 2=BLAKC 3=HISP 4=ASIAN 5=OTHER, 3
RACE5	4	1	-0.52839	0.13578	15.1435	<.0001	0.590	0.452 0.769	1=WHITE 2=BLAKC 3=HISP 4=ASIAN 5=OTHER, 4

Fig. 7.12 Results from Cox regression Model 2 adjusting gender and racial groups: Output of SAS Program 7.2.2

First, Type 3 test for all three categorical factors are presented, including the variable of interest LIFESMK and the two demographic factors. Since LIFESMK and GENDER are binary, the Type 3 test will be the same as the test for significance of the parameters for the variables. However, Type 3 test for RACE5 is unique. It provides a measure of RACE5 as one variable in affecting the outcome Y. Type 3 test indicated that RACE5 was an extremely significant influential factor (p < 0.001). Consistent with this result, several racial groups were associated with the same outcome Y, if analyzed by individual groups (see the results next).

Second, of the two demographic factors, the chi-square test indicated that the gender difference was not statistically significant with the estimated $\beta = 0.0401$, p > 0.05; but the impact of racial groups was extremely statistically significant (p < 0.001 from type 3 test). If the group "Other" was used as the reference, being White (RACE5 = 1, $\beta = -0.3010$, p < 0.05), Hispanic (RACE5 = 3, $\beta = -0.6046$, p < 0.001) and Asian (RACE5 = 4, b $\beta = 0.5284$, p < 0.001) were associated with a reduced risk of early onset of high blood pressure.

Last are the findings about lifetime smoking, the influential factor of our interest. The results from the Cox regression Model 2 showed that the adjusted $\beta_1 = 0.0769$ (p > 0.05); the corresponding HR (hazards ratio) = 1.080 (p > 0.05). The non-significant findings from Model 2 analysis indicated the need for further analysis to determine the validity of the association between lifetime smoking and the early onset of high blood pressure. The results from the bivariate analysis could be totally due to the heterogeneity of the study sample with regard to gender and race. Therefore, we cannot confirm the hypothetic smoking – early high blood pressure relationship suggested by the Cox regression Model 1.

Students with interest in further confirming the results from Model 1 can revise Model 2 to analyze the data for male and female gender and racial groups one at a time. Similar analyses can also be conducted using different smoking measures with data already acquired in Chap. 4 for bivariate analysis.

To analyze a subsample (i.e., for one gender or one racial group), SAS program provides a very useful command that has already been introduced in previous chapters. That is to add one line before the command **RUN**. Using the variable GENDER as an example, to analyze data for males only, simply add the following statement before the command **RUN**:

```
WHERE GENDER EQ 1;
```

7.7.5   Results from Cox Regression Model 3 Controlling for Confounder

Figure 7.13 displays the main findings from Model 3 analysis that controlled for the education as an important confounder. Frist, the data model-fit statistics (not included in the figure) indicate that Model 3 is better (smaller value of all the statistics) than that of Model 1. The data-model fit statistics for Model 1 (without EDUCATION) was -2LOG L = 21411 and Model 3 (with EDUCATION) was -2LOG L = 21382. Results from the global null hypothesis test indicated that chi-square = 29.06 using likelihood ratio test, $p < 0.001$.

Second, findings in Figure 7.13 indicate that the confounder variable (EDUCATION) was significantly associated with the hazard of high blood pressure

	Type 3 Tests		
Effect	DF	Wald Chi-Square	Pr > ChiSq
LIFESMK	1	5.6713	0.0172
EDUCATION	2	19.5016	< .0001

Analysis of Maximum Likelihood Estimates									
Parameter		DF	Parameter Estimate	Standard Error	Chi-Square	Pr > ChiSq	Hazard Ratio	95% Hazard Ratio Confidence Limits		Label
LIFESMK	1	1	0.12888	0.05412	5.6713	0.0172	1.138	1.023	1.265	EVER SMOKED 100 CIGARETTES IN ENTIRE LIFE 1=Y 2=N, 1
EDUCATION	1	1	-0.02749	0.08362	0.1081	0.7424	0.973	0.826	1.146	1= LESS THAN HIGH SCHOOL 2=HIGH 3=COLLEGE+, 1
EDUCATION	2	1	0.22641	0.06802	11.0782	0.0009	1.254	1.098	1.433	1= LESS THAN HIGH SCHOOL 2=HIGH 3=COLLEGE+, 2

Fig. 7.13 Results from Cox regression Model 3 controlling for education as confounder: Output of SAS Program 7.2.2

onset by age from type 3 test. However, a further check of the results by individual education levels indicated that relationship was bi-directional. Relative to participants with a college education or higher, high school education was a risk factor for early onset of high blood pressure (HR = 1.25, greater than 1.00 and p < 0.01), while less than high school education appeared to be a protective factor (HR=0.97, less than 1.00, p = 0.742), but the association was not statistically significant (p > 0.05).

Finally, the estimated beta coefficient for X_1 (LIFESMK), the variable of interest. The adjusted $\beta_1 = 0.1289$ and the HR [95% CI] = 1.138 [1.023, 1.265], p < 0.05. This result suggests that lifetime smoking remained to be a risk factor that can significantly increase the risk of early onset of hypertension among US adults.

Up to now, we can consider results from all three models described above together, including Model 1, Model 2, and Model 3. The positive result from Model 1 was not confirmed in Model 2 after the two demographic factors are considered; but confirmed in Model 3 after controlling the confounder. What remains to be examined is to see how the X~Y relation would be when both the demographic factors and the confounder are included - Model 4 analysis.

7.7.6 Results from Cox Regression Model 4 Considering Demographic and Confounding factors

Figure 7.14 displays the key findings from Model 4 in SAS Program 7.2 in which both the demographic factors in Model 2 and the confounding factor in Model 3 are included. Overall, the data fit the model quite well with the value of -2 LOG L reduced to 21304.06, and the likelihood ratio test of the global hypothesis that all beta = 0 was rejected with the estimated chi-square = 107.14, p < 0.0001. Type 3 test indicated racial groups (chi-square = 77.8, p < 0.001) and education (chi-square =6.85, p < 0.05) were statistically significant. To save space, these results are not shown.

Detailed results in Fig. 7.14 indicate that the adjusted $\beta_1 = 0.0549$ for X_1 (LIFESMK), the influential factor of interest. The adjusted hazard ratio = 1.056 based on the estimated β_1, indicated an increased risk of the variable with early high blood pressure onset, but the result was not statistically significant (p > 0.05). In other words, the hypothetic lifetime smoking and high blood pressure onset from the bivariate analysis in Model 1 as well as from Model 3 that controlled for the confounder of education did not pass the test from Model 4.

Similar to Chaps. 5 and 6, as a byproduct of the multiple Cox regression, results from Model 4 suggest that education and racial groups were two significant influential factor for early onset of high blood pressure.

							95% Hazard Ratio		
Analysis of Maximum Likelihood Estimates									
Parameter		DF	Parameter Estimate	Standard Error	Chi-Square	Pr > ChiSq	Hazard Ratio	Confidence Limits		Label
LIFESMK	1	1	0.05489	0.05702	0.9266	0.3358	1.056	0.945	1.181	EVER SMOKED 100 CIGARETTES IN ENTIRE LIFE 1=Y 2=N, 1
GENDER	1	1	0.04391	0.05463	0.6461	0.4215	1.045	0.939	1.163	1=MALE 2=FEMALE, 1
RACE5	1	1	-0.29480	0.12161	5.8769	0.0153	0.745	0.587	0.945	1=WHITE 2=BLAKC 3=HISP 4=ASIAN 5=OTHER, 1
RACE5	2	1	0.03693	0.12074	0.0935	0.7597	1.038	0.819	1.315	1=WHITE 2=BLAKC 3=HISP 4=ASIAN 5=OTHER, 2
RACE5	3	1	-0.58511	0.13022	20.1896	<.0001	0.557	0.432	0.719	1=WHITE 2=BLAKC 3=HISP 4=ASIAN 5=OTHER, 3
RACE5	4	1	-0.46984	0.13752	11.6731	0.0006	0.625	0.477	0.818	1=WHITE 2=BLAKC 3=HISP 4=ASIAN 5=OTHER, 4
EDUCATION	1	1	0.07207	0.08851	0.6630	0.4155	1.075	0.904	1.278	1= LESS THAN HIGH SCHOOL 2=HIGH 3=COLLEGE+, 1
EDUCATION	2	1	0.17441	0.07019	6.1743	0.0130	1.191	1.038	1.366	1= LESS THAN HIGH SCHOOL 2=HIGH 3=COLLEGE+, 2

Fig. 7.14 Results from Cox regression Model 4 considering gender and race, and controlling for education: Output of SAS Program 7.2.2

7.7.7 Conclusion Remarks on the Cox Regression Analysis

In this chapter, we introduced a new type of data - the time to event or TTE data, and new methods to analyze the data, including (1) survival analysis to quantify the characteristics of TTE and (2) multiple Cox regression to verify a hypothetic X~Y relationship by controlling for covariates. Like in other chapters for multiple regression analysis, data from the 2017 to 18 NHANES were used to demonstrate the data type and the analytical methods. Different from the methods in other chapters, we included both positive (significant) and negative (nonsignificant) results from verifying an X~Y relationship based the theory and bivariate analysis. The demonstration analysis ended with a failure to confirm the hypothetic relationship.

Negative findings in quantitative epidemiology are not uncommon. Observing a negative result does not mean the end but often a new beginning of the same research. We must learn to get used to seeing negative results and think of new approaches to overcome the challenge for valid scientific results.

7.8 Practice

7.8.1 Statistical Analysis and Computing

1. Repeat both the survival analyses and Cox regression analyses described in this chapter, including the use of K-M method and acturial method to estimate survival functions, and stratified analysis. The purpose is to gain familiarity with the methods and techniques from data processing to statistical analysis, tabulation and plotting of results, result interpretation and reporting.

2. Repeat the same analysis with data on age when first smoked cigarettes in life as TTE, including survival analysis, overall and by gender, race, and education; and a Cox regression analysis to test a variable you identified through bivariate analysis that may affect age of smoking onset.
3. Analyze any data of your choice using the same survival and proportional hazard regression modeling methods.

7.8.2   Update Research Paper

1. For students who used time-to-event data, please conduct your analysis using the methods introduced in this chapter.
2. Present your results in a table with reference to the Template Table 3 described in Sect. 5.7, Chap. 5.
3. Report your results in writing and draw conclusions.

7.8.3   Study Questions

1. Survival analysis has been used often to address three types of research questions, and what they are? Discuss your answer with real examples.
2. Two methods are used to estimate survival function, what are they, and which one is often used in which condition, and how does the result differ from each other?
3. What make the TTE data different from the data used in linear and logistic regression to examine the association between an influential factor X and an outcome variable Y?
4. The survival analysis is developed to examine deaths as the outcome. Can the method be used to examine other health outcomes? If yes, what information can we gain from using the method?
5. In addition to Cox regression, what are the other regression methods that can be used to verify a hypothetic X-Y relationship? List them all and describe the type of outcome variables suitable for each method.
6. What does censored data mean? Why the methods for analyzing TTE data can handle the missingness due to censoring?
7. What are the three conditions that must be met to use a Cox regression model to examine an influential factor and to quantify its impact on the hazards of onset of a study event?
8. How to determine if your TTE data are suitable for survival analysis?
9. Why is the Cox regression model also named as the proportional hazard regression model?

References

Ahmad, T., Munir, A., Bhatti, S.H., Aftab, M., Raza, M.A.: Survival analysis of heart failure patients: A case study. PLoS One. **12**(7), e0181001 (2017). https://doi.org/10.1371/journal.pone.0181001

Chen, X., Stanton, B., Shankaran, S., Li, X.: Age of smoking onset as a predictor of smoking cessation during pregnancy. Am. J. Health Behav. **30**(3), 247–258 (2006)

Cox, D.R.: Regression models and life-tables. J. R. Stat. Soc. Ser. B. **34**(2), 187–220 (1972)

Cutler, S.J., Ederer, F.: Maximum utilization of the life table method in analyzing survival. J. Chronic Dis. **8**(53), 457–481 (1958)

Dirick, L., Claeskens, G., Baesens, B.: Time to default in credit scoring using survival analysis: A benchmark study. J. Oper. Res. Soc. **68**, 652–665 (2017)

Donovan, J.E., Molina, B.S.: Childhood risk factors for early-onset drinking. J. Stud. Alcohol Drugs. **72**(5), 741–751 (2011)

Dyer, A.R., Stamler, J., Shekelle, R.B., Schoenberger, J.: The relationship of education to blood pressure: Findings on 40,000 employed Chicagoans. Circulation. **54**(6), 987–992 (1976)

Hingson, R.W., Heeren, T., Winter, M.R.: Age at drinking onset and alcohol dependence: Age at onset, duration, and severity. Arch. Pediatr. Adolesc. Med. **160**(7), 739–746 (2006)

Kaplan, E.L., Meier, P.: Nonparametric estimation from incomplete observations. J. Am. Stat. Assoc. **53**(282), 457–481 (1958)

Kendler, K.S., Myers, J., Damaj, M.I., Chen, X.: Early smoking onset and risk for subsequent nicotine dependence: A monozygotic co-twin control study. Am. J. Psychiatry. **170**(4), 408–413 (2013)

Keyfitz, N., Caswell, H.: Applied mathematical demography, pp. 29–207. Springer (2005)

Lee, E.T., Go, O.T.: Survival analysis in public health research. Annu. Rev. Public Health. **18**, 105–134 (1997)

Lim, Y.J., Kim, Y., Kong, M.: Comparative survival analysis of preoperative and postoperative radiotherapy in stage II-III rectal cancer on the basis of long-term population data. Sci. Rep. **8**, 17153 (2018). https://doi.org/10.1038/s41598-018-35493-2

Moolgavkar, S.H., Chang, E.T., Watson, H.N., Lau, E.C.: An assessment of the Cox proportional hazards regression model for epidemiologic studies. Risk Anal. **38**(4), 777–794 (2018)

Mudholkar, G.S., Srivastava, D.K., Kollia, G.D.: A generalization of the Weibull distribution with application to the analysis of survival data. J. Am. Stat. Assoc. **91**(436), 1575–1583 (1996)

Ross, M.K., Wei, W., Ohno-Machado, L.: "Big data" and the electronic health record. Yearbook Med. Inf. **9**(1), 97–104 (2014)

Spruance, S.L., Reid, J.E., Grace, M., Samore, M.: Hazard ratio in clinical trials. Antimicrob. Agents Chemother. **48**(8), 2787–2792 (2004)

Tomioka, K., Kurumatani, N., Saeki, K.: The association between education and smoking prevalence, independent of occupation: A nationally representative survey in Japan. J. Epidemiol. **30**(3), 136–142 (2020)

Chapter 8
Analysis of Two Influential Factors: Interaction and Mediation Modeling

The connected universe is complex, but a few parts can be disentangled.

In the previous three chapters, we focused on the use of quantitative methods to verify a hypothetic X ~ Y relationship supported by evidence from binary exploratory analysis for causal inference. In these chapters, methods of multiple linear, logistic, Poisson, and Cox (proportional hazards) regression were introduced for different types of outcome variables Y. One characteristic common for all these chapters is that they all focus on one influential factor (independent variable) X. Because of the heterogeneity inherited from population-based studies, an observed X ~ Y association could be biased if covariates are not considered. Multivariate modeling methods are often used to control covariates including demographic factors and confounders. Demographic factors are used to adjust the sample heterogeneity and confounders are used to control the interactions these variables with the X and Y.

In this chapter, we extend the analysis by adding one more independent factor X to the simple X ~ Y relationship. As a natural extension, the concepts, knowledge, and skills described in previous chapters for the simple one-X and one-Y relationship will be useful to help understand the complex two-X and one-Y relationship. In Chap. 5, we demonstrated that as the number of independent variables X increases, complexity of the X ~ Y relationship increases exponentially. In this chapter, we will focus on four possible relationships between two independent variables and one outcome variable, including (1) independent effect of two influential factors X_1 and X_2; (2) interactive effect of two influential factors $X_1 \times X_2$; (3) mediation effect with X_2 bridging the relationship between X_1 and Y; and (4) colliding effect in which one of the two *Xs* is the outcome of the other *X* and *Y*.

8.1　Relationships Between Two Influential Factors and One Outcome

Up to now, we can understand that in a closely connected universe, it is highly challenging to quantitatively examine if a hypothetic X ~ Y relationship is causal even if it is theory-based and/or supported by pilot data. The multivariate modeling methods described in previous chapters provide an approach to confirm a simple X ~ Y relationship even if the relationship is conceived or developed based on strong theories and/or supported by data from pilot studies. A natural extension is to examine two influential factors on one outcome.

8.1.1　Importance of Two Influential Factors

All health outcomes can be considered as multifaceted, including disease, health status, and health-related behaviors. Although affected by many factors, it is unfeasible to examine all of them at once despite the availability of large amount of data and advanced multivariate methods. The main reason is that all influential factors may also be connected with each other, forming a causal network system. To date, few if any of the analytical methods are capable to gain insight into a network causal relationship by disentangling all the relations in the network. This is why the practical approach has been adopted for any etiological studies to focus on the simple one-X and one-Y relationship as detailed in Chaps. 5, 6, and 7.

Simultaneously studying two influential factors is a natural extension of the simple one-X and one-Y relationship. For example, in Chap. 5, we demonstrated a significant positive relationship between an influential factor X (years of smoking) and the outcome Y (systolic blood pressure) after adjusting for the covariate of gender (Fig. 5.7). In the analysis, the demographic factor gender was used as a covariate. For the same analysis, we can reframe the study to examine: (1) If blood pressure is affected by years of smoking and gender? (2) If blood pressure and years of smoking differ between males or females? (3) Is the higher blood pressure among males than among female attributed to more males smoking than females?

Likewise, in Chap. 6, the same X (years of smoking) was demonstrated to be significantly associated with another outcome Y (diagnosed with high blood pressure) after controlling for BMI (Fig. 6.9). If we reframe the same analysis as an approach to simultaneously examine the impact of BMI and years of smoking on high blood pressure, it will help us to answer the questions like: (1) Are both factors related to high blood pressure independenlty7? (2) Does the smoking-high blood pressure relationship differ for people with different BMI levels? (3) Likewise, does the BMI-high blood pressure relationship differ for people with different durations of smoking?

The questions described in the previous two paragraphs cannot be addressed using the simple one-X and one-Y approach described in Chaps. 5, 6, and 7. New analytical strategies must be used. As described at the beginning of this chapter, with two influential Xs, there are four different X ~ Y relationships: (1) independent impact of two factors X_1 and X_2 on the outcome Y; (2) interactive effect of the two factors $X_1 \times X_2$ on the outcome Y; (3) mediation effect with one X bridging the effect of the other X on the outcome Y, and (4) colliding effect in which one X is the outcome of the other X and the outcome Y. In this chapter, we will focus on these four relationships.

8.1.2   Independent Impact of Two Influential Factors

The first and most straight forward relationship between two influential factor Xs and one outcome Y is that the two Xs exert their effect independently on the outcome Y. As shown in Fig. 8.1, conceptually, this relationship means the two Xs exert the influences on Y parallelly, and there is no interference with each other. Geometrically, the independence means the two Xs interact with each other at 90 degree to affect Y.

Fig. 8.1 Independent relationship between two influential factor Xs and one outcome Y

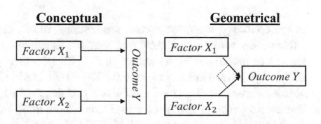

Statistically, the independent relationship of two Xs with one Y in Fig. 8.1 can be expressed using the following regression model:

$$Y = \alpha + \beta_1 X_1 + \beta_2 X_2 + e \tag{8.1}$$

Model 8.1 is a typical linear regression reflecting one of the theoretical models from Model 5.2 described at the beginning of Chap. 5. If the impact of each of the two Xs on the outcome Y is *in theory* independent from each other, the two estimated β coefficients will quantify the fully impact of the two Xs on each Y, individually.

In epidemiology, this type of causal relationships with two influential factors independently affecting an outcome is not common. In many cases when two or more variables are included in one model, only the independent portion of the effect of individual factors has been quantified with the rest unintentionally neglected.

8.2   Impact of Two Intertwined Influential Factors

In epidemiology, it is not hard to find many scenarios in which two influential factors interact with each other to exert their effect on the outcome Y. For example, the risk of mortality of a population can be affected by levels of education and access to health care. Weight gain for youth and young adults can be attributed to the interaction between personal behavior and genetic differences. Poor mental health of migrant populations can be attributed to the interactive influence of both acculturation and occupation. The list is endless.

Interactions of two influential factor Xs with each other to affect an outcome Y has been discussed intensively in almost all epidemiology textbooks. Results from interaction analysis will deepen our understanding of the potential causal mechanisms and supporting effective interventions for disease treatment and prevention and health promotion. Consequently, inclusion of an examination of interactions between two influential factors can increase the odds for a research paper to be accepted for publication in a peer reviewed journal.

8.2.1   Conceptual Model of Interaction

In epidemiology, when two factors are assumed to be interactive with each other in affecting an outcome variable, one variable is named as the main factor X and another as moderator W. As shown in Fig. 8.2 (top panel), *an interactive relationship is defined as a model in which the X ~ Y relationship is checked by a third variable, moderator W*. This model indicates that the single X ~ Y relationship, as seen in previous chapters, is now no longer considered to be independent but depends on the influence of another factor W. Here the W serves conceptually like a switch to control a dim light. Changing in W just like turning the dim light switch, it can increase, decline, or totally turn of the X ~ Y relationship. State in another way, the X ~ Y relationship is *conditioned* on a third variable W.

Fig. 8.2 Conceptual and analytical model for interaction between two influential factors on outcome Y with one factor named as X and another as W

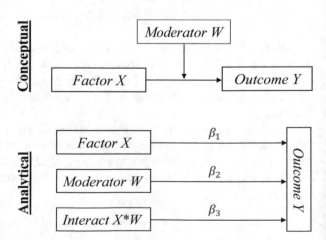

8.2.2   Statistical Modeling of an Interactive Relationship

Following the conceptual model in the upper panel of Fig. 8.2, analytical models are developed to quantify the interaction between X and W to affect Y. One of the analytical models is also presented in Fig. 8.2 (lower panel). Following the model, in an interaction analysis, three independent components are used to disentangle the impact of the two influential factors X and W, on the outcome Y:

1. The independent effect of X, which is captured by the model parameter β_1;
2. The independent effect of W, which is captured by β_2; and
3. The effect of interaction between X and W, which is captured by β_3.

With the analytical model described geometrically in Fig. 8.2, and the quantitative methods described in Chap. 5, the following multiple regression is used for interaction analysis:

$$Y = \alpha + \beta_1 X + \beta_2 W + \beta_3 \left(X \times W \right) + e, \tag{8.2}$$

Here the term $X \times W$ is used to capture the interaction between X and W. Different from Model 8.1, there is no independence assumption of the two influential factors X and W; on the contrary, Model 8.2 allows the two variables to interact with each other in addition to the effect from each of the two factors. This regression model thus makes it possible to simultaneously quantify the three effects described above, including two independent effects and one interactive effect from the two influential factors.

8.2.3   Main Effect and Effect of Interaction

With the interaction model 8.2, the estimated model parameters β_1 and β_2 are termed as *the main effect* of X and W respectively, while the estimated β_3 as *the interactive effect*. If the estimated β_3 is statistically significant allowing for type I error, the hypothesis of X – W interaction is supported after controlling for the main effects of the two factors. If the estimated β_3 is not statistically significantly different from zero, Model 8.2 becomes Model 8.1, and we can claim that the impact of X and W are independent from each other.

To further the understanding of model 8.2, let use review the results in Fig. 5.7 from Chap. 5. In the top part of the figure, the estimated β coefficient was 0.1824 for years of smoking and −3.9480 for gender. The analysis can be extended to become an interaction model by treating years of smoking as X, gender as W, and adding another term of $X \times W$. In this model, in addition to determine the main effect of both years of smoking and gender, the effect from the interaction of the two variables will be quantified. We will use this as an analytical example in Sect. 8.3.

8.2.4   Inclusion of Other Covariates

As in Chaps. 5, 6, and 7, covariates can also be added to model 8.2 when conducting analyses to assess the interaction of two influential factors on an outcome measure using the following multiple regression model:

$$Y = \alpha + \beta_1 X + \beta_2 W + \beta_3 (X \times W) + \beta_4 cov X_1 + \ldots + e. \qquad (8.3)$$

As one of the multiple regression models, the guidelines previously described in Chaps. 5, 6, and 7 are applicable for covariate selection and result interpretation when Model 8.3 is used in data analysis.

8.2.5   Reported Interaction Studies with Survey Data

Two-variable interaction models as described in Fig. 8.2 and Model 8.2 are commonly used in examining the impact of two influential factors on an outcome with survey data. For example, a meta-analysis with 17 case-control studies conducted in Europe and America confirmed that in addition to the significant and independent influences of alcohol and tobacco, there is a joint effect of the two variables on the risk of head and neck cancers, particularly for the oral cavity cancer and the head and neck cancer among women at younger ages (Hashibe et al. 2009). Another example is that a 10-year cohort study in Spain with a large sample size (n = 54,466) demonstrated that in addition to a dose-response relationship between BMI and risk of death, BMI can significantly modify the mortality risk from cardiovascular diseases attributed to other conventional risk factors such as total cholesterol, diabetes, and hypertension (Barroso et al. 2018). A last example is that a literature review of published studies indicated that sleeping problems are interacted with anxiety and stress, leading to depression among youth who are addicted to internet gaming (Lam 2014).

It is clear that when an interactive approach is used to examine two factors and their impact on an outcome, new and important information can be obtained. In addition to confirming the independent effect of two factors, evidence can be obtained regarding the interaction between the two. Such information is valuable for deepening our understanding of the etiology of a medical, health or behavioral problem. The information is sometimes also essential for disease treatment, prevention and health promotion. In the three examples described above, findings of the first example indicate that use of tobacco and alcohol together will have a synergetic effect on the risk of head and neck cancer. This result suggests the importance to control both tobacco and alcohol for cancer prevention. Findings from the second example suggest that BMI can alter the impact of conventional risk factors related to cardiovascular disease. Such findings suggest the importance of body weight control in cardiovascular disease prevention and control in addition to the conventional risk factors. Similar information can also be derived from the third example on sleep problems and mental health for addictive internet gaming.

8.2.6 Gene-Environmental Interaction

Gene (G)-environmental (E) interaction represents another category of studies that examine two variables at the same time on an outcome. In such studies, the measure of a gene is often treated as the moderator W. Change in a gene (i.e., mutation) will alter the capacity of the body to deal with risk exposure (such as toxicants from tobacco, alcohol, and environment pollutants), thus modifying the effect of the exposure (most often toxicants) on a health outcome (i.e., cancer incidence) or a health-related behavior (i.e., addiction). This approach has been widely used in studying diseases and health behaviors (Hunter 2005; Caspi and Moffitt 2006). In an early study, the author of this book showed significant interaction between smoking during pregnancy and polymorphisms in metabolic genes CYP1A1 and GSTM1 on lung function in young children (Chen et al. 2011a, b). First, child lung function is negatively associated with maternal smoking during pregnancy. Furthermore, the reduction in child lung function is greater for mothers who carry the polymorphic CYP1a1*2a and GSTM1 genes, which reduce the capacity to metabolize toxicants.

There are many strengths associated with studies taking a G-E interaction approach. Almost all health-related issues can be considered as resulted from interactions between the physical body and the living environment. Physical body is determined to a large extent by the human genes inherited through millions of years of evolution. As a result, findings from a G-E interaction study will, in theory, shed light on the etiology of almost all medical, health, and behavioral problems. Furthermore, evidence derived from G-E interactions is essential to search for biological and chemical agents for disease prevention and treatment, and health promotion.

8.2.7 Interaction of an Influential Factor with a Demographic Factor

In etiological studies, influential factors can be broadly categorized into two groups: *modifiable* and *non-modifiable*. Non-modifiable factors can hardly be changes and they are not uncommon, such as gene, age, gender, skin color, race, birthplace, family history etc. Although many non-modifiable demographic factors can hardly be altered, they may be associated with a health outcome. Analysis of the interaction of each of these factors with other influential factors can provide information useful to advance etiology and to inform disease treatment, prevention, and health promotion.

If an X ~ Y relation differs for subgroups of a population marked by a demographic factor, such as gender, age, and racial group, such information of interaction can be used to tailor intervention strategies targeting the high-risk subgroup for the best effect. For example, an epidemiological study with the most recent data indicated that the association between opioid overdose and suicide varied from being the lowest for the racial group of Hispanics, to moderate for Whites, and to the highest for Blacks (Lippold et al. 2019). This finding provides data supporting extra efforts on substance reduction among Whites and Blacks for effective suicide prevention to curb the increasing trend of suicide death in the United States. Interaction analysis of gender and racial groups has been used in assessing health disparities to promote health for everyone in a population (Ward et al. 2019).

8.2.8 Interactions with Modifiable Influential Factors

On the contrary, modifiable factors are those that can be altered, and these factors are countless, including large arrays of factors of socioeconomic, behavioral, and intrapersonal biological and psychological factors as described in Chap. 4 (Fig. 4.4 and the related text). Interactions between any two of these factors as well as their interaction with the non-modifiable factors will generate rich information to enhance our knowledge basis about diseases, health status and health-related behaviors and support evidence-based disease treatment and prevention and health promotion.

8.3   Interaction Analysis with Real Data

With knowledge from previous sections, we will turn to interaction analysis with real data in this section. As a demonstration, two types of analyses will be conducted, one focusing on the interaction of one modifiable influential factor with one unmodifiable demographic factors and another focusing on the interaction of two modifiable influential factors. With regard to gene-environmental interactions, no demonstration analysis will be provided because of the need for solid knowledge genetics and molecular biology.

8.3.1   Data Sources and Variables

Data will be derived from DATCH5, the dataset used in Chap. 5. As a demonstration, two outcome variables will be used: (1) High blood pressure (HBPX, yes/no) defined based on the measured blood pressure and (2) systolic blood pressure (SYSTBP, mmHg), the average of three consecutive measures. Three influential factors are: EDUCATION (less than high school, high school and more than high school), BMI (computed using self-reported height and weight), and self-image (SELF_IMAGE, feel too thin, average, or too fat). Three demographic factors are: AGE (in year), GENDER (male-female gender), and RACE3 (White, Black, and Other).

8.3.2 SAS Program for Data Processing

SAS Program 8.1 is for data processing. The program first reads DATCH5 used in Chap. 5 into a temporary dataset TMP for further processing. A list of 10 variables plus the SEQN (for later use) are taken from DATCH5. More variables are included for students to practice. A permanent dataset DATCH8 is then created by defining and coding the variables.

```
************************************************************************************;
SAS PROGRAM 8.1 DATAYPREPARATION FOR PRACTICING INTERACTION ANALYSIS
************************************************************************************;
* CREATE DATCH8 BY SELECTED VARIABLES FROM DATCH5;
LIBNAME SASDATA "C:\QUANTLAB\A DATA\";
DATA TMP; SET SASDATA.DATCH5;
KEEP AGE GENDER RACE5 EDUCATION SMKYRS COTININE BMI DIASBP SYSTBP HBPX WHQ030 SEQN;
RUN;
* CHECK SELECTED VARIABLES;
PROC CONTENTS; RUN;
PROC FREQ DATA = TMP; TABLES AGE WHQ030; RUN;
* CREATE DATCH8 BY EXCLUDING SUBJECTS WITH MISSING DATA ON AGE;
DATA SASDATA.DATCH8; SET TMP;
IF AGE NE .;
SELF_IMAGE = WHQ030; IF WHQ030 EQ 9 THEN SELF_IMAGE = .;
* RECODE RACE5 TO RACE3;
RACE3 = RACE5; IF RACE5 GT 3 THEN RACE3=3;
LABEL  SELF_IMAGE = "1=TWO THIN, 2=AVERAGE, 3=TOO FAT",
       RACE3      = "1=WHITE 2=BLACK 3=OTHER";
* CHECK DATA, VARIABLES, AND MISSING
PROC CONTENTS; RUN;
PROC FREQ DATA= SASDATA.DATCH8; TABLES RACE3 SELF_IMAGE EDUCATION SMKYRS; RUN;
************************************************************************************;
```

It is worth noting that extra variables were included in the new dataset. These variables include COTININE (serum biomarker for exposure to tobacco) and DIASBP (diastolic blood pressure). They are included for students to practice these methods. This program can also be used as a template to select/add variables to meet research needs of yours.

8.3.3 SAS Program for Interaction Analysis

SAS Program 8.2 is prepared to demonstrate how to conduct interaction analysis using regression models 8.2 and 8.3. The program consists of four parts representing the steps and approaches of interaction analysis for different conditions. Part 1 simply shows the process to creating the work dataset A for analysis; Part 2 demonstrates the steps to analyze the interaction between an influential factor and a demographic factor for a continuous outcome; Part 3 shows the same analysis for a binary outcome; part 4 presents the interaction analysis of two influential factors.

Prior to the designated interaction analyses, a simple correlation analysis is often conducted to check the relationships among all the key variables to be used, including the outcome, the two influential factors, and covariates. After correlation analysis, Model 1 is used assuming the two influential factors are independent. Results from this step of analysis also serve as a background check to demonstrate the need for interaction effect. Model 2 is for interaction with no covariates and Model 3 is for interaction plus covariates. When conducting the interaction analysis, three terms must be included in the model, the two influential factors X and W and the interaction term X*W.

```
********************************************************************************
SAS PROGRAM 8.2 ANALYSIS OF INTERACTION WITH DEMOGRPAHIC FACTORS
********************************************************************************;
** PART 1. CREATE A WORK DATASET FOR ANALYSIS;
DATA A; SET SASDATA.DATCH8;
* CREATE AND LABEL A NEW VARIABLE FOR INTERACTION;
EDU_GENDER = EDUCATION * GENDER;
SMKYR10 = SMKYRS/10;          * RESCALING;
SMKYR10_BMI = SMKYR10 * BMI;
LABEL  EDU_GENDER = "EDUCATION GENDER INTERACTION",
       SMKYR10 = "SMOKING YEARS WITH 10 YEARS AS UNIT",
       SMKYR10_BMI = "SMOKING YEARS AND BMI INERATION";
RUN;

** PART 2 ANALYSIS FOR CONTINUOUS Y;
* CHECK CORRELATION AMOLNG KEY VARIABLES;
PROC CORR DATA = A;
VAR SYSTBP EDUCATION GENDER AGE RACE3; RUN;
* MODEL 1. INDEPENDENT ASSOCIATION;
PROC REG DATA = A;
MODEL SYSTBP = EDUCATION GENDER;
RUN;
* MODEL 2. INTERACTION WITHOUT COVARIATTES;
PROC REG DATA = A;
MODEL SYSTBP = EDUCATION GENDER EDU_GENDER;
RUN;
* MODEL 3. INTERACTION PLUS COVARIATES - ALTERNATIVE MODELS;
PROC REG DATA = A;
*MODEL SYSTBP = EDUCATION GENDER EDU_GENDER AGE;
*MODEL SYSTBP = EDUCATION GENDER EDU_GENDER RACE3;
MODEL SYSTBP = EDUCATION GENDER EDU_GENDER AGE RACE3;
RUN;

** PART 3. ANALYSIS FOR BINARY OUTCOME Y;
* MODEL 1. INDEPENDENT ASSOCIATION;
PROC LOGISTIC DATA = A;
CLASS HBPX RACE3;
MODEL HBPX (EVENT = '1') = BMI RACE3;
RUN;
* MODEL 2. INTERACTION WITHOUT COVARIATES;
PROC LOGISTIC DATA = A;
CLASS HBPX RACE3;
MODEL HBPX (EVENT = '1') = BMI RACE3 BMI*RACE3;
RUN;
* MODEL 3. INTERACTION PLUS COVARIATES - ALTERNATIVE MODELS;
PROC LOGISTIC DATA = A;
CLASS HBPX RACE3 GENDER;
MODEL HBPX (EVENT = '1') = BMI RACE3 BMI*RACE3 AGE GENDER SELF_IMAGE;
RUN;

** PART 4. ANALYSIS OF TWO INFLUENTIAL FACTORS;
PROC REG DATA = A;
* MODEL 1. INDEPENDENT ASSOCIATION;
MODEL SYSTBP = BMI SMKYR10;
* MODEL 2. INTERACTION WITHOUT COVARIATES;
MODEL SYSTBP = BMI SMKYR10 SMKYR10_BMI;
* MODEL 3. INTERACTION PLUS COVARIATES;
MODEL SYSTBP = BMI SMKYR10 SMKYR10_BMI AGE GENDER RACE3;
RUN;
********************************************************************************;
```

It is worth noting that in Part 1 of SAS Program 8.2, the variable SMKYR10 is created by dividing the original SMKYRS with 10. This rescaling is used so that the estimated regression coefficient for this factor will not be numerically too small.

In addition, two more new variables EDU_GENDER and SMKYR10_BMI are created by mathematically *multiplying* the two related variables. Creation of these two new variables is needed for interaction analysis using SAS procedure **PROC REG** for linear regression.

8.3.4   Results of Interaction Analysis with a Continuous Outcome

Part 2 of SAS Program 8.2 demonstrates the steps for interaction analysis of continuous (SYSTBP) outcome and interaction of an influential factor EDUCATION with a demographic factor GENDER. To confirm the result from the interaction analysis, two covariates are included, AGE and RACE3.

Figure 8.3 displays the main results from the simple correlation analysis from SAS Program 8.2, part 2. The results indicate that the five variables were significantly correlated with each other. Particularly, the correlations between the Y(SYSTBP), X (EDUCATION), and W(GENDER), the three key variables were all statistically extremely significant at the $p < 0.01$ level.

Pearson Correlation Coefficients Prob > |r| under H0: Rho=0 Number of Observations					
	SYSTBP	EDUCATION	GENDER	AGE	RACE3
SYSTBP MEASURED SYSTOLIC BLOOD PRESSURE, MEAN,	1.00000 4187	-0.11321 <.0001 4182	-0.08512 <.0001 4187	0.43952 <.0001 4187	0.00740 0.6320 4187
EDUCATION 1=LESS THAN HIGH 2=HIGH SCHOOL 3=COLLEGE+,	-0.11321 <.0001 4182	1.00000 5125	0.03034 0.0299 5125	-0.05563 <.0001 5125	-0.08566 <.0001 5125
GENDER GENDER 1=MALE 2=FEMALE,	-0.08512 <.0001 4187	0.03034 0.0299 5125	1.00000 5134	-0.02305 0.0987 5134	0.02275 0.1031 5134
AGE AGE IN YEAR,	0.43952 <.0001 4187	-0.05563 <.0001 5125	-0.02305 0.0987 5134	1.00000 5134	-0.08994 <.0001 5134
RACE3 1=WHITE 2=BLACK 3=OTHER	0.00740 0.6320 4187	-0.08566 <.0001 5125	0.02275 0.1031 5134	-0.08994 <.0001 5134	1.00000 5134

Fig. 8.3 Correlation among all related variables for interaction analysis: Output of SAS Program 8.2, Part 2

8.3.5　Results for Independent Association

Results from Model 1 in SAS Program 8.2 is a simple regression analysis with the two predictable variables X and W (detailed SAS output not shown). As expected, results from the independent association analysis (no interaction term) indicate that the outcome Y was negatively associated education with the estimated $\beta = -3.1597$ (p < 0.001) and gender (1 = male, 2 = female) with the estimated $\beta = -3.0998$ (p < 0.001). If the influence of these two factors on high blood pressure are independent from each other, the analysis will be completed.

However, if influences of the two variables are related to each other, or there is an existence of an interaction between the two, the estimated regression coefficients will be biased. For example, results from the correlation suggest a significant and positive correlation between education and gender (r = 0.0303, p < 0.05). This result suggests the need for an interaction analysis of these two variables.

8.3.6　Interactions Between Education and Gender

Figure 8.4 displays the results from Model 2 and Model 3 in SAS Program 8.2, the two interaction models. The top part of Fig. 8.4 shows the result from the interaction analysis without considering covariates. What can be seen first is that the main effect of both education and gender were no longer statistically significant for the

Parameter Estimates							
Variable	Label	DF	Parameter Estimate	Standard Error	t Value	Pr > |t|
Intercept	Intercept	1	127.29440	2.94818	43.18	<.0001
EDUCATION	1=LESS THAN HIGH 2=HIGH SCHOOL 3=COLLEGE+,	1	1.14672	1.37068	0.84	0.4029
GENDER	GENDER 1=MALE 2=FEMALE,	1	2.81133	1.87377	1.50	0.1336
EDU_GENDER	EDUCATION GENDER INERACTION	1	-2.87686	0.86850	-3.31	0.0009

Parameter Estimates							
Variable	Label	DF	Parameter Estimate	Standard Error	t Value	Pr > |t|
Intercept	Intercept	1	101.77878	2.84708	35.75	<.0001
EDUCATION	1=LESS THAN HIGH 2=HIGH SCHOOL 3=COLLEGE+,	1	0.65479	1.23340	0.53	0.5955
GENDER	GENDER 1=MALE 2=FEMALE,	1	1.73990	1.68687	1.03	0.3024
EDU_GENDER	EDUCATION GENDER INERACTION	1	-2.10640	0.78199	-2.69	0.0071
AGE	AGE IN YEAR,	1	0.49337	0.01572	31.38	<.0001
RACE3	1=WHITE 2=BLACK 3=OTHER	1	0.74066	0.29917	2.48	0.0133

Fig. 8.4 Interaction of education with gender with and without control age and race: Output of SAS Program 8.2, part 2, models 2 and 3

outcome of systolic blood pressure (p > 0.05 for both) after the education-gender interaction is included. This suggests that the results from Model 1 were biases because the interaction between the two factors were not considered.

Further view of the results reveals a significant interaction between education and gender (EDU_GENDER) as it relates to systolic blood pressure, the estimated $\beta = -2.8769$ (p < 0.01) for the interaction term. This analytical result suggests that instead of an independent association, education and gender were associated with systolic blood pressure interactively. In other words, the education-systolic blood pressure relationship is conditioned on another variable – gender (see Fig. 8.2 and related text). The bottom part of the SAS output shows that the interaction effect remained statistically significant after adjusting for age and racial groups. The adjusted $\beta = -2.1064$ (p < 0.01).

Considering the same analytical approach described in Chap. 5 with gender and other demographic factors, interaction analysis provides new information about the relationship between an influential factor X, levels of education, on the outcome variable Y, systolic blood pressure. The education-blood pressure relationship is *not independent* but v*aries depending on the variable gender*. This is the power of inter-action analysis in epidemiology – advancing etiology by disentangling the complex causal relationship.

8.3.7   Interaction Analysis for a Binary Outcome

In this example, the outcome variable was HBPX (high blood pressure, yes/no), determined based on the measured systolic and diastolic blood pressure. Two influential factors are BMI and racial group (RACE3, White, Black, Other). Three covariates are AGE, GENDER and SELF_IMAGE. These variables are all included in the dataset for analysis. Age and gender are well-known to be risk factors for hypertension. Self-image was also included as a covariate since this variable is closely related to BMI (Ahadzadeh et al. 2018). As described in Chap. 6, logistic regression is used for the binary outcome.

Figure 8.5 displays the result from Model 1 in which BMI and racial group (RACE3) were modeled as independent influential factors on the outcome, high blood pressure (HBPX). As expected, high blood pressure was significantly associated with BMI (estimated $\beta = 0.0177$, p < 0.01) and racial groups (RACE3) with reference to the racial group Other, the estimated $\beta = -0.2016$ for White (RACE3 = 1); and estimated $\beta = 0.0324$ for Black (RACE3 = 2), p < 0.01.

If a study focuses on the body mass index – high blood pressure relationship controlling for racial groups, the analysis is now completed. However, there might be an interaction between race and body weight. If an interaction exists, we have to conduct further analyses.

Analysis of Maximum Likelihood Estimates						
Parameter		DF	Estimate	Standard Error	Wald Chi-Square	Pr > ChiSq
Intercept		1	-2.1202	0.1633	168.5313	<.0001
BMI		1	0.0177	0.00535	10.9287	0.0009
RACE3	1	1	-0.2106	0.0568	13.7359	0.0002
RACE3	2	1	0.3244	0.0561	33.3998	<.0001

Fig. 8.5 Independent effect of Body Mass Index (BMI) and racial group (RACE3) on high blood pressure (HBPX): Output of SAS Program 8.2, part 3, model 1

Figure 8.6 displays the results from Model 2, Part 3 of SAS Program 8.2 in which the interaction between BMI and RACE3 was included. The result that should catch our attention is that despite a negative interaction between BMI and RACE3, none of the two BMI − RACE3 interaction terms was statistically significant ($p > 0.05$ for all). The interaction remained non-significant after inclusion of the three covariates AGE, GENDER, and SELF_IMAGE (results now shown).

Analysis of Maximum Likelihood Estimates						
Parameter		DF	Estimate	Standard Error	Wald Chi-Square	Pr > ChiSq
Intercept		1	-2.1228	0.1635	168.6606	<.0001
BMI		1	0.0179	0.00536	11.0939	0.0009
RACE3	1	1	-0.1356	0.2337	0.3369	0.5616
RACE3	2	1	0.3873	0.2294	2.8495	0.0914
BMI*RACE3	1	1	-0.00261	0.00764	0.1166	0.7327
BMI*RACE3	2	1	-0.00214	0.00739	0.0842	0.7717

Fig. 8.6 Interaction between BMI and racial group (RACE3) on high blood pressure (HBPX): Output of SAS Program 8.2

The non-significant result in this example thus indicates that the BMI and high blood pressure association was not affected by racial groups. In other words, we have reason to use the findings in Fig. 8.5 as our final result. If the purpose of a study is to examine only the BMI and high blood pressure relationship, we can conclude that BMI is a risk factor for high blood pressure, the relationship showed no racial differences since the result remained to be statistically significant after controlling for racial groups using logistic regression models.

A little bit extension, if a study aims at examining two influential factors X_1 and X_2, and obtained a non-significant interaction of both Xs with a moderator (like racial groups in this example), such a result would suggest that the impact of the influential factors is independent from each other.

8.3.8   Interaction Analysis for Continuous X, W and Y

This part demonstrates the analysis of interaction between two influential factors on the outcome variable, all the three variables being continuous. In the example, the BMI and the smoking measured are used as the two influential factors. Smoking and BMI are known to be related with each other and both are also related to high blood pressure. As a demonstration, the three variables were defined as follows: SYSTBP, the measured systolic blood pressure (mmHg) was used as Y; SMKYR10 and BMI were used as the two influential factors W and X; plus an interaction term SMKYR10_BMI (X*W).

Figure 8.7 displays the results from Model 1 (top) and Model 2 (bottom) from SAS Program 8.2, Part 4. As expected, results from Model 1 indicate a significant and independent association of the two factors with the outcome, the estimated $\beta = 0.3698$, $p < 0.01$ for BMI and estimated $\beta = 1.6653$, $p < 0.01$ for SMKYR10. If the goal of a study is to examine the influence of the two variables without considering the interaction between the two variables, the analysis is done. However, there might be interactions between BMI and smoking, additional analysis must be conducted.

Parameter Estimates							
Variable	Label	DF	Parameter Estimate	Standard Error	t Value	Pr > |t|
Intercept	Intercept	1	111.94907	1.25349	89.31	<.0001
BMI	BODY MASS INDEX USING REPORTED DATA	1	0.36983	0.04191	8.82	<.0001
SMKYR10	SMOKING YEARS WITH A 10-YEAR UNIT,	1	1.66527	0.14768	11.28	<.0001

Parameter Estimates							
Variable	Label	DF	Parameter Estimate	Standard Error	t Value	Pr > |t|
Intercept	Intercept	1	108.55592	1.53298	70.81	<.0001
BMI	BODY MASS INDEX USING REPORTED DATA	1	0.48858	0.05206	9.38	<.0001
SMKYR10	SMOKING YEARS WITH A 10-YEAR UNIT,	1	4.09565	0.65119	6.29	<.0001
SMKYR10_BMI	SMOKING YEARS AND BMI INERATION	1	-0.08413	0.02196	-3.83	0.0001

Fig. 8.7 Results from Model 1 for independent association and Model 2 for interaction: Output of SAS Program 8.2 part 4

Interactions between smoking and BMI are frequently reported in the literature. This is also supported by results from the simple correlation as in Part 2 of SAS Program 8.2. If there is an interaction between the two variables, the estimated β coefficients from the independent association analysis in the top part of Fig. 8.7 will be biased (i.e., either over- or under-estimated) or not exist at all as seen in Fig. 8.4 for the education – gender interaction (EDU_GENDER).

The low part of Fig. 8.7 displays the results with Model 2 with an interaction term (SMKYR10_BMI), and the estimated $\beta = -0.0841$, $p < 0.01$ for the interaction. This result suggests an extremely significant negative interaction between the two influential factors. After considering the interaction, the adjusted $\beta = 0.4886$ for BMI, $p < 0.01$ and the value of the regression coefficient was greater than the previous estimate of 0.3698 from Model 1. The adjusted $\beta = 4.0956$ for SMKYR10 ($p < 0.01$) after control the main effect of BMI and the BMI-smoking interaction. Further, the adjusted of the adjusted regression coefficient is more than twice the estimate of 1.6653 from Model 1.

After controlling for the three demographic factors covariates, AGE, GENDER, and RACE3, results (detailed SAS output not shown) from Model 3 show that in addition to a significant negative interaction with the estimated $\beta = -0.0632$ ($p < 0.01$), the adjusted $\beta = 0.4560$ ($p < 0.01$) for BMI; and the adjusted $\beta = 1.6411$ ($p < 0.01$) for SMKYR10. As the *main effect* of the two influential factors, these two adjusted β s measure the independent part of their association with the outcome of blood pressure after the interaction effect between the two is considered.

As an example, we can now conclude that through bivariate and multivariate analysis, years of smoking and BMI are two risk factors for high blood pressure since years of smoking and BMI measures were both positively associated with measured systolic blood pressure. In addition to the independent effect, there was a significant and negative interaction between the two. Both the two main effects and the interaction effect remained significant after age, gender, and racial groups are statistically adjusted using multivariate regression method.

8.4   Positive and Negative Interactions and Interaction Plot

Understanding the direction of an interaction is essential to understand the causal mechanisms and to applying the results in practice. To introduce the concept of interaction at the beginning of this chapter, figures (i.e., Fig. 8.2) and equations (i.e., Models 8.2 and 8.3) were used. However, none of them tells what a positive or a negative interaction mean. The analysis with real data in Sect. 8.3 revealed that interaction between two influential factors X on the outcome Y did show the direction of an interaction between two influential factors on the outcome Y. Although all three examples included in the section showed a negative interaction, positive interaction is also common in epidemiological studies.

In this section, we will describe show to understanding the meaning of the direction of an interaction using equations and plots. Interaction plots are often included in published empirical studies to visualize the study findings.

8.4.1   Concept of Positive and Negative Interaction

In the first two sections of this chapter, we introduced and discussed in detail about the concept of interaction between two influential factors. In Sect. 8.2, we described the interaction mathematically (Model 8.2) in which one variable X was used as the influential factor, and another variable W as a moderator. With these notations, the impact of these two variables on Y was expressed as: $Y = \alpha + \beta_1 X + + \beta_2 W + \beta_3 (X * W)$, plus an error term.

In this model, parameter β_3 quantifies the interaction between X and W; and β_1 and β_2 are measures of the main effects for X and W, respectively. The concept of positive and negative interaction is thus determined by the sign of an estimated β_3.

Positive interaction: if the estimated β_3 is positive; and
Negative interaction: if the estimated β_3 is negative.

In the three analytical examples in Sect. 8.3, the estimated β_3 was negative for all, including the interactions between education and gender, BMI and racial groups, and BMI and smoking. Positive β_3 is also reported often in the literature. For example, in a study to examine the health status of the heart, the variable emotional reactivity is significantly and positively modified (interacted) the effect of the variable pleasant feeling on heart rate with estimated $\beta_3 = 0.2$, $p < 0.05$ (Cornelius et al. 2018).

8.4.2   Plot of Interaction for Visual Comprehension

In addition to the abstractive concepts described above, a visualization of the interaction is commonly used to enhance our understanding of the meaning of interaction. Starting with the model $Y = \alpha + \beta_1 X + \beta_2 W + \beta_3 (X * W)$, with some simple mathematical manipulation, this model can be expressed as follows:

$$Y = \alpha + \left(\beta_1 + \beta_3 W \right) X + \beta_2 W \qquad (8.4)$$

Model 8.4 represents another approach to express the $X \sim Y$ relationship with an interaction. With Model 8.4, $\alpha + \beta_2 W$ can be considered as the intercept and the $(\beta_1 + \beta_3 W)$ can be considered as slope to express the $X \sim Y$ relationship. Model 8.4 provides a means to plot the X~Y relation given different values of W. We have already discussed intensively early in this chapter that an interaction between X and

W can be considered as a conditional relation between X and Y at different levels of W (see Sect. 8.2 and Fig. 8.2), Model 8.2 is another approach to present the conditional relationship.

With completion of an interaction analysis, all parameters for Model 8.4 including α, β_1, β_2 and β_3 are estimated and thus they are known constants. In the case of positive interaction, the estimated β_3 will be positive. A positive β_3 will increase the value of $(\beta_1 + \beta_3 W)$, the slope of Model 8.4. In this case, as W increases, the slope that describes the $X \sim Y$ will also increase (see Fig. 8.8).

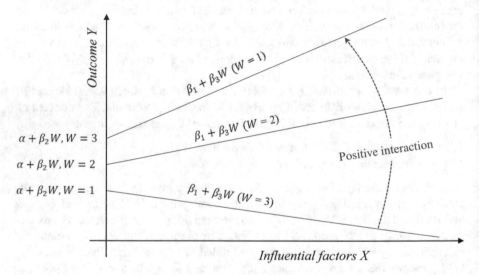

Fig. 8.8 Positive interaction enhances the $X \sim Y$ relation as W increases

As the figure depicted, if the estimated β_3 is positive for the moderator W, the interaction will enhance the effect of the $X \sim Y$ relationship. The same relationship holds if the position of X and W is switched. This phenomenon gives the positive interaction as the *synergetic effect* between the two variables. Interested students can try to prove the relationship by switching X and W.

After the positive interaction is comprehended, a negative interaction is just a reverse of it. Figure 8.9 depicts a negative interaction using the same Model 8.4 and the notations. When the estimated β_3 is negative for the moderator W, it will reduce the slope $(\beta_1 + \beta_3 W)$ by subtracting estimated coefficients. Given the same estimates for other parameters, as the value of W increases, the slope will decline. This relationship also holds when the position of X and W are switched. Therefore, negative interaction is also termed as *antagonistic effect* between two influential factors.

Students are encouraged to plot the interaction effects observed in the previous section, using the methods (i.e., Model 8.4) described above. This can be completed using an excel sheet in three steps.

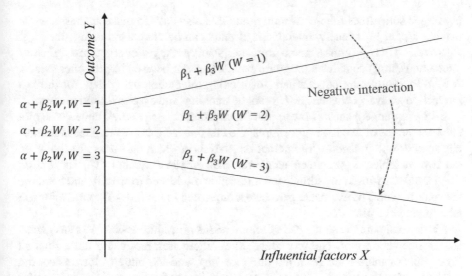

Fig. 8.9 Negative interaction suppresses the $X \sim Y$ relation as W increases

Step 1: Use the estimated model parameters and Model 8.4 to estimate the intercept and slope with different values for the observed W. For example, if gender is used as moderator, only two values are needed with 1 for male and 2
for female; if race is used, the value for W can be 1 (White), 2 (Black), and 3
(Other). However, for continuous variables such as BMI and Smoking, several typical values can be selected, such as mean, mean $\pm$ 0.5 SD and
mean $\pm$ 1 SD.

Step 2: Create data for plotting. In the spreadsheet, create a column for X first, and
then manually enter values for X from the smallest to the largest. Using education
as an example, you only need to enter three values: 1, 2,and 3. Add columns for
Y and then compute Y using X and the estimated intercept and slope in the previous step. After the estimated Y are computed for all Ws across X, you are ready
to plot.

Step 3: Plotting. Select the scatter plot (line plot) from excel to plot the data.
Properly adjust the values for both X and Y to achieve the best visual effect.
Also, edit the title and both X- and Y-axis for easy understanding and
interpretation.

8.4.3   SAS Program for Interaction Plot – An Example

Plotting interaction is very informative for readers to understand how two factors
interact with each other to affect an outcome of interest. In addition, interaction plot
is routinely required by academic journals for peer reviewed publications. Manual

plotting is sometimes time-consuming, and it is also easy to make mistakes while making a plot. Fortunately, interaction plotting can be conducted using statistical software. URL (https://cran.r-project.org/web/packages/interactions/vignettes/interactions.html) contains a program from R that can be used to plot interactions. A SAS Program is introduced here for plotting interaction using data for the last interaction analysis between BMI, years of smoking, and systolic blood pressure.

SAS Program 8.3 shows how to plot interaction between two variables. The plot involves the use of two SAS procedures, the first one is **PROC GLM**. This is eventually another SAS procedure for interaction analysis in which the interaction between the two variables is expressed using the mathematical symbol "|". The option ODS SELECT is used to estimate the interaction model and to specify and generate the contour plot. The estimated parameters are stored in the file GLMMODEL for use later to draw the plot.

The second part shows the use of another SAS procedure **PROC PLM** to generate the interaction plot. The procedure draws interaction plot using the estimated parameters of interaction from the previous step, and the output plot reflects the principles discussed in Figs. 8.8 and 8.9. In addition to the linear plot, contour plot is generated. Contour plots are not often used in published studies and they are shown here.

```
**************************************************************************************
SAS PROGRAM 8.3 VISUALIZATION OF INTERACTIONS USING PROC GLM FROM SAS;
**************************************************************************************;
* CONTOUR PLOT;
PROC GLM DATA = A;
MODEL SYSTBP = BMI | SMKYR10 AGE/SOLUTION;
ODS SELECT PARAMETERESTIMATES CONTOURFIT;
STORE GLMMODEL; RUN;
* LINEAR PLOT;
PROC PLM RESTORE=GLMMODEL NOINFO;
EFFECTPLOT SLICEFIT(X=BMI SLICEBY=SMKYR10)/CLM;
RUN;
**************************************************************************************;
```

Figure 8.10 displays the linear plot generated using SAS Program 8.3. The plotted figure is well marked. The title indicates that it is a model to assess the interaction of two variables on the outcome **SYSTBP** (systolic blood pressure). Each line represents a measure of years of smoking with 10 years as the unit. Different years of smoking are colored such that the blue line = non-smoking, orange line = 17.5 years of smoking, green line = 35 years of smoking, brown line = 52.5 years of smoking, and purple line = smoking for 70 years.

Consistent with the negative interaction between BMI and years of smoking ($\beta_3 = -0.0841$), as years of smoking increased, the slope measuring the systolic blood pressure and BMI relationship declined. When the years of smoking = 0 (blue line), the slope is the sharpest, indicating the strongest association between BMI and systolic blood pressure. As the years of smoking increased, the slope of the line declined, indicating weakening of the association between BMI and systolic blood pressure. The BMI-blood pressure relationship remained positive until the years of smoking reached 70 years.

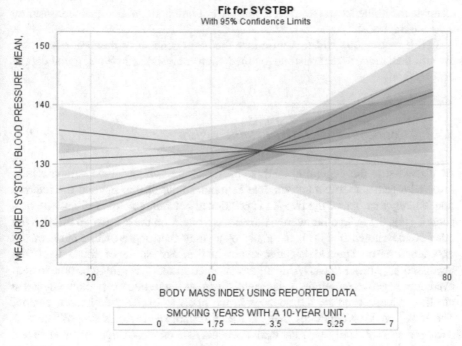

Fig. 8.10 Interaction plot showing the <u>negative</u> interaction between BMI and years of smoking on systolic blood pressure: Output from SAS Program 8.3

One issue worthy noting here is that the plot program does not allow for the inclusion of covariates, therefore the results in Fig. 8.10 can be biased as demonstrated earlier in this chapter. However, SAS Program 8.3 provides real data analysis example for interaction plotting.

8.5   Mediation Modeling Analysis: An Introduction

After interaction analysis, let us move to another interesting method to analyze two related variables with an outcome – mediation analysis. Mediation analysis is a method first proposed by scholars in psychology and behavioral sciences (Baron and Kenny 1986; Hayes 2009). This method was adapted later by epidemiologists (Chen et al. 2011a, b; Vanderweele et al. 2014). Efforts to disentangle the complex relationship among multiple influential factors and an outcome has challenged epidemiologists since the beginning of etiological studies. In addition to interaction analysis, mediation analysis adds another alternative.

The analysis of interaction for two influential factors in the first half of this chapter did provide new insights into causal relationships by considering the interaction of two variables, including the interaction of one influential factor and one demographic factor and two influential factors. Mediation will be another approach to examine the influence of two factors that are not interactional but chained, forming a mediation model.

In this section, we will first introduce the basic concept of mediation analysis. We will then move to demonstrate the mediation analysis method using real data in next section.

8.5.1   Concept of Mediation Relationship

As discussed at the beginning of this chapter, when two variables X_1 and X_2 are involved together to affect an outcome Y, another relationship beyond the interaction is likely that one of the two Xs is positioned between the other X and the outcome Y (Fig. 8.11). In other words, the effect of one X on the Y must go through the other X. As shown in Fig. 8.11, many of us may feel depressed because of the experience of unexpected negative event in life. For some of those who feel depressed, they may start smoking cigarettes since smoking is said to be able to help overcome negative emotions. It is established that cigarettes exert their effect via nicotine, which stimulate the neurons in the brain to excite a depressed person. Therefore, smoking cigarettes may also lead to poor quality of sleep. When conducting a research study, we may want to collect data on these three variables to test the mediation hypothesis. Following all the methods we learned up to now, various analytical approaches can be used to examine the relationship between the two influential factors of cigarette smoking and depression on quality of sleep, including the single-X and single-Y approach shown in Chap. 5 and the interaction approach between the two Xs on Y as presented earlier in this chapter. However, if a mediation relationship is assumed as shown in Fig. 8.11, new analytical strategies must be applied to verify the study hypothesis.

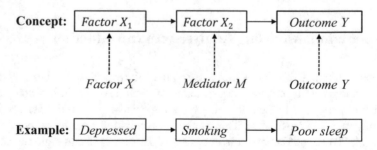

Fig. 8.11 Introduction to mediation with two influential factors Xs and one outcome Y

8.5.2   Mediation Modeling

The mediation relationship described above looks innovative, but all the statistical methods we learned so far cannot be used directly for data analysis to address the model. All the methods we learned can only assess one-step relationships from an

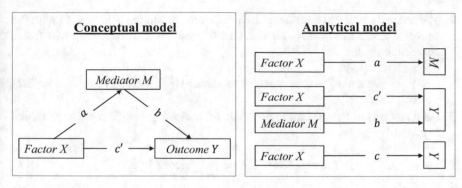

Fig. 8.12 The conceptual and analytical models of mediation analysis in etiological studies for quantitative epidemiology

influential factor to an outcome. In addition, an X ~ Y relationship presented in Fig. 8.11 may not be fully mediated by the factor M. In other words, in addition to the mediation part, there might be some direct relationship between X and Y. This speculation leads to the concept of mediation modeling (left part of Fig. 8.12).

In the conceptual mediation model (left part of Fig. 8.12) the impact of an influential factor X on the outcome Y is divided into two parts.

1. The *indirect effect*: the part of the effect of X on Y that is mediated by M. The effect from X to M is measured using the coefficient *a*, the effect from M to the Y is measured using the coefficient *b*, the indirect or mediation effect is thus calculated as:

$$Mediation\ effect = a \times b. \tag{8.5}$$

2. The *director effect*: the net effect of the X on the Y after the mediation effect is controlled, and this effect is expressed as c'.

The model in Fig. 8.12 provides a mechanism to detect both direct and indirect effect, enhancing the ability to disentangle the complex two-X and one-Y relationship. If results from statistical analysis indicated no direct effect, the conceptual model depicted in Fig. 8.12 will be the same as the model presented in Fig. 8.1.

With the conceptual model, an analytical model can be developed using the methods introduced in Chap. 5. The right part of Fig. 8.12 depicts the analytical models for mediation analysis, corresponding to the conceptual model in the left part of the figure. The analytical part consists of three regression models:

1. Association between X and M, the first part of the mediation effect, this relation can be expressed using a regression model:

$$Mediator\ M = intercept + a(influential\ factor\ X) + e \tag{8.6}$$

2. Associations between both the influential factor X and the mediator M with the outcome Y, and this relationship can be analyzed using the following two-factor regression model:

$$Outcome\,Y = intercept + b\left(Mediator\right) + c'\left(factorX\right) + e \qquad (8.7)$$

3. As a last part of the mediation analysis, the following simple regression model is added:

$$Outcome\,Y = intercept + c\left(factorX\right) + e, \qquad (8.8)$$

where the regression coefficient c is used to measure *the total effect* of the independent variable X on the outcome Y without considering the mediator M. Mathematically, the following relation holds among all the four estimated effects:

$$c = c' + \left(a \times b\right). \qquad (8.9)$$

Following Model 8.9, the total effect c of the influential factor X on the outcome Y is simply a sum of the direct effect c' and the indirect effect (a times b) With the estimated regression coefficient a, b, and c, the following two measures are often derived: (1) percent of the indirect effect $= \dfrac{a \times b}{c} = \%$; and (2) percent of the direct effect $= 100\% - \%$ indirect effect.

With data for X, M, and Y, all the model parameters a, b, c, and c' can be estimated using the linear regression methods introduced in Chap. 5.

8.5.3   *Confounders, Multiple Mediators and Covariates*

Although it takes a while to introduce the mediation modeling analysis, the model is not that complex relative to the interaction analysis introduced in the first part of this chapter. The main challenge is not the data analysis but the formation of a mediation model, considering the complex relations associated with the concept of confounders, moderators and mediators.

As discussed in Chap. 5, a confounder is a factor that is associated with both X and Y with the direction of connection ignored. From Fig. 8.12, a mediator is also associated with both X and Y with the direction of association imposed based on the literature or theoretical analysis. Therefore, with mediation analysis, some if not all confounders will no longer be problematic for etiological studies. On the contrary, a confounder could be a moderator as in previous sections or a mediator as in this part of the chapter. If a study has demonstrated the mediation effect with real data, the study uses the confounder as a key variable rather than simply controlling it. Therefore, mediation analysis will deepen our understanding of the etiology of a medical, health or a health-related behavioral problem.

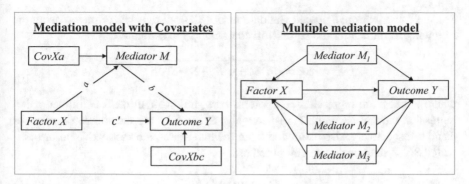

Fig. 8.13 Mediation modeling with covariates (left) and mediation model with multiple mediators (right)

Furthermore, demographic factors (i.e., age, gender, racial groups) can be added to a mediation model as covariates. The left part of Fig. 8.13 depicts a mediation model with covariates. In the model, CovXa represents covariates that affect the X-M association and CovXbc affecting the relationship between X and M on Y. These covariates can be added to the regression models 8.6 to 8.8 to obtain the adjusted a, b, c, and c' for mediation modeling.

As a natural extension, the mediation model presented in Fig. 8.12 can be extended to including multiple mediators. The right part of Fig. 8.13 presents a conceptual model of a mediation model with three mediators. Multiple mediators are used in epidemiological literature (Chen et al. 2011a, b; Yu and Chen 2020), including multiple mediators with chained mediation analysis (Yu and Chen 2020). As a taste of further development in this line of research, moderated (interaction) mediation modeling analysis is also developed and used in studies to address more complex causal relationships (Preacher et al. 2007).

8.5.4   Significant Test of the Mediation Effect

The significance of all model parameters in a mediation analysis can be obtained directly from the regression models with one exception: the mediation effect that is computed using formula 8.5. Formula 8.5 is not a statistical model, and therefore it cannot be used to test the significance of the computed indirect effect.

In developing the mediation modeling method, a statistical method called *Sobel test* (Baron and Kenny 1986) was developed to assess the significance of the estimated indirect effect. As the name suggests, the test is based on the previous work by a statistician Michael E. Sobel at Columbia University. In the mediation analysis, the indirect effect $a \times b$ is equal to the total effect c, minus the direct effect c'. Assuming that the difference in the two regression coefficients (c−c') following the

Student t distribution, a pooled standard error (SE) can thus be estimated using the following formula after the regression coefficients are estimated:

$$SE = \sqrt{b^2 S_a^2 + a^2 S_b^2 + S_a^2 \cdot S_b^2},$$

(8.10)

where a and b are regression coefficients (raw, not standardized) estimated using regression models 8.6 and 8.7, respectively; S_a^2 and S_b^2 are the standard errors for a and b respectively, also estimated from the two regression models. With the estimated SE, Z statistic can be computed as:

$$Z = (a \times b) / SE$$

(8.11)

With the estimated Z, statistical inference will be made based on the following criteria:

$p < 0.05$ if the estimated $Z > 1.96$; and $p < 0.01$ if the estimated $Z > 2.58$

The Sobel test is simple and can be completed manually. The Sobel test works the best if data for M and Y in the mediation analysis follow the normal distribution (continuous variable or categorical variables with a very large sample). If not normally distributed, advanced methods are used. One highly recommended method is bootstrapping that can be conducted using the published method/software (Preacher and Hayes 2004).

8.6   Mediation Analysis with Real Data

To demonstrate the methods, mediation modeling analysis will be conducted using data from the same source: the 2017–18 NHANES. More variables from the dataset used in Chap. 5 (DATCH5) are included by expanding the dataset DATCH8 that previously created and used for interaction analysis. In mediation analysis, the results would be more robust if the study sample is more homogenous. We will also demonstrate this point in the analysis examples presented in this section. As a demonstration, the mediation role of cigarette smoking in bridging the relationship between depression and sleeping problems will be used as an example.

8.6.1   Participants and Variables

To ensure internal validity, participants aged 20–64 are included. These participants represent the population at the working age range and their sleeping behavior differs from young children as well as those 65 years and older who are retired (Myllyntausta and Stenholm 2018). We also limit the participants to Whites knowing the large racial differences in smoking (Jamal et al. 2018) and mental health problems (Bailey et al. 2019). These selection criteria will increase the homogeneity of the study sample, in favor of etiological studies to make statistical inference without many concerns about differences in demographic factors. This approach can be used because of the large sample size of the 2017–18 NHANES data.

The influential factor X: *Depressive symptoms in the past two weeks* measured using the PHQ-9 questionnaire. This variable was described in detail in a previous chapter of this book.

Outcome variable Y: *Reported hours of sleep during the weekend.* Data available about hours of sleep during the weekdays and weekends are included and tested, and the measure for the weekend provides better results.

The mediator M: *Days smoked in the past 30 days.* A number of variables are available, but this is used because of the concurrent and short-term impact of smoking and sleeping problems

Covariates: *Age in year* and *gender (male and female)* as CovXa (for X-M relationship) and CovXac (for W and M as they are associated with Y), considering potential heterogeneity of the two relationships with regard to age and gender.

8.6.2   SAS Program for Data Process

Data from two sources are used for this demonstration. The first is for demographic factors, smoking behavior and depression, and they were derived from the dataset DATCH5 used in Chap. 5. Data on sleeping problems will be derived directly from the original dataset SLQ_J.XPT directly downloaded from the NHANES website. SAS Program 8.4 shows the steps to process the data.

```
*******************************************************************************
SAS PROGRAM 8.4 DATA PROCESSING FOR MEDIATION ANALYSIS;
*******************************************************************************;
** 1. OBTAIN DATA ON DAYS OF SMOKING AND DEPRESSON FROM DATCH5 USED IN CHAPTER 5;
LIBNAME SASDATA "C:\QUANTLAB\A_DATA\";
DATA TMP1; SET SASDATA.DATCH5;
* CODE SYSTEM MISSING AS ZERO FOR DAYS OF SMOKING IN THE PAST 30 DAYS;
IF SMKDAYS EQ. AND SMKYRS EQ 0 THEN SMKDAYS = 0;
KEEP SMKDAYS DEPRESS SEQN;
PROC CONTENTS; RUN;

** 2. GET DATA ON SLEEPING PROBLEMS FROM A NEW NHANES DATASET SLQ_J;
* READ, CONVERT AND PROCESS THE ORIGINAL SLQ_J FOR TWO SMOKING MEASURES;
LIBNAME XPTDATA XPORT " C:\QUANTLAB\A_DATA\ORIGINAL\SLQ_J.XPT" ACCESS=READONLY;
PROC COPY INLIB=XPTDATA OUTLIB= SASDATA; PROC CONTENTS; RUN;
DATA TMP2; SET LIB.SLQ_J;
SLPWKDS = SLD012;
SLPWKND = SLD013;
LABEL   SLPWKDS = "AVERAGE HOURS OF SLEEP DURING WEEK/WORK DAYS",
        SLPWKND = "AVERAGE HOURS OF SLEEP DURING WEEKEND DAYS";
KEEP SLPWKDS SLPWKND SEQN; PROC CONTENTS; RUN;

** 3. EXPAND THE DATCH8 BY ADDING THE TWO NEWLY CREATED TWO TMP DATASETS;
* READ DATCH8 TO BE EXPANDED;
DATA TMP3; SET SASDATA.DATCH8; PROC CONTENTS; RUN;
* SORT TMP1 TMP2 AND TMP3 RESPECTIVELY;
PROC SORT DATA=TMP1; BY SEQN; RUN;
PROC SORT DATA=TMP2; BY SEQN; RUN;
PROC SORT DATA=TMP3; BY SEQN; RUN;
* EXPAND DATCH8 BY MERGING ALL THREE TOGETHER;
DATA SASDATA.DATCH8; MERGE TMP1 TMP2 TMP3; BY SEQN; PROC CONTENTS; RUN;
*******************************************************************************;
```

SAS Program 8.4 is straightforward, and it consists of three parts. Part 1 is for getting the two key variables DEPRESS and SMKDAYS from DATCH5, the dataset that was created and used for analysis in Chap. 5. Part 2 is for processing of the original data from NHANES to obtain two variables, SLPWKDS and SLPWKND, measuring hours of sleep during the week/workdays and weekend days. Part 3 is for expanding the dataset DATCH8 that was created and used early in this chapter for interaction analysis.

8.6.3   Steps for Mediation Modeling Analysis

Mediation analysis is usually completed in four steps: First, a mediation model must be presented and used as a guidance to construct the regression model, to read and organized the analytical results, and to prepare and compute the final results based on the regression results. Although the three regression models for mediation analysis are simple, results from the model are not and cannot be directly used in reporting. It is very easy getting confused when collecting results to compute the final results for mediation modeling, and to report the findings.

Second, the mediation analysis often starts with a simple descriptive and correlation analysis to understand and select the variables for analysis. The best approach in this step is a simple linear correlation analysis with all related variables included. This is very similar to all the other multivariate analyses included in Chaps. 5, 6, and 7. The output of such analysis is often presented as a correlation coefficient matrix. Carefully review the results to see if the proposed mediation model is supported. If the three correlations between X and M, X and Y and M and Y are statistically significant, the proposed mediation model is supported; otherwise, no mediation analysis is needed.

Third, if results from the previous step of analysis suggest the existence of a mediation relationship, run the three regression models to obtain all the regression coefficients. Use the proposed mediation model, like the one presented in Fig. 8.12 (the left part) as guidance to link the estimated regression coefficients to the mediation model parameters a, b, c, and c'; and compute the indirect effect and conduct significance test.

Last, the analysis should be furthered to include covariates if the study sample is highly heterogeneous.

8.6.4   A Hypothetical Mediation Model for Demonstrative Analysis

Following the steps described above, we start the demonstration analysis using a hypothetical model based on literature search and/or pilot data. Figure 8.14 presents a hypothetical mediation model based on literature and findings from the analysis presented in Chap. 5 of the book. In the model, depression was used as X and smoking was used as M. This is based on the fact that after feeling depressed, a common

Fig. 8.14 A hypothetical mediation model to be tested using SAS Program 8.5 and 2017–18 NHANES data

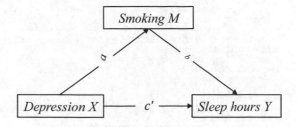

coping mechanism is for an individual to pick up a cigarette and smoke. This relationship has been repeatedly reported in the literature.

Hours of sleep were modeled as Y since both depression and smoking may interfere with normal sleep, reducing sleep quality, while hours of sleep provide one measure of the quality of sleep.

8.6.5 SAS Program for Mediation Modeling Analysis

Following the steps described above and the *hypothetical mediation model* as shown in Fig. 8.14, SAS Program 8.5 is prepared as a template for mediation analysis. This program consists of five parts.

In part 1 of the program, a work dataset B is created from the newly created data DATCH8 that was created using SAS Program 8.4. In this step, participants were also selected using the two criteria that are used to define the study population: (1) less than 65 years and (2) of White race.

Part 2 of the program shows the use of a simple correlation analysis to (1) obtain the descriptive measures (i.e., mean and SD) for all variables and (2) to assess the bivariate relationship among the key variables for mediation analysis and covariates. As a demonstration, two covariates, AGE and GENDER, were included.

It is worth noting that two variables measuring the same variable of sleep hours were included, and they are: SLPWKND and SLPWKDS. As described in Chap. 2, one variable can be measured using different indicators; the purpose here to include two alternative measures for one outcome variable is to demonstrate the selection of one among the two in favor of testing the proposed mediation model.

```
********************************************************************************
SAS PROGRAM 8.5 MEDIATION ANALYSIS WITH DATASET CREATED FROM SAS PROGRAM 8.4;
********************************************************************************;
** 1. CREATE A WORK DATASET AND SELECT STUDY PARTICIPANTS FROM A TOTAL OF 6161;
DATA B; SET SASDATA.DATCH8;
* SELECT THOSE AGED 20-64;
IF AGE LT 65;
* SELECT WHITES;
IF RACE5 EQ 1;
PROC CONTENTS; RUN;
** 2. SIMPLE CORRELATION ANALYSIS TO OBTAIN MEAN, SD, AND CORRELATION;
PROC CORR DATA = B;
VAR SLPWKND SLPWKDS SMKDAYS DEPRESS AGE GENDER;
RUN;
** 3. MEDIATION MODELING WITH NO COVARAITES;
PROC REG DATA = B;
* MODEL X ON MEDIATOR USING EQUATION 8.5;
MODEL SMKDAYS = DEPRESS /STB;
* MODELING X AND MEDIATOR ON Y USING EQUATION 8.6;
MODEL SLPWKND = DEPRESS SMKDAYS/STB;
* MODEL TOTAL EFFECT OF X ON Y USING EQUATION 8.7;
MODEL SLPWKND = SMKDAYS/STB;
WHERE DEPRESS NE .;  * ANALYSIS FOR SUBJECTS WITH NO MISSING ON DEPRESS;
RUN;
** 4. MEDIATION MODELING WITH GENDER AS COVARAITE;
PROC REG DATA = B;
MODEL SMKDAYS = DEPRESS /STB; *GENDER NOT ASSOCIATED WITH DEPRESS, NOT ADDED;
MODEL SLPWKND = DEPRESS SMKDAYS GENDER/STB;
MODEL SLPWKND = SMKDAYS GENDER/STB;
WHERE DEPRESS NE .;  * ANALYSIS FOR SUBJECTS WITH NO MISSING ON DEPRESS;
RUN;
** 5. MEDIATION MODELING WITH AGE AS COVARIATE;
PROC REG DATA = B;
MODEL SMKDAYS = DEPRESS /STB; *AGE NOT RELATED WITH DEPRESS AND SMOKING, NOT ADDED;
MODEL SLPWKND = DEPRESS SMKDAYS AGE/STB;
MODEL SLPWKND = SMKDAYS AGE/STB;
WHERE DEPRESS NE .;  * ANALYSIS FOR SUBJECTS WITH NO MISSING ON DEPRESS;
RUN;
********************************************************************************;
```

Part 3 consists of three regression models, showing the core part of mediation modeling analysis. From these three models, the parameters a, b, c, and c' can be estimated. With these estimated parameters, indirect effect can be computed, and a significant test can be conducted using the Sobel test.

Parts 4 and 5 show how to add covariates to a mediation model. Be advised, instead of putting all covariates, adding one covariate at a time and then comparing the results with the model without covariates is recommended. Performing the analyses this way, will help check the impact of individual covariates and can avoid over-controlling covariates by dropping the non-significant covariates.

Lastly, in all parts of analysis from 3 to 5, the statement WHERE DEPRESS NE . is used to ask the computer to conduct analysis only for participants with no missing data.

8.7 Results and Interpretation from Mediation Analysis

8.7.1 Results of Simple Correlation Analysis

Figure 8.15 displays the output of SAS Program 8.5 part 2 for descriptive statistics and correlation. From the top part of the figure, it can be seen that the mean and SD (Std Dev) of the six variables appeared to be reasonable. The mean of GENDER = 1.54 indicates that this variable was coded as 1 = male and 2 = female. The sample size N varied for different variables, suggesting missing values for various variables. For example, N = 755 for DEPRESS, the smallest among all, suggesting lots of missing while N = 825, was the largest for three variables (i.e., AGE, GENDER and SMKDAYS). These variables have no missing data in the dataset (see Chap. 9 for missing data).

The lower part of Fig. 8.15 displays the correlation among all six variables. Frist, of the two variables measuring sleep, the correlations of SLPWKND (hours of sleep during weekend days) with the other two variables (SMKDAYS and DEPRESS) were

Simple Statistics							
Variable	N	Mean	Std Dev	Sum	Minimum	Maximum	Label
SLPWKND	817	8.18299	1.62863	6686	2.00000	13.00000	AVERAGE HOURS OF SLEEP DURING WEEKEDN DAYS
SLPWKDS	820	7.54329	1.53737	6186	2.00000	14.00000	AVERAGE HOURS OF SLEEP DURING WEEK/WORK DAYS.
SMKDAYS	825	10.64242	13.93281	8780	0	30.00000	DAYS SMOKED IN THE PAST 30 DAYS 0-30.
DEPRESS	755	3.85828	4.68020	2913	0	25.00000	DEPRESSIVE SYMPTOMS PHQ SCALE SCORE
AGE	825	39.84242	12.03643	32870	20.00000	60.00000	AGE IN YEAR.
GENDER	825	1.53576	0.49902	1267	1.00000	2.00000	GENDER 1=MALE 2=FEMALE.

Pearson Correlation Coefficients Prob > |r| under H0: Rho=0 Number of Observations						
	SLPWKND	SLPWKDS	SMKDAYS	DEPRESS	AGE	GENDER
SLPWKND AVERAGE HOURS OF SLEEP DURING WEEKEDN DAYS	1.00000 817	0.52474 <.0001 816	-0.12709 0.0003 817	-0.07350 0.0442 750	-0.18527 <.0001 817	0.09402 0.0072 817
SLPWKDS AVERAGE HOURS OF SLEEP DURING WEEK/WORK DAYS.	0.52474 <.0001 816	1.00000 820	-0.03887 0.2662 820	-0.06211 0.0890 751	-0.12136 0.0005 820	0.10184 0.0035 820
SMKDAYS DAYS SMOKED IN THE PAST 30 DAYS 0-30.	-0.12709 0.0003 817	-0.03887 0.2662 820	1.00000 825	0.22988 <.0001 755	0.00851 0.8071 825	-0.07836 0.0244 825
DEPRESS DEPRESSIVE SYMPTOMS PHQ SCALE SCORE	-0.07350 0.0442 750	-0.06211 0.0890 751	0.22988 <.0001 755	1.00000 755	-0.00257 0.9439 755	0.05682 0.1188 755
AGE AGE IN YEAR.	-0.18527 <.0001 817	-0.12136 0.0005 820	0.00851 0.8071 825	-0.00257 0.9439 755	1.00000 825	-0.04856 0.1634 825
GENDER GENDER 1=MALE 2=FEMALE.	0.09402 0.0072 817	0.10184 0.0035 820	-0.07836 0.0244 825	0.05682 0.1188 755	-0.04856 0.1634 825	1.00000 825

Fig. 8.15 Descriptive statistics and correlation among variables used for mediation analysis: Output of SAS Program 8.5 part 2

stronger than the SLPWKDS (hours of smoking during work/weekdays) and all statistically significant. This result provides evidence supporting the selection of the SLPWKND as the outcome Y for mediation analysis.

Second, the correlation of the three key variables X (DEPRESS), M (SMKDAYS), and Y (SLPWKND) are in the right direction. The depression measure is positively correlated with the smoking measure ($r = 0.2299$, $p < 0.01$) while both the depression ($r = -0.0735$, $p < 0.05$) and smoking measure ($r = -0.1271$, $p < 0.01$) were negatively correlated with the hours of sleep measure. With these results, the data is ready for mediation modeling using the three selected variables.

Last, among the two demographic factors, GENDER was significantly correlated with M (SMKDAYS) and Y (SLPWKND) but not with X (DEPRESS); while AGE was significantly correlated only with Y (SLPWKND). These results will be used to set up the mediation models with covariates.

8.7.2 Mediation Analysis Results Without Covariates

Data model fit statistics for the three linear regression for mediation analysis, including variance test indicated a well fit of our data to the models described in SAS Program 8.5 part 3 (results not shown). Figure 8.16 displays the main results from the three regressions corresponding to models 8.6, 8.7, and 8.8.

Using the standard regression coeffients, the top part of Fig. 8.16 indicates that the estimated $a = 0.2237$, $p < 0.01$ for the M (SMKDAYS) to Y (SLPWKND) relation. Results in the middle part of Fig. 8.16 show that the estimated $b = -0.1371$, $p < 0.01$

Parameter Estimates							
Variable	Label	DF	Parameter Estimate	Standard Error	t Value	Pr > |t|	Standardized Estimate
Intercept	Intercept	1	7.97059	0.64255	12.40	<.0001	0
DEPRESS	DEPRESSIVE SYMPTOMS PHQ SCALE SCORE	1	0.67097	0.10690	6.28	<.0001	0.22368

Parameter Estimates							
Variable	Label	DF	Parameter Estimate	Standard Error	t Value	Pr > |t|	Standardized Estimate
Intercept	Intercept	1	8.39416	0.08474	99.05	<.0001	0
DEPRESS	DEPRESSIVE SYMPTOMS PHQ SCALE SCORE	1	-0.01521	0.01317	-1.15	0.2487	-0.04283
SMKDAYS	DAYS SMOKED IN THE PAST 30 DAYS 0-30,	1	-0.01623	0.00439	-3.70	0.0002	-0.13709

Parameter Estimates							
Variable	Label	DF	Parameter Estimate	Standard Error	t Value	Pr > |t|	Standardized Estimate
Intercept	Intercept	1	8.26481	0.07783	106.20	<.0001	0
DEPRESS	DEPRESSIVE SYMPTOMS PHQ SCALE SCORE	1	-0.02610	0.01295	-2.02	0.0442	-0.07350

Fig. 8.16 Main results of the mediation analysis testing the model in Fig. 8.14: Output of SAS Program 8.5 part 3

for the M (SMKDAYS) to Y controlling for depression; c' = −0.0428, p > 0.05 for the direct effect of X (DEPRESS) on Y (SLPWKND) controlling for M. The last part of Fig. 8.16 indicates the total effect c = −0.0735, measuring the X − Y relationship without controlling any other factors.

Be advised, in practice it can easily be confused to link various regresson coefficients to the coefficients a, b, c, and c' in a proposed mediation model. This is particularly true for beginners. If experiencing difficulties in recognizing which regression coefficient is for what part of the medaition path, please use Fig. 8.14, the hypothetical mediation model as a guidance.

8.7.3   Compute Indirect Effect, % Direct and Indirect Effect

From the results in Fig. 8.16, the estimated a = 0.2299 and b = −0.1268. Based on the definition and Eq. 8.5, the indirect (mediation effect) is estimated as (use 5 decimal points for computing to ensure 4 valid decimals from round up):

$$Mediation(indirect)effect = a \times b = 0.22368 \times -0.13709 = -0.03066.$$

Verification: The indirect effect = −0.03066, the direct c' = −0.01587, the estimated
   total effect c would be:
Total effect c = −0.03066–0.01587 = −0.07349. This is exactly the total effect estimated using the regression model (the last part of Fig. 8.16).

Compute the percentage of direct and indirect effect:

% direct effect = −0.04283/−0.07349 = 58.28%
% indirect effect = −0.03066/−0.07349 = 41.72%

8.7.4   Sobel Significance Test

All model coefficients from the mediation analysis were tested for sampling error with p value estimated except the indirect effect. Statistical tests must be conducted to assess if the estimated indirect effect is significantly different from zero using the Sobel test as described earlier. To conduct the Sobel test, we first need to estimate the SE of the indirect effect using formula 8.10. To use the formula, the following are to be derived from the SAS output in Fig. 8.16 (be advised, using raw regression coefficients for a and b):

a = 0.68154, the raw regression coefficient measuring the X-M relation;
S_a = 0.01015, the standard error of a;
b = −0.01496, the raw regression coefficient measuring the X-M relation controlling
   for M; and
S_b = 0.00417, the standard error of b

Computing the following intermediate statistics for estimating SE with the four parameter estimates presented above:

$a^2 = 0.68154 \times 0.68154 = 0.464497,$
$b^2 = -0.01496 \times -0.01496 = 0.000224,$
$S_a^2 = 0.10515 \times 0.10515 = 0.011057,$ and
$S_b^2 = 0.00417 \times 0.00417 = 0.000017.$

Computed using formula 8.10:

$$SE = \sqrt{0.04697 + 0.000224 + 0.011057 + 0.000017} = 0.00325.$$

Estimate the Sobel statistic Z using Eq. 8.11:

$$Z = a*b / SE = 0.68154 * -0.00417 / 0.00325 = 3.1399.$$

Make statistical inference with the estimated Z statistic: Since the estimated Z = 3.1339, greater than 2.58, thus p < 0.01 following the criteria presented after Eq. 8.11. Based on the result, it can be concluded that the indirect effect between depression and sleep mediated through smoking was statistically extremely significant.

8.7.5　Mediation Result Presentation and Interpretation

With mediation analysis, a figure is often used to present the final result. Figure 8.17 shows an example with result and related information included. A figure title clearly states the result. Instead of X, M, and Y, using the actual name of the related variables can usually enhance the presentation of the study findings. In most case, a note is also added to the table to describe the indirect effect (significant test result) that cannot be easily put in the figure.

With the statistical analysis and the computed results and the figure presented above, it is the time to state the findings and to draw conclusions. The following is an exemplary statement:

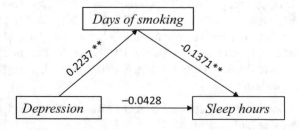

Fig. 8.17　Days of smoking during the weekend mediating the depression-hours of sleeping during the weekend. US Whites 20–64, N = 750, 2017–18 NHANES. (Note: Indirect effect = −0.0307, p < 0.01 from Sobel test; **: p < 0.01)

"Results from the mediation modeling analysis support the hypothetical model that people who suffer from depression would be more likely to smoke; and increased smoking will reduce the hours of sleep during the weekend days. Our analysis indicates that approximately 42% of the depression and poor sleep relationship is mediated through smoking, suggesting the importance of smoking cessation to improve quality of sleep."

"In addition to smoking, the estimated *direct effect* of depression on hours of sleep accounted for about 48% of the total effect. Although the effect was statistically not significant, additional studies are needed to examine this effect."

8.7.6 Analyses with Gender Included as a Covariate

In the analytical example presented above, studies are limited to White participant in working age range for a more homogenous study sample to ensure adequate internal validity. However, other covariates, such as gender and age, may still need to be considered. Further, results in Fig. 8.15 suggested significant correlations of these two factors with the other variables included in the mediation modeling analysis.

Figure 8.18 presents the results from SAS Program 8.5 part 4, in which gender was included as a covariate. The top panel of the figure shows the model to assess the effect of X (DEPRESS) on M (SMKDAYS) on the Y (SLPWKND). As it can be seen here, the variable GENDER was not included in the model since results in Fig. 8.15 indicated no significant association of this variable with depression. In other words, it acts parallel with depression to affect days of smoking. To avoid over

			Parameter Estimates					
Variable	Label	DF	Parameter Estimate	Standard Error	t Value	Pr > |t|	Standardized Estimate
Intercept	Intercept	1	7.97059	0.64255	12.40	<.0001	0
DEPRESS	DEPRESSIVE SYMPTOMS PHQ SCALE SCORE	1	0.67097	0.10690	6.28	<.0001	0.22368

			Parameter Estimates					
Variable	Label	DF	Parameter Estimate	Standard Error	t Value	Pr > |t|	Standardized Estimate
Intercept	Intercept	1	7.96563	0.20324	39.19	<.0001	0
DEPRESS	DEPRESSIVE SYMPTOMS PHQ SCALE SCORE	1	-0.01737	0.01317	-1.32	0.1876	-0.04891
SMKDAYS	DAYS SMOKED IN THE PAST 30 DAYS 0-30.	1	-0.01530	0.00440	-3.48	0.0005	-0.12928
GENDER	GENDER 1=MALE 2=FEMALE.	1	0.27707	0.11951	2.32	0.0207	0.08404

			Parameter Estimates					
Variable	Label	DF	Parameter Estimate	Standard Error	t Value	Pr > |t|	Standardized Estimate
Intercept	Intercept	1	7.78627	0.19806	39.31	<.0001	0
DEPRESS	DEPRESSIVE SYMPTOMS PHQ SCALE SCORE	1	-0.02784	0.01291	-2.16	0.0314	-0.07841
GENDER	GENDER 1=MALE 2=FEMALE.	1	0.31482	0.11990	2.63	0.0088	0.09549

Fig. 8.18 Regression results for mediation analysis using the hypothetical model in Fig. 8.14, output of SAS Program 8.5 part 4

adjustment, this variable was not included as a covariate. Without a covariate, this part of the result is identical to the corresponding part in Fig. 8.16.

Results presented in the middle and bottom panel of Fig. 8.18 differed from those in top panel of Fig. 8.18 after inclusion of gender as covariate. First, the effect of gender was positively and statistically significant in both models, suggesting the need to adjust for gender difference in the mediation analysis. Overall, the inclusion of GENDER did not change the mediation effect model. Students can also do the computing to check if the indirect effect remains to be significant with the adjusted model.

It is worth noting that after adjusting gender, results in the bottom panel of the figure indicate increases in the total effect c (from -0.0735 to -0.0784), consistent with the positive effect of gender on the regression coefficient (refer to Chap. 5 for details). With the adjustment of gender, the direct effect c' for depression also increased from -0.0428 to -0.0489. On the contrary, the estimated b from M (SMKDAYS) to Y (SLPWKND hours of sleep) reduced from -0.1371 to -0.1293.

In formal studies, adjusted results must be reported. This will be kept as part of the practice.

8.7.7 Analyses Adjusting for Age as Well as Both Gender and Age as Covariates

Likewise, additional analyses can also be conducted to include other demographic factors. SAS Program 8.5 part 5 shows the method to adjust age as a covariate. To save space, the results are not reported here. Students can use it as a practice. Certainly, models can also be constructed to include both gender and age as covariates. This will also be kept for practice.

As expressed in this book, the author is very careful about adding too many demographic factors and confounders into a model for analysis. A best practice for etiological studies with a large-scale of survey data is to identify a relatively more homogenous sample with regard to the study question first; then focus on the core variables to plan the analysis to test the study hypothesis.

8.8 Collider Effect of Two Influential Factors

8.8.1 Definition of Collider and Collider Effect

A relatively new concept discussed in the modern causal inference and epidemiology is the *collider effect*. It is the last one among the four relations covered in this book that involve two independent variables Xs and one outcome Y. Following the general understanding of covariates/confounders, a collider is a variable that is statistically associated with both X and Y; however as shown in Fig. 8.19, a confounder

Fig. 8.19 Conceptual model for the collider effect

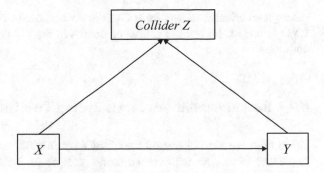

can be a collider only if it is eventually caused by X and Y. Instead of W for interaction and M for mediation, a collider is names as Z.

Recalling the mediation and interaction model, if a collider is included as either a moderator or a mediator, the statistical software will still generate all the statistics programed in the software, the results would be totally wrong. This is because no statistical software can tell the direction of any correlation. Therefore, it is important to be aware of the potential impact in etiological studies.

With the interaction and mediation modeling analysis introduced up to now, it is not hard to avoid models with a collider Z either used as a W or M if knowledge informs that Z is the outcome of X and Y. However, this could be an issue for pure data-driving studies with no or limited knowledge on the relationship among three variables. In other words, with adequate knowledge of epidemiology, it will not be hard to avoid misusing a Z as either W or M.

8.8.2 Collider Bias

Collider bias is another term that has been discussed in epidemiology these days (Banack and Kaufman 2014). Collider bias is referred to the case in which X and Y are not related with each other. However, if a collider Z is included in model like a mediation (see Fig. 8.19), the X ~ Y relation can become significant. One typical case about the collider bias reported in the literature is regarding the obesity paradox in which obesity was demonstrated to be a protective factor for cardiovascular disease (CVD) because of collider bias (Banack and Kaufman 2014). In their example with NHANES III data (2006) for 17,636 participants aged 20–80, when data were analyzed together, there was a positive relationship between obesity and risk of total mortality with OR = 1.24 (95% CI: 1.11, 1.39). However, when the same data were stratified by causes of deaths, the estimated OR = 0.79 (95% CI: 0.68, 0.61) for assessing the risk of obesity on CVD mortality, obesity is negatively associated with CVD.

The problem of the obesity-CVD paradox described above is termed as collider bias, also known as the selection collider bias. In this case, obesity (X) and total death (Y) are causally associated with CVD deaths. Obesity is a risk factor for total death and death from CVD; although total deaths are not the cause of CVD death in theory, numerically, deaths from CVD is proportionate with the total deaths since CVD is one of the leading causes of deaths in the US and many other developed countries.

8.9   Recommendations to Analyzing Two Influential Factors

Up to now, we have discussed a total of four possible scenarios in analyzing two influential factors Xs with one outcome Y. Each of the four should be addressed with a different approach.

If two influential factors each affect the outcome independently, do nothing. The method to check if such a relationship exist is to simply run a correlation of the two influential factors X_1 and X_2 and the outcome Y. If X_1 and X_2 are not related to each other and both X_1 and X_2 are related to Y, take the independent analysis approach.

If two influential factors X_1 and X_2 are related with each other while both of them are in turn related to Y as from the simple correlation analysis, three posibilities are likely: interaction, mediation, and colliding. The method to separate the three will be largely based on our knowledge about these variables. Therefore, it is very important to have a hypothesis (theory)-driven study in epidemiology.

If X_1 and X_2 have an interaction relationship, i.e., the relationship between X_1 on Y depends on the value of X_2, interaction analysis would be the choice; and the same is true if the $X_2 \sim Y$ relationship depends on X_1.

If a mediation mechanism exists in which X_1 bridges the $X_2 \sim Y$ relation or X_2 bridges the $X_1 \sim Y$ relation, a mediation effect model would be the choice for analysis. Construction of a mediation model requires adequate knowledge of the study question.

If one of the two influential factors is a collider, this means this variable is caused by the other influential factor and the outcome. In any case, avoid conducting any modeling analysis using such data. In particular, never include a collider as a confounder in a multiple regression model.

8.10   Practice

8.10.1   Statistical Analysis and Computing

1. Repeat all the interaction analysis models presented in this chapter to gain familiarity with the method and understanding the results.
2. Conduct interaction analysis with other variables included in the examples in the book and understand the results
3. Repeat all the mediation modeling analyses presented in this chapter to gain familiarity with the method and understanding the results. Complete the analyses that are included in the SAS program even where analytical results are not presented.

4. Conduct mediation modeling analyses for other variables included in the chapter that were not used in the demonstration analysis.
5. Conduct moderation and mediation modeling analysis with research questions of your own choice to test and practice your analytical skills.

8.10.2 Research Paper Update

1. Think of incorporating the interaction and/or mediation modeling to strengthen your own study project.
2. It is not required to incorporate the two methods into your own study. If you do not want to incorporate these two methods into your study, you are encouraged to practice the methods yourself.
3. Update your paper from the beginning to the end to reflect the addition of the new method and new results if you did incorporate new analyses for your study. For example, the paper title can be revised to highlight the new analytical methods (i.e., interaction or mediation); the abstract must be revised to reflect the new findings; all other parts of the paper, including the introduction, methods, results, and discussion should be updated.
4. Prepare for the final presentation. For most students, this could be the last step to finalize the research project. It is now that time to prepare the presentation to share your findings with your peers.

8.10.3 Study Questions

1. How many possibilities exist when studying two influential factors with one outcome in epidemiology?
2. Describe interaction using your own words.
3. Instead of controlling covariates, interaction and mediation presents two approaches to disentangle the complex relationships among three factors with two as the influential factors and one as the outcome. Comment on these two analytical approaches.
4. Define the collider effect. How should you avoid using colliders in interaction and mediation analysis?
5. Do we need to control/adjust for a collider in etiological studies?
6. In addition to controlling confounders, we learned how to turn confounders into influential factors through interaction and mediation analyses. Please use some examples to demonstrate the power of these two types of analyses.
7. What is positive interaction? What is negative interaction?
8. What is the total effect, direct effect, and indirect effect?
9. What is the condition to use the Sobel test in assessing the indirect effect in mediation analysis?

References

Ahadzadeh, A.S., Rafik-Galea, S., Alavi, M., Amini, M.: Relationship between body mass index, body image, and fear of negative evaluation: moderating role of self-esteem. Health Psychol. Open. **5**(1), 2055102918774251 (2018). https://doi.org/10.1177/2055102918774251

Bailey, R.K., Mokonogho, J., Kumar, A.: Racial and ethnic differences in depression: current perspectives. Neuropsychiatr. Dis. Treat. **15**, 603–609 (2019)

Banack, H.R., Kaufman, J.S.: The obesity paradox: understanding the effect of obesity on mortality among individuals with cardiovascular disease. Prev. Med. **62**, 96–102 (2014, May)

Baron, R.M., Kenny, D.A.: The moderator-mediator variable distinction in social psychological research – conceptual, strategic, and statistical considerations. J. Pers. Soc. Psychol. **51**(6), 1173–1182 (1986)

Barroso, B., Goday, A., Ramos, R., Marín-Ibañez, A., Guembe, M.J., Rigo, F., Tormo-Díaz, M.J., Moreno-Iribas, C., Cabré, J.J., Segura, A., Baena-Díez, J.M., et al.: Interaction between cardiovascular risk factors and body mass index and 10-year incidence of cardiovascular disease, cancer death, and overall mortality. Prev. Med. **107**, 81–89 (2018)

Caspi, A., Moffitt, T.: Gene–environment interactions in psychiatry: joining forces with neuroscience. Nat. Rev. Neurosci. **7**, 583–590 (2006)

Chen, X., Abdulhamid, I., Woodcroft, K.: Maternal smoking during pregnancy, polymorphic CYP1A1 and GSTM1, and lung-function measures in urban family children. Environ. Res. **111**(8), 1215–1221 (2011a)

Chen, X., Dinaj-Koci, V., Brathwaite, N., Cottrell, L., Deveaux, L., Gomez, P., et al.: Development of condom-use self-efficacy over 36 months among early adolescents: a mediation analysis. J. Early Adolesc. **32**(5), 711–729 (2011b)

Cornelius, T., Birk, J.L., Edmondson, D., Schwartz, J.E.: The joint influence of emotional reactivity and social interaction quality on cardiovascular responses to daily social interactions in working adults. J. Psychosom. Res. **108**, 70–77 (2018)

Hashibe, M., Brennan, P., Chuang, S.-C., Boccia, S., Castellsague, X., Chen, C., et al.: Interaction between tobacco and alcohol use and the risk of head and neck cancer: pooled analysis in the international head and neck cancer epidemiology consortium. Cancer Epidemiol. Biomark. Prev. **18**(2), 541–550 (2009)

Hayes, A.F.: Beyond Baron and Kenny: statistical mediation analysis in the new millennium. Commun. Monogr. **76**(4), 408–420 (2009)

Hunter, D.: Gene–environment interactions in human diseases. Nat. Rev. Genet. **6**, 287–298 (2005). https://doi.org/10.1038/nrg1578

Jamal, A., Phillips, E., Gentzke, A.S., Homa, D.M., Babb, S.D., King, B.A., Neff, L.J.: Current cigarette smoking among adults – United States, 2016. Morb. Mortal. Wkly Rep. **67**(2), 53–59 (2018)

Lam, L.T.: Internet gaming addiction, problematic use of the internet, and sleep problem: a system review. Curr. Psychiatry Rep. **16**, 444 (2014). https://doi.org/10.1007/s11920-014-0444-1

Lippold, K.M., Jones, C.M., Olsen, E.O., Giroir, B.P.: Racial/ethnic and age group differences in opioid and synthetic opioid–involved overdose deaths among adults aged ≥18 years in metropolitan areas – United States, 2015–2017. Morb. Mortal. Wkly Rep. **68**(43), 967–973 (2019)

Myllyntausta, S., Stenholm, S.: Sleep before and after retirement. Curr. Sleep Med. Rep. **4**(4), 278–283 (2018)

Preacher, K.J., Hayes, A.F.: SPSS and SAS procedures for estimating indirect effects in simple mediation models. Behav. Res. Methods Instrum. Comput. **36**, 717–731 (2004)

Preacher, K.J., Rucker, D.D., Hayes, A.F.: Addressing moderated mediation hypotheses: theory, methods and prescriptions. Multivar. Behav. Res. **42**(1), 185–277 (2007)

Vanderweele, T.J., Vansteelandt, S., Robins, J.M.: Effect decomposition in the presence of an exposure-induced mediator-outcome confounder. Epidemiology. **25**(2), 300–306 (2014)

Ward, J.B., Gartner, D.R., Keyes, K.M., Fliss, M.D., McClure, E.S., Robinson, W.R.: How do we assess a racial disparity in health? Distribution, interaction, and interpretation in epidemiological studies. Ann. Epidemiol. **29**, 1–7 (2019)

Yu, B., Chen, X.: Relationship among social capital, employment uncertainty, anxiety, and suicidal behaviors: a chained multi-mediator mediation modeling analysis. Arch. Suicide Res. Online. (2020, July 22). https://doi.org/10.1080/13811118.2020.1793044

Chapter 9
Data Quantity, Missing Data, and Imputing

Ignore a problem and you will miss the chance to solve it.

Data quality is the key for quantitative epidemiology. Errors in data can occur in all steps of research from research design to data collection, data processing, and statistical analysis. Data errors can be reduced but cannot be avoided. Therefore, investigators must pay attention to this issue. Most data errors can hardly be fixed after data are collected and stored on a computer, but there is one exception – missing data. Although missing data are not exactly an error, the impact of missing data cannot be ignored. Missing data are common in quantitative analysis of survey data. Different from other data errors, methods are developed to help check the data for missingness, including the missing pattern as well as the method fill in the missing data when appropriate. In this chapter, we will discuss issues related to missing data, as well as methods to check and fill in the missing data.

9.1 Data Quality and Bias in Epidemiology

No one will disagree that valid results of a study depend on the quality of data, and this is particularly important for epidemiology. As discussed in Chaps. 1 and 2, a research project consists of a series of closely connected steps carefully engineered to ensure the success of the research. Measures to ensure data quality often included in all research steps starting with the study design and ending with the data analysis.

9.1.1 Quality Data

Data quality can be defined as *the closeness of the observed values of a* variable *to the character the variable is intended to measure*. Data quality can be assessed at the individual research participant level. For qualitative measures, if a male gender

© The Author(s), under exclusive license to Springer Nature Switzerland AG 2021
X. Chen, *Quantitative Epidemiology*, Emerging Topics in Statistics and
Biostatistics, https://doi.org/10.1007/978-3-030-83852-2_9

is mismarked as female, a healthy participant is misclassified as sick, a smoker is grouped with nonsmokers, such data will have no quality. For quantitative measures, such as an incorrect measurement of blood pressure or incorrect use of a measurement unit (such as lb. vs. kg) will reduce data quality.

Data quality can also be assessed at the study sample level. Data quality would not be high if the study sample does not correctly reflect the study population despite quality data from individual participants. Data quality would be problematic if the tools used to collect data are lack of reliability, sensitivity, and/or validity. Data quality would also not be high if many variables in a dataset have missing data due to refusal of participation, withdrawal during the middle of a study, and/or skipped many survey questions during the data collection.

9.1.2 Data Error and Biases

Data errors are often associated with the concept of bias that has been intensively discussed in epidemiology. Typical examples include selection bias, respondent bias, and personnal bias. Selection bias is referred to as the discrepancy between the study sample we obtained and the true sample we intend to have. Selection bias thus can occur (1) if the study population we defined substantially differs from the true population we intend to study, (2) errors due to random sampling, and (3) errors due to volunteering participation during recruitment and withdrawing during data collection process.

Respondent bias is referred to as errors that originated from the study participants when they responded to survey questions in data collection. Errors due to respondent bias are most common and the error often occur in the following conditions: (1) incorrect or incapable of reading and/or comprehending a survey question, (2) errors in memory or memory loss, (3) error in recall, also known as recall bias, (4) purposefully editing responses for sensitive/intrusive questions to avoid social punishment or to gain social rewards, and (5) skipping questions as a right permitted by law.

Personnal bias is referred to as errors made by researchers, particularly persons involved in (1) data collection, known as data collector bias, (2) data processing, known as data processing bias, and (3) statistical analysis. Of these biases, data collector bias is the most common. Data collector bias can occur due to a lack of training for data collection, poor adherence to the data collection protocols, errors when manually entering data into a computer, errors when recoding variables, mismatching during data merging, and so forth.

9.2 Missing Data and How Do They Occur?

Missing data is an issue almost all epidemiologists who rely on quantitative data have to address. Missing data can occur in various different conditions. Although nothing can be done to prevent missing data after the data are collected, knowledge about contributing factors to missing data will inform researchers to know the data that have already been collected, and to think of methods to deal with the missing.

Many factors may contribute to missing data in research studies. We will focus on the following three: (1) factors related to study participants for voluntary participation and withdraw, (2) missing data due to issues related to data collection instruments/survey questionnaires, and (3) missing data accidently occurred in data processing.

9.2.1   Missing Data Related to Study Participants

Missing data related to study participants consist of the main source for missing. By law to protect human subjects, all research projects with a plan to collect data directly from human participants must warrant the rights for them to refuse to participate in data collection even after they have been consented to; they can also skip any questions they do not feel conformable answering or simply do not want to answer.

If a person refuses to participate at the beginning, there would be no missing data in the dataset since this person will not be included in the study and will be replaced with another person who agrees to participate. However, if a person agreed to participate but refuses to answer a question simply because he/she does not want to or does not feel comfortable answering, this person has the right to skip the question. Consequently, missing data are generated.

In longitudinal studies with follow-up assessments, if a participant agreed to participate and provided data at one wave of data collection, he/she can, permitted by law, refused to participate in subsequent assessments. In some cases, participants who withdrew from one wave of data collection re-joined the study later as their right. In both cases, missing data for all variables will occur during the wave(s) when these participants were absent.

Attrition is another source of missing data in multi-wave longitudinal studies. In this case, participants have missing data not because they do not want to participate, but because they cannot. Typical examples of attrition include that a participant (1) was moved to other places or migrated to other countries, (2) was died or too sick at the time for data collection, (3) had a time conflict for data collection, or (4) was simply due to lost to follow-up (e.g., contact information changed). This type of missing is termed as missing due to attrition.

9.2.2   Missing Related to Survey Questionnaire and Delivery

Questions in a survey instrument/questionnaire and survey delivery method consist of two important sources for missing data. In epidemiological studies, missing data will occur if a study needs to collect data by asking sensitive or intrusive questions. Depending on the cultural and social backgrounds, many questions can be perceived as sensitive or intrusive. For example, questions are considered sensitive or intrusive if they are related to age, sex, immigration status, income, self-image, dating and sexual behavior, tobacco, and alcohol and illicit drug use and abuse.

When coming across a sensitive or intrusive question, concerns of potential harms to one's own interest may be raised by disclosure of the information with regard to the survey question. If a participant thinks the question is too sensitive or too intrusive, he/she may decide to skip the question since this is the right all study participants are entitled to. Missing data occurs when a participant skips a survey question.

In addition to sensitive and intrusive questions, another issue is the comprehension of a survey question. Sometimes, a survey question can be too "hard" for participants with limited education to understand and they may also skip the question, leading to missing data. Occasionally, when a survey question adopted from studies conducted in another country is not appropriate, this can also lead to missing data. For example, most people in low-income countries do not drive and any survey questions that are related to using a car may lead to missing data.

Missing data can also occur accidently when data are collected using the traditional paper-and-pencil method. This is particularly problematic when the blank spaces between individual questions are small, answer options are not appropriately aligned with individual questions, or using a separate answer sheet like in the standardized exams. In addition to errors, missing data can occur simply because of accident errors in matching the selected response to the question. This type of missing data will be minimized using computerized survey or online survey.

A number of methods are used in administer survey questions, including the conventional paper-and-pencil method, computer-assisted interview, audio computer-assisted self-interview and online. Missing data are more likely to occur using paper-and pencil method and less likely to occur using the modern computer-based method or online.

9.2.3 Missing Due to Error in Data Entering and Processing

Missing data can also be generated during data processing and recoding. As we have experienced in processing the data for statistical analysis since Chap. 2 in this book, missing data can be generated accidently when new variables are created, and datasets are merged to create a new dataset for analysis.

First, missing data due to error can occur when survey data on papers are manually entered into a computer. Manual data entering is time-consuming and boring. Reductions in work efficiency may lead to both wrong and missing data. As a quality control measure, a dual-enter protocol is often used for manual data entry in which two persons independently enter the data into a computer. After the data entry is completed, a comparison will be made, and identified discrepancies between the two datasets will be resolved by checking with the original data.

Second, missing data can result when new variables are created in data processing. As demonstrated in various chapters in this book, when creating a new variable, a logic condition is often used. Missing data can be generated accidently if the condition is not specified correctly. As an illustrative example, in some studies, the variable gender is coded such that 1 means male and 0 means female; while in other studies, 1 means male and 2 means female. If gender is used as a condition to code a new variable and 2 is used as female, ignoring that 0 is for female, a large number of missing data will be generated for the newly coded variable.

In addition to conditional coding, missing data can be generated when combining two datasets with different sample sizes. We have described this issue in Chap. 7 when learning the Cox proportional hazard regression model. To conduct the analysis, datasets from two different sources with different sample sizes were combined. To avoid generating a large number of missing data, a special data procedure in the data step of the SAS program was devised and used (see SAS Program 7.2, Chap. 7).

Among various types of missing data, missing during error in manual data entry and data processing can be corrected. For example, dual-entry protocol can be used to correct missing data and other data errors. Be careful in data processing, dataset combination, and variable coding to avoid accidental errors.

9.3   Potential Impacts of Missing Data

Among various data errors, missing data is an error that can be observed directly. Understanding the impact of missing data is thus important for an epidemiologist to assess data quality and to think of methods to deal with it. In this section, we will discuss two main impacts of missing data: statistical power and internal validity.

9.3.1   Reducing the Statistical Power

One obvious impact of missing data is the *reduction of statistical power*. Statistical power is the ability to find a hypothetic relation if such relation really exists. More details about statistical power will be covered in Chap. 10. As a rule of thumb, a larger sample size will ensure greater statistical power. When subjects with missing data are excluded, the sample size will be reduced, so does the statistical power.

Few statistical methods can handle missing data. Therefore, observations with missing data are to be excluded. By exclusion of observations with missing data, the effective sample size will be reduced, thus lowering the statistical power. If extra samples were added during the period of study design and subjects with missing are limited, it may not be an issue to exclude observations with missing data. However, if increasing the sample size is associated with substantial increases in cost for data collection, it is very likely that there is little room for excluding participants with missing data.

In many large-scale national studies, the sample size is often very large, ranging from several thousands to tens of thousands. In such cases, the impact of missing data on statistical power could be minor. However, for various studies with a focus on special issues, the costs for data collection are either very high or limited by the budget of a study. In this case, study samples are often determined through careful power analysis (covered in Chap. 10) to achieve the required statistical power. In this case, the impact of missing data on statistical power will be significant, a small reduction in the sample size may make a study inadequately powered to find a real X ~ Y relationship.

9.3.2   Reducing the Internal Validity

Relative to statistical power, another impact of missing data is that it may affect causal inference because of differential missing. *Differential missing* is referred to the cases in which the rate of missing differ for participants with and without the health outcome of interest. This type of missing will make the proportion of the study sample with and without the health outcome differ from the true proportion of the study population.

Differential missing can occur in different conditions. For example, in clinical-based studies, participants with the disease of study are less likely to withdraw (wanting more knowledge and care), leading to lower missing rates for the patients than for the healthy controls; while in community-based studies, participants with the disease of study are more likely to withdraw (disclosure concerns), leading to higher missing rates for the patients than for the healthy controls.

Differential missing data will lead to incorrect estimates of an X ~ Y association, reducing the internal validity of a study. To ensure quality research, efforts must be used to reduce differential missing in all steps of a research study from study design to participant recruitment, data collection, data quality assessment, statistical analysis, result interpretation and causal inference.

9.4   Patterns of Missing Data

Correcting missing data requires adequate knowledge regarding the patterns and statistical mechanisms about the missing data. In this section, we will first introduce several anticipated patterns of missing data, and then discuss three well-known mechanisms of missing: Missing completely at random, missing at random and missing not at random. These three mechanisms are essential for imputing missing data.

9.4.1 Observed Missing Patterns

From the discussions in Sect. 9.2, three typical missing patterns in a dataset are anticipated: Missing Pattern 1 – missing data for all or almost all variables of an observation; Missing Pattern 2 - missing data for a variable for all or almost all observations; and Missing Pattern 3 - missing data scattered around for some variables and/or some observations.

Missing Pattern 1: Fig. 9.1 is a hypothetical dataset showing Missing Pattern 1 in which missing data are present for all or almost all variables of an observation. In the figure, the first column **OBS** represents observations. The first observation is labeled as **A01**, the second as **A02**,... The first row presents 12 variables in the dataset, including **AGE, SEX, RACE, EDU** (education), **INC** (income), **MRG** (marriage), **HGH** (height), **WGT** (weight), **MET** (metabolic syndrome), **HBP** (high blood pressure), and **CVD** (cardiovascular diseases).

OBS	AGE	SEX	RACE	EDU	INC	MRG	HGT	WGT	MET	HBP	CVD
A01	18	1	5	2	25	0	165	70	0	0	0
A02	22	1	1	1	40	0	180	90	0	1	0
A03	.	.	.	.	.	.	.	.	.	.	.
B00	38	1	1	1	36	1	160	58	1	0	0
A04	44	2	4	3	41	0	175	83	0	0	1
B05	65	1	.	.	.	.	.	.	.	.	.
A00	46	2	1	3	40	1	155	63	0	1	0
C08	37	2	3	2	28	1	172	75	1	1	0
C02	50	1	2	1	36	0	190	110	0	1	1

Fig. 9.1 Missing Pattern 1: Missing data for all or almost all variables for an observation (*EDU* education, *INC* income, *MRG* marriage, *HGH* height, *WGT* weight, *MET* metabolic syndrome, *HBP* high blood pressure, *CVD* cardiovascular disease)

In the figure, observation (**A03**) has data missing for all variables and the observation (**B05**) has data only for **AGE** and **SEX** and data are missing for the rest of the variables. The first case could be caused by refusing to participate after agreeing to at the beginning of the study, and the second case could be caused by withdrawing after answering the questions on age and sex.

This missing pattern appears frequently in many large-scale and national survey studies. Since data are missed for almost all variables among a certain number of observations, observations with this type of missing are often excluded from analysis.

Missing Pattern 2: Fig. 9.2 depicts this pattern of missing in which missing data are presented for a few variables of all or almost all observations. Pattern 2 of missing data is more common than Pattern 1 in epidemiology. This pattern of missing is particularly common in studies addressing very special topics, such as HIV/AIDS

OBS	AGE	SEX	RACE	EDU	INC	MRG	HGT	WGT	MET	HBP	CVD
A01	18	1	5	2	.	0	165	70	0	0	0
A02	22	1	1	1	.	0	180	90	.	1	0
A03	35	1	3	3	.	1	152	61	.	1	0
B00	38	1	1	1	.	1	160	58	.	0	0
A04	44	2	4	3	.	0	175	83	.	0	1
B05	36	1	1	2	.	1	165	70	.	1	0
A00	46	2	1	3	.	1	155	63	1	1	0
C08	37	2	3	2	.	1	172	75	.	1	0
C02	50	1	2	1	.	0	190	110	.	1	1

Fig. 9.2 Missing Pattern 2: Missing data of a variable for all or almost all observations (*EDU* education, *INC* income, *MRG* marriage, *HGH* height, *WGT* weight, *MET* metabolic syndrome, *HBP* high blood pressure, *CVD* cardiovascular disease)

and other sexually transmitted infections, and research related to the gender minority of individuals in the LGBTQ+ community.

Type 2 missing occurs most likely because of the following reasons:

1. The question is too sensitive to all or almost all participants and no one, or only a few participants, provided data for the variable.
2. The question is not relevant. For example, questions asking about attending bars or driving cars in low-income countries.
3. Potential system errors such as errors in data entry, data transforming across different platforms (i.e., transfer from excel spread sheet to SAS dataset, SPSS dataset, or csv dataset) and merging, etc.

Missing Pattern 3: Fig. 9.3 depicts this type of missing pattern. Missing Pattern 3 is characterized by the missing data points that are scattered across both observations and variables. For example, observation **A04** has missing data for **AGE**, observation **B00** has missing data for **RACE**, observation **A01** has missing data on **MRG** (marriage), and observation **B05** has missing data on **HGT** (body height) and **WGT** (body weight), etc.

This pattern of scattered missing is most common in real studies and the missingness can be caused by many factors as discussed early in this chapter. This is also the type of missing data that can be filled with imputing methods if the missing data follows certain mechanisms, such as missing at random which will be discussed next.

OBS	AGE	SEX	RACE	EDU	INC	MRG	HGT	WGT	MET	HBP	CVD
A01	18	1	5	2	25	.	165	70	0	0	0
A02	22	1	1	1	40	0	180	90	1	.	0
A03	35	1	3	3	18	1	152	61	0	1	0
B00	38	1	.	1	36	1	160	58	1	0	0
A04	.	2	4	3	41	0	175	83	1	0	1
B05	36	1	1	2	25	1	.	.	0	1	.
A00	46	1	1	3	.	1	155	63	0	1	0
C08	37	2	3	2	28	1	172	75	0	1	0
C02	50	1	2	1	36	0	190	110	1	1	1
C06	61	1	.	1	.	1	173	90	1	0	1
B14	40	2	3	1	62	1	165	75	1	0	1

Fig. 9.3 Missing Pattern 3: Scattered missing data for some variables among some observations (*EDU* education, *INC* income, *MRG* marriage, *HGH* height, *WGT* weight, *MET* metabolic syndrome, *HBP* high blood pressure, *CVD* cardiovascular disease)

9.5 Mechanisms of Missing

One purpose of understanding missing data is to think of methods to deal with them in order to reduce/minimize the impact of missing data on the internal validity of a study, and to fill in the missing data wherever possible. In the literature on missing data, three mechanisms are well investigated, and they are: missing completely at random, missing at random, and missing not at random (Rubin 1976; Enders 2010).

9.5.1 Missing Completely at Random (MCAR)

As the name suggests, missing completely at random (MCAR) is referred to the conditions in which the probability of missing for any variable of any observation is independent of all the variables of interest in the dataset. In other words, the causes of missing data are not related to the collected data but due to some other cause that cannot be controlled by the investigators as well as the study participants. An example of MCAR is that a measurement scale was broken at the time when a participant came to measure body weight. This participant would thus end up with missing data. This participant had missing data on body weight simply because of a bad luck that the scale was broken. Another example of MCAR is when a participant could not be able to complete a part of the assessment on the scheduled date and time because of a bad weather, a disease, an injury, or a disaster (i.e., fire, flooding, and earthquake).

Although MCAR is rarely in the real world, this concept has been often discussed in the context of missing data as the reference to demonstrate other mechanisms of missing. Furthermore, since the data are missed at random, statistically, the missingness will not qualitatively affect the analytical results for causal inference. In other words, ignorance of such missing data will not affect the interval validity of a study. If there are only a few numbers of observations with missing data that are MCAR, simply exclude them. If exclusion of the observations with missing data will significantly reduce the sample size, the missing data can be filled with simple methods, such as mean of the variable. The imputing with sample mean will be discussed in the next section.

It is challenging to determine if the missingness in a collected dataset meets the criteria of MCAR. Based on the definition of MCAR, the author of this book proposes an empirical method to evaluate the data. As shown in Fig. 9.4, the following steps can be used to assess if missing data for the variable **AGE** is MCAR.

1. Create a variable **MISS** based on the missing data for **AGE**: **MISS** = 0 if **AGE** in the data has no missing and **MISS** =0 if data for **AGE** is missed.
2. Conduct a simple correlation analysis of the newly created variable **MISS** with all other variables in the data set.
3. Decision-making: If the estimated correlation coefficient r between the new variable **MISS** and any other variables in the dataset was not statistically significant at $p < 0.05$ level, the missing for **AGE** can be considered as MCAR.

OBS	AGE	MISS	SEX	RACE	EDU	INC	MRG	HGT	WGT	MET	HBP
A01	18	0	1	5	2	25	.	165	70	0	0
A03	35	0	1	1	1	40	0	180	90	1	.
B00	38	0	1	3	3	18	1	152	61	0	1
A04	.	1	1	.	1	36	1	160	58	1	0
B05	36	0	2	4	3	41	0	175	83	1	0
A00	46	0	1	1	2	25	1	.	.	0	1
C08	37	0	1	1	3	.	1	155	63	0	1
C02	50	0	2	3	2	28	1	172	75	0	1
B14	40	0	1	2	1	36	0	190	110	1	1
A16	.	1	1	.	1	.	1	173	90	1	0
B09	27	0	2	3	1	62	1	165	75	1	0

Fig. 9.4 Illustration to assess if missing data for AGE is completely at random (MCAR)

It is worth noting that the method described above is very exploratory, and no rigorous statistical tests have been conducted to verify the method. Interested researchers can test and finalize the method.

9.5.2 Missing at Random (MAR)

The second and the most commonly discussed, practically widely used mechanism is missing at random (MAR). MAR is a very intriguing, even misleading term. When discussing the term MAR, we eventually mean that the missed values of a variable can be expressed with information from all variables included in the dataset. Because of the relationship between the missed data and the observed data, data can be generated (imputed) randomly to fill in the missing data. It is in this regard, that the missing values seemed to have occurred randomly since randomly generated data are used to replace missing data.

Missing at random (MAR) is the foundation for imputing missing data using various established methods. However, it is worth noting that MAR is simply an assumption to justify methods used to impute data; it is not an intrinsic property of the collected data at hand. Different from MCAR that requires the missingness is independent of all variables in the dataset, MAR assumes that the missed values are highly correlated with all variables in the dataset with data, thus variables without missing data can be used to predict the missed values for the variables with missing data. We will discuss more about MAR in later sections of this chapter for imputing missing data. Since the missing values are randomly imputed, it implies that the missingness occurred at random or MAR.

9.5.3 Missing Not at Random (MNAR)

Opposite of MCAR, missing not at random (MNAR) is referred to the condition where missing data did not occur randomly, but are related to values of the study variables and/or the research topic. For example, participants with lower education are more likely to have missing data on education; participants with HIV infections are more likely to not report their infection status or even drop out from the study; a person with depression is more likely to not answer questions that measure depression; and overweight participants are more likely to have missing data on body measurement or drop out of the study. In all these conditions, the missing data generated are not random, and they can be termed as MNAR.

Data error due to MNAR is highly problematic because exclusion of such data will lead to biased results, jeopardizing the internal validity of a study. One way to assess the MNAR for a dataset is to contact the participants and ask the reason for missing. If the reason is not related to the variable with missing but some random factors as in MCAR, the missing will not be MNAR; otherwise, the missing will be MNAR.

Brief analyses can also be conducted to check missing values by demographic and socioeconomic factors. If missing occurred randomly, the frequency of subjects with missing value of a variable should more or less be similar across demographic and socioeconomic groups. If the frequency of missingness varies substantially across groups, the missingness is very likely to not be random.

In theory, MNAR can never be MCAR; but MNAR can be MAR if the missingness meets the criteria – the missed values for the variable are closely related to all the variables in a dataset with no missing values.

9.6   Methods for Missing Data Imputing and Analysis

Missing data are a common issue, and they can have significant effects on the analytical results, leading to inaccurate and even invalid conclusions. There is no consensus with regard to whether the missing data should be imputed or if subjects with missing data should be excluded. This is because missing data is a special type of error, and we do not know what the value for the missing data would be; while the missed data are imputed, new errors may be introduced.

However, in many cases in practice, maintaining sample size to ensure adequate statistical power is needed to prove a study hypothesis. Furthermore, relevant methods have been developed for use to fill in the missing data with reasonable assumptions. Typical examples include mean imputing, imputing with k-nearest neighbors (Cheng et al. 2019), imputing with random forest method (Tang and Ishwaran 2017), and multiple imputing (Sterne et al. 2009). In addition, rigorous analytical approaches are developed to test if the imputed data are valid, such as sensitivity analysis by comparing results with and without the imputed data. In this section, we will briefly introduce two methods: mean imputing, which is the simplest, and multiple imputing (MI), which is widely used.

9.6.1   *Check the Missing Data Before Imputing*

To impute missing data, the very first step is to check missing data in the dataset using the patterns we discussed in Sect. 9.4. With data on hand, this can be completed using SAS Procedure **PROC FREQ**. In addition to frequencies of the observed values, this procedure also generates frequency for a variable with missing data. As mentioned early, if only a few observations, say <5% with missing data on one or two variables, and exclusion of these observations would not significantly reduce sample size, the best approach would be to simply drop these observations and go back to data analysis.

If the number of observations with missing data for some key variables is big, say greater than 5%, excluding these observations will reduce sample size substantially, and power analysis (Chap. 10) indicates that the effective sample size will not be adequate to achieve 80% statistical power for your study, imputing missing values would be one approach to maintain the sample size to save the study.

It is worth noting that the SAS Procedure **PROC FREQ** is not efficient to evaluate the combined missingness of more than one variable simultaneously. For example, the **PROC FREQ** is not efficient to assess if a participant has missing data on age, gender, and race, which may also be very useful. Fortunately, this issue can be solved with **PROC MI**, which will be introduced in Sect. 9.7 for real data analysis.

9.6.2   Mean Imputing

The simplest way to impute the missing value is to fill in the missed values with the mean of the same variable with observed data. For example, by checking your data, you noted that 6 of the total 128 observations have missing data for the variable **AGE**. In this case, you first compute the mean age with data from the 122 observations with data, and then replace the missing data with the mean.

When imputing the missing value with mean, it serves as a way mainly to maintain the sample size, since the imputed data do not provide any information (no change in SD) about the participants with missing data. If MCAR, the missing values can be considered as a subsample randomly selected from the total sample, the mean computed with observations without missing data would be a good approximate of the observations with missing data; otherwise, replacement of missing values with the sample mean may lead to biased results.

9.6.3   Multiple Imputing

Multiple imputing (MI) is a widely accepted method to impute missing data. This method is based on the MAR assumption. First, a predictive relationship must be seen between the missed values of the variables and the observed values of all the variables in the dataset. Second, more than one set of complete data will be generated randomly through a special random process, such as Markov Chain Monte Carlo (MCMC) simulation. The name MI is used to reflect the imputed results of more than one, or multiple complete datasets imputed randomly (usually 3–5 datasets). Third, conduct analysis using the multiple imputed datasets one at a time. After completion of the analysis, results from the multiple datasets will be summarized to get the final results.

The advantage of the MI method is that it uses all the information contained in the dataset with complete data; the imputed data are randomly generated, thus all observations are independent from each other. This is different from the mean imputing in which the mean of a variable for missing data is computed with the data of the same variable for other participants (i.e., not independently but closely related). In addition to the mean, missing data imputed using MI also brings in the variation for the observations with missing data.

For the MI method to work well, the overall data quality must be high to ensure high quality of the imputed data. Furthermore, the more variables in the dataset and the larger the study sample, the better the imputed data. This logic is obvious since the imputed data are generated based on the data for subjects without missing data. High data quality is the foundation of the imputed data and more observations in the data will provide more information to impute the missed data.

9.6.4 Sensitivity Analysis

Given so many limitations to the imputed data, analytical approaches are imposed to ensure if the results using the imputed data are biased. One of the most accepted methods is sensitivity analysis (Héraud-Bousquet et al. 2012; Carpenter et al. 2007). The procedure is simple. For all the statistical analyses conducted, including simple descritpive analysis, student tests, variances analysis and regression, conduct the same analysis for the data without imputing and the data with the imputing and then make a comprison of the results from the two sources of data. Results with the imputed data would be valid if there are no obvious differences in the point estimates (i.e., mean, rate, ratio, OR, RR, and regressin coefficients), although significance levels (i.e., p values or type I error) may differ between the two with p values for the imputed data smaller than those without the imputed data.

9.7 Example of Imputing with SAS PROC MI

Data imputing is complex and such tasks are often implemented by a statistician with formal training in data science. As a part of quantiative epidemiology, we will introduce missing data imputing using the statistical software SAS. The data and SAS programs presented here will serve for two purposes: 1) Assist investigators to imputing missing data for practice or for small projects; and 2) prepare beginniers to learn other advanced techniques for missing data imputing as discussed earlier in this chapter.

9.7.1 Data Source and SAS Program for Imputing

As a demonstration of the method, dataset DATCH7 created for use in Chap. 7 will be used. A total of 9 variables are included and they are: age, gender, racial groups, education, high blood pressue and age of onset of high bloold pressure, if censored, lifetime smoking, and number of cigarettes smoked per day in a typical day. Detailed description of these variables was provided when these variables were first used in this book. We use these variables because they are familiar to us and many of these variables contain missing data.

SAS Program 9.1 shows the steps for imputing, and it includes data processing, checking the missing pattern, and imputing missing data with mean and multiple imputing (MI) method. Part 1 is for data preparation. The LIBNAME tells the location of dataset DATCH7. A work dataset A is created to keep the nine variables listed using the key word KEEP. As usual, the **PROC CONTENTS** is used to check the dataset, including total observations, and a alphabetic list of all variables as detailed in Fig. 9.5.

Alphabetic List of Variables and Attributes			
#	Variable	Type	Len	Label
1	AGE	Num	8	AGE IN YEAR,
5	AGEHYPR	Num	8	AGE OF HYPERTENTION ONSET,
7	CENSORED	Num	8	
4	EDUCATION	Num	8	1= LESS THAN HIGH SCHOOL 2=HIGH 3=COLLEGE+,
2	GENDER	Num	8	1=MALE 2=FEMALE,
6	HBP	Num	8	HIGH BLOOD PRESSURE 1=YES 0 = NO,
8	LIFESMK	Num	8	EVER SMOKED 100 CIGARETTES IN ENTIRE LIFE 1=Y 2=N,
3	RACE5	Num	8	1=WHITE 2=BLAKC 3=HISP 4=ASIAN 5=OTHER,
9	SMKNUMS	Num	8	AVERAGE # CIGARETTES SMOKED PER DAY 1-60

Fig. 9.5 Variables in dataset A for imputing: Output of SAS Program 9.1, Part 1

```
*********************************************************************************
* SAS PROGRAM 9.1 MISSING DATA AND IMPUTING THE MISSED VALUES
*********************************************************************************;
** PART 1 DATA PREPARATION: DATA FROM ALL CHAPTERS CAN BE USED;
*  READ DATA FEOM DATCH7 AND SELECT NINE (9) FOR DEMONSTRATION;
LIBNAME SASDATA "C:\QUANTLBA\A_DATA";
DATA A; SET SASDATA.DATCH7;
KEEP AGE GENDER RACE5 EDUCATION AGEHYPR HBP CENSORED LIFESMK SMKNUMS;
* CHECK DATA;
PROC CONTENTS DATA = A; RUN;

** PART 2 SAS PROGRAM CODES TO CHECK THE MISSING PATTERN BY SETTING NIMPUTE = 0;
PROC MI DATA=A SEED=1234 NIMPUTE=0
        OUT=MI_A0;  *IMPUTED DATA NAMED AS MI_A0;
RUN;

** PART 3 REPLACE MISSING VALUE WITH MEANS OBTAINED FROM PART 2 ABOVE;
DATA SASDATA.COMPLETE; SET A;
IF AGE        EQ . THEN AGE=44.3;
IF GENDER     EQ . THEN GENDER=2;
IF RACE5      EQ . THEN RACE5=3;
IF EDUCATION  EQ . THEN EDUCATION = 2;
IF AGEHYPR    EQ . THEN AGEHYPR = 41.1;
IF SMKNUMS    EQ . THEN SMKNUMS=1.75;
RUN;
* CHECK THE DATA TO SEE IF MISSING VALUES ARE IMPUTED;
PROC FREQ DATA = LIB.COMPLETE; RUN;

** PART 4 MULTIPLE IMPUTING;
*  IMPUTING MISSING WITH MONTE CARLO MARKCO CHAIN METHOD;
PROC MI DATA=A SEED=1234 NIMPUTE=5
   OUT=SASDATA.MI_DAT5;        *IMPUTED DATA NAMED AS MI_DAT5;
     MCMC;
RUN;
* CHECK DATASETS AND NUMBER OF VARIABLES;
PROC CONTENTS DATA = SASDATA.MI_DAT5; RUN;
* FREQUENCY CHECK;
PROC FREQ DATA = SASDATA.MI_DAT5;
TABLES GENDER; RUN;
*********************************************************************************;
```

In Part 2 of the program, SAS Procedure **PROC MI** is used to help check the pattern of missing data in the newly created work dataset **A**. The program is written in the standard syntax with SEED=1234 to ensure the imputed results can be replicated if the same dataset is used again for practice or in real research studies. In addition to 1234, any other number works. The key word NIMPUTE in SAS specifies the number of datasets to be imputed. This is because in mulitple imputing, as the name suggests, more than one dataset can be imputed. When NIMPUTE=0, it asks the computer not to impute any missing data but simply to check the missing pattern, and compute the mean for all variables with and without missing. The command OUT is used to name the imputed dataset. Since no dataset will be imputed, we simply put the sentence here to assist you in getting familiar with the syntax.

The remaing two of SAS Program 9.1 parts are simple, Part 3 shows how to fill in the missing data based on results from Part 2 and Part 4 shows how to do multiple imputing. The key word MCMC is used to specify the method of Markov Chain Monte Carlo method for imputing, one of the most advanced methods for random imputing (Schunk 2008). From Part 3, a dataset named "**COMPLETE**" is created and saved in the same data folder A_DATA; and from part 4, a dataset named MI_DAT5 that contains 5 sets of imputed data aggregated together is also saved in the A_DATA folder.

9.7.2 *Check the Dataset and Missing Patterns*

By executing part 1 of SAS Program 9.1, if everything goes correctly, you will find that the dataset A contains 5134 observations and 9 variables. Figure 9.5 lists the nine variables as indicated. All variables are approriately labeled except the variable **CENSORED** that was not labeled in Chap. 7. Interested students can use **PROC FREQ** command to check missing data as we previously practiced in other chapters.

A major part of the SAS output from SAS Program 9.1 part 2 is the missing pattern. As shown in Fig. 9.6, the SAS program checked not only missing for individual variables as those fom **PROC FREQ**, but also shows the various combinations of missing data. In the figure, X indiates no missing and . indicates missing. Clearly, Group 1 includes all subjects with no missing, N = 3573, and accounts for 69.59% or about 70% of the total sample. Group 2 contains observations with missing data only on the variable SMKNUMS, the number of cigarettes smoked per day on a typical day; and a total of 912 observations with missing data on this variable account for 17.76% of the total sample.

Likewise, Group 3 presents observations with missing data on AGEHYPR, the measure of age when first having high blood pressure. Statisics in Group 4 indicate observations with missing data on both SMKNUMS and AGEHYPR. Group 5 shows the statistics for observations with missing data on another variable EDUCATION; and Group 6 shows the statistics for observations with missing data on EDUCATION and the two variables presented in Group 4. Detailed statistics for other variable combinations with missing data are presented in Groups 7 to 10.

Group	AGE	GENDER	RACE5	EDUCATION	AGEHYPR	HBP	CENSORED	LIFESMK	SMKNUMS	Freq	Percent
1	X	X	X	X	X	X	X	X	X	3573	69.59
2	X	X	X	X	X	X	X	X	.	912	17.76
3	X	X	X	X	.	X	X	X	X	16	0.31
4	X	X	X	X	.	X	X	X	.	8	0.16
5	X	X	X	.	X	X	X	X	X	6	0.12
6	X	X	X	.	.	X	X	X	.	1	0.02
7	.	.	.	.	X	X	X	X	X	231	4.50
8	.	.	.	.	X	X	X	X	.	154	3.00
9	.	.	.	.	.	X	X	X	X	144	2.80
10	.	.	.	.	.	X	X	X	.	89	1.73

Fig. 9.6   Missing pattern: Output of SAS Program 9.1, Part 2

Last, from the results in Fig. 9.6, there are three variables with no missing data, and they are HBP (reported high blood pressure), **CENSORED** (if censored), and LIFESMK (lifetime smoking). These results are anticipated since these three variables were defined by us in the previous chapters. When defining these variaable, observations with missing values were properly recoded.

It is worth noting that results in Fig. 9.6 is generated using a very simple SAS syntax; however the results provide very detailed information on missing patterns. These results are essential for us to understand the missing pattern. such information is of fundamental significance for an investigator to know the data, to determine whether to impute the missing data or not, and to plan for the key task: quantitative analysis.

Simply as an illustration, the missing data would be reduced by 17.17% (87.35% observations will have complete data) if the variable SMKNUMS measuring smoking is not used for the study. In practice, this variable can be replaced by other variables that measure smoking behaviors. Number of cigarettes smoked per day appears to be a good quantitative measure, but unfortunately it contains too many observations with missing data.

9.7.3   Statistics of the Variables with and Without Missing Values

Another part of the output from SAS Program 9.1, the table "Group Means" in Fig. 9.7 displays a set of important statistics about the data on hand. The first row of the table shows the mean value of the subsample of 3573 observations with complete data. These values are those previously used in Part 3 of SAS Program 9.1 to create dataset "COMPLETE" using the sample mean. In that imputing step, the

Group	Group Means								
	AGE	GENDER	RACE5	EDUCATION	AGEHYPR	HBP	CENSORED	LIFESMK	SMKNUMS
1	44.332494	1.552197	2.469353	2.073328	41.141058	0.292471	0.707529	1.750910	2.733837
2	50.893640	1.393640	2.280702	1.995614	45.714912	0.421053	0.578947	1.000000	
3	54.437500	1.500000	1.937500	1.687500		1.000000	0	1.625000	5.187500
4	64.625000	1.250000	2.375000	1.875000		1.000000	0	1.000000	
5	52.000000	1.666667	2.833333		43.500000	0.333333	0.666667	1.833333	0.166667
6	67.000000	1.000000	5.000000			1.000000	0	1.000000	
7					55.354978	1.000000	0	1.844156	1.926407
8					54.409091	1.000000	0	1.000000	
9						0.083333	0.916667	1.777778	3.291667
10						0.089888	0.910112	1.000000	

Fig. 9.7 Means for variables with and without missing: Output of SAS Program 9.1, Part 2

group means were taken from this table and rounded for use. Particularly, gender is rounded up to 2 since in the original data, 1 was used for male and 2 for female; the sample mean for gender = 1.55, rounding up to 2.

It is worth noting that the computed mean for all variables differs for different groups with different missing data combinations. For example, in Group 3, the mean age = 54.4 for the subsample of participants excluding observations with missing data on AGEHYPR and the same mean was 44.3 in Group 1 with the complete observations of all variables. This result indicates large differences in the sample without missing data and the sample with missing data on AGEHYPR.

There is a question for all readers: Is it appropriate to use the mean of all subjects without missing (the first row in Fig. 9.7) or to select the mean in different rows (groups) to fill in the missing data? Why and why not?

9.7.4   The Complete Data After Replacement of the Missing Values with Sample Mean

Although data errors cannot be fixed after data are collected, there are some remedies for missing data. Imputing missing data with sample mean is one of such methods. By executing Program 9.1 Part 3, one dataset named "COMPLETE" will be generated.

After this step of computing, nothing will appear in the SAS output. However, in the SAS Log window, you can get some information about the imputed dataset, such as total observed (n = 5134) and total variables (9). If you want to check if all observations/variables with missing data are imputed, the simplest approach is to use the **PROC FREQ** DATA = = LIB.COMPLETE command. There should not be any missing data in the dataset.

9.7.5 Datasets with Multiple Imputing (MI)

Imputing missing data with the sample mean is simple but not frequently used in research because of its limitations. Multiple imputing is preferred for large scale and more formal studies. SAS Program 9.1 part 4 shows the method to conduct MI using the example dataset. By executing the program, in addition to missing patterns and sample mean as in Fig. 9.6, several sets of information are produced.

Since MI assumes missing at random (MAR), the missing values are generated based on the data for all variables with no missing data. The table "EM (Posterior Mode) Estimates" in Fig. 9.8 displays the estimated mean and covariances of all variables using the imputed data with no missing data. These statistics are estimated using the EM (expectation-maximization method, a computing algorithm), and it tells us the correlation of all variables in the dataset that are used to estimate the missed values.

EM (Posterior Mode) Estimates										
TYPE	_NAME_	AGE	GENDER	RACE5	EDUCATION	AGEHYPR	HBP	CENSORED	LIFESMK	SMKNUMS
MEAN		47.080745	1.516708	2.422460	2.050786	43.079677	0.362485	0.637515	1.585314	4.629831
COV	AGE	232.762764	-0.091034	-0.486377	-0.547322	184.383931	3.390283	-3.390283	-0.928159	12.901680
COV	GENDER	-0.091034	0.249173	-0.001820	0.013257	-0.039626	-0.009188	0.009188	0.047438	-0.585824
COV	RACE5	-0.486377	-0.001820	1.463389	0.021701	0.101355	-0.034841	0.034841	0.097506	-1.476849
COV	EDUCATION	-0.547322	0.013257	0.021701	0.431723	-0.367118	-0.013749	0.013749	0.056081	-0.720334
COV	AGEHYPR	184.383931	-0.039626	0.101355	-0.367118	195.285862	0.846047	-0.846047	-0.597026	8.393095
COV	HBP	3.390283	-0.009188	-0.034841	-0.013749	0.846047	0.230640	-0.230640	-0.025324	0.351165
COV	CENSORED	-3.390283	0.009188	0.034841	0.013749	-0.846047	-0.230640	0.230640	0.025324	-0.351165
COV	LIFESMK	-0.928159	0.047438	0.097506	0.056081	-0.597026	-0.025324	0.025324	0.242250	-2.704635
COV	SMKNUMS	12.901680	-0.585824	-1.476849	-0.720334	8.393095	0.351165	-0.351165	-2.704635	47.034835

Fig. 9.8 Mean and covariances of all variables for the imputed data: Output of PROC MI

The table "Variance Information (5 Imputations)" in Fig. 9.9 displays the between-imputation variance, within-imputation variance, total variance, and other related statistics. These parameter estimates, including measures for multiple imputing efficiency are useful for biostatisticians to draw statistical reference when all 5 imputed datasets are used (Rubin 1996).

The table "Parameter Estimates (5 Imputations)" also in Fig. 9.9 displays the estimated mean and standard errors with imputed data for all the 9 variables used in imputing. For example, the mean age = 47.05 with imputed data. This mean age is greater than 44.33 (Fig. 9.7) for the subsample of 3573 observations without missing values.

Variance Information (5 Imputations)							
	Variance				Relative Increase in Variance	Fraction Missing Information	Relative Efficiency
Variable	Between	Within	Total	DF			
AGE	0.008675	0.045416	0.055826	111.94	0.229221	0.200262	0.961490
GENDER	0.000008037	0.000048698	0.000058343	141.54	0.198046	0.176483	0.965907
RACE5	0.000028210	0.000285	0.000319	329.61	0.118731	0.111122	0.978259
EDUCATION	0.000011214	0.000084264	0.000097720	201.35	0.159693	0.145764	0.971673
AGEHYPR	0.002985	0.038092	0.041674	485.44	0.094030	0.089305	0.982452
SMKNUMS	0.001085	0.009197	0.010498	245.92	0.141550	0.130656	0.974534

Parameter Estimates (5 Imputations)										
Variable	Mean	Std Error	95% Confidence Limits		DF	Minimum	Maximum	Mu0	t for H0: Mean=Mu0	Pr > |t|
AGE	47.052005	0.236275	46.58385	47.52016	111.94	46.978473	47.209653	0	199.14	<.0001
GENDER	1.519070	0.007638	1.50397	1.53417	141.54	1.516490	1.523762	0	198.88	<.0001
RACE5	2.420226	0.017860	2.38509	2.45536	329.61	2.411717	2.425173	0	135.51	<.0001
EDUCATION	2.051247	0.009885	2.03176	2.07074	201.35	2.048572	2.055458	0	207.50	<.0001
AGEHYPR	43.035550	0.204142	42.63444	43.43666	485.44	42.988194	43.127239	0	210.81	<.0001
SMKNUMS	4.634793	0.102462	4.43298	4.83661	245.92	4.598131	4.669888	0	45.23	<.0001

Fig. 9.9   Statistics of the imputed data: Output of SAS Program 9.1, Part 4

9.7.6   Understanding the Imputed Data

After executing the **PROC CONTENTS** DATA = SASDATA.MI_DAT5 in Part 4 of SAS Program 9.1, you will note that one new variable _imputation_ is added to the table "Alphabetic List of Variables and Attributes" (not shown here). This variable was generated by the computer automatically, and it labels individually imputed datasets. Although all the imputed five data sets are pooled together as one, and individual dataset are indexed by this variable and thus can be identified and used for analysis separately as needed.

9.7.7   Integers and Decimal Points in Imputing

When checking the imputed data, you may realize that some variables with imputed values look odd if you use **PROC FREQ DATA = MI_DAT5, TABLES = GENDER** to check the distribution. For example, the imputed values for gender have negative values, values with decimals, and values greater than 2 although this variable in the original data was measured only using 1 (male) and 2 (female). The same or similar imputed values can be found for almost all variables with missing data.

To control the imputed values for different variables, more specifications can be imposed. SAS Program 9.2 presents an example. Relative to SAS Program 9.1 Part 4, a total of four more program lines are added. First, the key word VAR is used to list all nine variables. Second, an additional 3 lines of programs are used to specify the imputed data with MINIMUM for minimum values, MAXIMUM for maximum values and ROUND for round up. These specifications must be lined up with the order of the variables specified with VAR. For example, 20 and 80 are used as the minimum and maximum for the variable AGE with round up = 1(on decimal); and 1 and 5 are specified as the minimum and maximum values for the variable with round up set at 0 (no decimal or integer).

```
**********************************************************************************
SAS PROGRAM 9.2 CONTROLLING IMPUTED VALUES FOR INDIVIDUAL VARIABLES:
VALUES 1 2 FOR GENDER, VALUES 1 2 3 FOR EDUCATION, AND VALUES 0 1 FOR HBP
**********************************************************************************;
PROC MI DATA = A SEED = 37851 NIMPUTE = 3 OUT = SASDATA.MI_DAT3
MINIMUM = 20   1 1 1    12 0 0 1 0
MAXIMUM = 80   2 5 3    80 1 1 2 30
ROUND   = 0.1 1 1 1 0.1 1 1 1 1; *1 FOR INTEGER, 0.1 FOR ONE DECIMAL;
MCMC CHAIN = MULTIPLE DISPLAYINIT INITIAL = EM;
VAR AGE GENDER RACE5 EDUCATION AGEHYPR HBP CENSORED LIFESMK SMKNUMS;
RUN;
**********************************************************************************;
```

As an example, the number of imputed datasets is set at NIMPUTE = 3. With this program, the imputed values for all variables with missing will be consistent with the values in the original data with regard to the type integer or values with decimal point.

SAS Program 9.2 will be used as part of the practice and no detailed description of the results will be provided. It is worth noting that the SAS program will become increasingly complex as more variables are included in the variable list for imputing. An important suggestion before imputing missing data is to first create a dataset that contains only the variables you will use for a research study, and then impute the missing data.

9.8   Use of the Imputed Data and Sensitivity Analysis

If missing data are simply replaced by the sample mean, there is only one imputed dataset with completed data. When missing data are imputed using the multiple imputing method, more than one data set are produced in addition to the original data without imputing. As a routine, usually 5 imputed datasets with complete data are generated for use. Different methods are established and have been used to analyze these two types of data.

9.8.1   Analysis Data with Missing Replaced by Sample Mean

As previously discussed, when the missing values are imputed using sample means, there are two datasets for use, one for the original dataset with missing values not imputed and one imputed dataset in which no missing data exists for all variables. With mean-imputed data, statistical analysis can be completed using the following steps:

Step 1: Conduct all planned statistical analyses using *the imputed data*. Results from this step of analysis are used as the final if results from next two steps are supportive;

Step 2: Conduct the same analyses with the original data without imputing. When conducting such analyses, observations with missing data are automatically excluded. Results from this step of analysis provide information on the results if missing data are ignored;

Step 3: Make comparisons of the results from Step 1 with those from Step 2, and check if the results with imputed data are supported.

The comparison of analytical results between the datasets with and without imputing is known as *sensitivity analysis*. Rigorous sensitivity analysis often involves sophisticated statistical modeling, and it has been used in clinical trials (see Carpenter et al. 2007; Heraud-Bousque et al. 2012). As a demonstration of the concept, we limit the sensitivity analysis to a simple comparison of results from Step 1 with those from Step 2.

9.8.2   Examples of the Result and Comparisons

To illustrate the method, the original data DATCH7 and the imputed dataset COMPLETE generated through SAS Program 9.1 are used. The following simple descriptive statistics are computed, including: (1) Distribution of gender, race, and education; (2) mean age and mean number of cigarettes smoked. As an illustration, the estimated results are presented in Table 9.1, the left three columns.

Results in the table indicate that the three categorical variables, Gender, Race and Education, are very sensitive to missing imputing. This is because with the imputed data, the estimated distribution of the three variables differed substantially from those without imputing. For example, with the imputed data, the computed percentage of females increased from 51.9% to 57.7%, a net increase of 5.8%. In addition, the sex ratio of 57.7% female estimated using the imputed data substantially different from gender the ratio commonly observed in the population, which is close to 50%.

Relative to the three categorical variables, the two continuous variables seemed less sensitive to the imputing missing data with regard to the sample mean. The estimated result for the variable age with the imputed data, although differed from that without imputing, the difference is only 0.1 years, which can be ignored within

Table 9.1 Comparison of results with no imputing and imputed with sample mean and MI

Variable	No imputing	Mean imputing	Difference	MI imputing[a]	Difference
Gender, n (%)					
Male	2170 (48.1)	2170 (42.3)	0 (−5.8)	2454 (47.8)	288 (−0.3)
Female	2346 (51.9)	2964 (57.7)	618 (5.8)	2680 (52.2)	334 (0.3)
Race, n (%)					
White	1326 (29.4)	1326 (25.8)	0 (−3.6)	1450 (28.2)	124 (−1.2)
Black	1116 (24.7)	1116 (21.7)	0 (−3.0)	1305 (25.4)	189 (0.7)
Hispanic	1115 (24.7)	1733 (33.8)	618 (12.1)	1315 (25.6)	200 (0.9)
Asian	723 (16.0)	723 (14.1)	0 (−1.9)	808 (15.7)	85 (−0.3)
Other	236 (5.2)	236 (4.6)	0 (−0.6)	256 (5.0)	20 (−0.2)
Education, n (%)					
Less than high	856 (19.0)	856 (16.7)	0 (−2.3)	989 (19.3)	133 (0.3)
High school	2545 (56.4)	3170 (61.8)	625 (5.4)	2895 (56.4)	350 (0.0)
College or more	1108 (24.6)	1108 (21.6)	0 (3.0)	1250 (24.3)	142 (0.3)
Age in year					
Mean (SD)	45.7 (14.5)	45.6 (13.6)	−0.1 (−0.9)	47.1 (15.1)	1.4 (0.6)
# cigarettes per day					
Mean (SD)	43.1 (14.0)	43.0 (13.6)	−0.1 (−0.4)	43.1 (13.9)	0 (0.1)

[a]Note: Results are from one of the three MI imputed datasets MI_DAT3 generated using SAS Program 9.2

the adult population. In addition, differences in the estimated standard deviation with the imputed data is 0.9 smaller than that without imputing.

Similar results are also observed for the other variable, number of cigarettes smoked per day.

9.8.3   Analysis with Multiple Imputed Datasets

Different from the imputed missing data with the sample mean, multiple datasets are generated using the MI method. Methods to analyze such data are more complex and can also be conducted in three steps.

Step 1: Conduct analysis for all sets of imputed data one at a time and save the results;

Step 2: Combine and integrate the results from all analyses of the multiple datasets to obtain the final results;

Step 3: Sensitivity analysis – comparison of differences between the results in Steps 1 and 2 as seen in Sect. 9.8.2 and Table 9.1.

Completion of analysis with multiple datasets generated through MI needs specialized training and will not be covered in this book. It is worth noting that individual imputed datasets from MI are independent from each other. In theory, each imputed dataset can be used for statistical analysis for a project. Although these imputed datasets are included in one dataset, individual datasets are indexed using the computer-generated variable `_imputation_`. We can select any one of the datasets for analysis.

As an example, the first dataset from `MI_DAT3` is used for analysis. The results for the five variables are presented in the last two columns of Table 9.1. It is clear that the observations with missing values imputed for the three categorical variables are distributed in different levels. This is quite different from the mean imputing that are limited only to one subgroup. For example, with mean imputing, 258 observations with missing data are added to females, while none are added to males. Consequently, with MI imputed data, the % distribution of the 3 demographic variables do not differ much from those without imputing. In other words, relative to mean imputing, MI is less sensitive.

9.8.4   Two Caveats for Analyzing the MI Imputed Data

Experience from the author's own research indicates that in most cases, differences are rather small in the results estimated using anyone dataset selected from the multiple MI imputed datasets. To avoid complicated modeling, one simple way to obtain results from multiple imputed datasets is to conduct analysis for all datasets one at a time and compute the average of the results as final. For example, if dataset `MI_DAT5` is used to estimate mean age, mean age will first be computed using each of the five datasets. With the five estimates of mean age, the mean of these five means can be manually computed as the final estimate of the variable age.

In practice, this process is time-consuming. Depending on actual data, the difference of a statistic (i.e., the computed mean) between individual imputed datasets is rather small. Sometimes, results from one set of imputed data can be used simply like the mean imputing. If you are less confident, simply run the same analysis for different imputed datasets and assess the differences between them.

9.9   Practice

9.9.1   Statistical Analysis and Computing

1. Run SAS Program 9.1 yourself to gain efficiency in using SAS program **PROC MI** for imputing missing data, including imputing with sample mean and multiple imputing using the MCMC methods.
2. Run SAS Program 9.2 and gain efficiency in controlling the imputed values while using **PROC MI** for imputing.
3. Create a dataset that contains the variables of your own choice and use the same methods to impute data.
4. Conduct sensitivity analysis by comparing results from the imputed data with the results without imputing and try to draw conclusions.

9.9.2 Research Paper Update

1. Use the imputing methods in this chapter to check the data you used for your own project. Carefully examine missing patterns detected using various methods, including **PROC FREQ** and **PROC MI**.
2. Decide whether to impute the missing data or not. If imputing, use the appropriate imputing method.
3. Impute data and update all the statistical analyses with the imputed data. Conduct sensitivity analysis to support your results.
4. Update your paper, including the Methods section to add missing and imputing, and justification for the imputing method selection and how the imputation was conducted (i.e., using SAS **PROC MI**, number of data sets imputed, etc.), update analytical results, and all numbers throughout the paper to reflect the changes after the imputed data were used.

9.9.3 Study Questions

1. What are the three missing patterns often observed in quantitative epidemiology?
2. Name 4–6 conditions in which missing values can occur in epidemiological studies. Discuss what can be done to avoid missing during data collection?
3. What does the term missing completely at random (MCAR) mean? Which conditions may lead to MCAR? How to assess if the missingness of a variable is completely at random.
4. What are the major impacts of missing values on a research study?
5. What does the term missing at random (MAR) mean? Why the term MAR is misleading? Why is MAR a prerequisite (assumption) for imputing missing values?
6. What does sensitivity analysis mean when missing values are imputed for statistical analysis?
7. Should we always impute missing values? Why and why not?

References

Carpenter, J.R., Kenward, M.G., White, I.R.: Sensitivity analysis after multiple imputation under missing at random: a weighting approach. Stat. Methods Med. Res. **16**(3), 259–275 (2007)

Cheng, C., Chan, C., Sheu, Y.: A novel purity-based k nearest neighbors imputing method and its application in financial distress prediction. Eng. Appl. Artif. Intell. **81**, 283–299 (2019)

Enders, C.K.: Applied Missing Data Analysis. Guilford Press (2010)

Héraud-Bousquet, V., Larsen, C., Carpenter, J., et al.: Practical considerations for sensitivity analysis after multiple imputation applied to epidemiological studies with incomplete data. BMC Med. Res. Methodol. **12**, 73 (2012). https://doi.org/10.1186/1471-2288-12-73

Rubin, D.B.: Inference and missing data. Biometrika. **63**(3), 581–590 (1976)

Rubin, D.B.: Multiple imputation after 18+ years. J. Am. Stat. Assoc. **91**, 473–489 (1996)

Schunk, D.: A Markov chain Monte Carlo algorithm for multiple imputation in large surveys. Adv. Stat. Anal. **92**, 101–114 (2008)

Sterne, A.C., White, I.R., Carlin, J.B., Spratt, M., Royston, P., Kenward, M.G., et al.: Multiple imputation for missing data in epidemiological and clinical research: potential and pitfalls. BMJ. **338**, b2393 (2009). https://doi.org/10.1136/bmj.b2393

Tang, F., Ishwaran, H.: Random Forest missing data algorithms. Statistical Anal. Data Min. **10**(6), 363–377 (2017)

Chapter 10
Sample Size, Statistical Power, and Power Analysis

Planning and designing a research project is both a science and an art.

In epidemiology, all most all of us are familiar with or at least have heard of the terms sample size and statistical power. However, if faculty and students in epidemiology are asked about it, only a few may have conducted the relevant analyses themselves to determine the sample size and to assess the statistical power for a project. In routine statistical analysis, the task is to extract information from data – give me the data and I will give you the results. In sample size and power analysis, however, an *if-than process* is repeated for a number of times to make a decision. Sample size and power analysis thus can be considered as a process involving both science and art.

10.1 Introduction to Power Analysis

Power analysis is both an science and an art (Cohen 1988). It is very different from the statistical methods routinely used for data analysis to test study hypotheses. For all the statistical methods, data are provided to the computer and the analytical results are expected with limited researcher-computer interactions. In assessing and imputing missing data in Chap. 9, we had some taste of the researcher-computer interactions in controlling the output. When researcher-computation interaction is involved, outcome from such analysis will no longer be unique. With the same data and analytical method, different results can be generated, each of which is meaningful. In power analysis, it heavily depends on researcher-computer interaction; and the goal is not to search for unique result but provide data for decision making.

© The Author(s), under exclusive license to Springer Nature Switzerland AG 2021   301
X. Chen, *Quantitative Epidemiology*, Emerging Topics in Statistics and
Biostatistics, https://doi.org/10.1007/978-3-030-83852-2_10

10.1.1   The Concept of Statistical Power

The word power is often associated with power in politics or power plant for electricity. However, statistical power has nothing to do with political power or electrical power. One analogy of statistical power similar to medical and health sciences is the power of a microscope. The power of a microscope determines its capacity to see small objects. Microscopes with greater powers are more capable to find smaller objects than microscopes with less powers.

In quantitative epidemiology, statistical power is *a measurement of the strength* of a research project with a sample size N to test a study hypothesis (Cohen 1988; Ott and Longnecker 2015). Statistical power is thus a measure of the capability of a research project to find the expected outcome if it really exists. For example, to prove if physical activity is a protective factor for cardiovascular disease, we may plan a research project by recruiting 1000 adult subjects. Before implementing the project, we want to know the statistical power of the project to detect the protective effect of physical activity with the sample if the effect exists.

Statistical power is thus defined in principle as the probability to reject a null hypothesis given that the alternative hypothesis is true and is quantitatively measured using $(1 - \beta)$:

$$Power = \Pr\left(reject\ H_0 \mid H_1 is\ true\right) = 1 - \beta, \tag{10.1}$$

where β is the probability for type II error, or the likelihood to accept a false null hypothesis (or false negative).

Equation 10.1 is the foundation supporting the development of methods for power analysis. Parameter β is closely related to another very important parameter α for type I error (incorrect rejection of a true null hypothesis or false positive). As a review, Table 10.1 summarizes the relationship between statistical power, type I and type II error, true and false positive and negative.

Table 10.1 indicates that statistical power $(1 - \beta)$ is described with the probability of type II error β. Thus, estimated statistical power varies from 0 to 1. In designing a study project, type I error is typically set at $\alpha < 0.05$, corresponding to $p < 0.05$ in data analysis for statistical inference. Statistical power is often described in percentages. A study project is considered adequately powered if the estimated statistical power $(1 - \beta) \geq 80\%$.

Table 10.1 Statistical power as it is related to type I and type II error, true and false positive, and true and false negative

Study Findings	Positive in reality	Negative in reality	Total
Results suggest positive	Power (1-β) True positive	Type I error (α) False positive	Subjects detected positive
Results suggest negative	Type II error (β) False negative	No error (1-α) True negative	Subjects detected negative
Total	100.00%	100.00%	100.00%

10.1.2   Geometric Presentation of Statistical Power

Statistical power of a study project can be visually comprehended using Student t-test to compare two sample means as an example.

Figure 10.1 describes the relationship in Table 10.1 with geometric curves to describe the hypothesis test and statistical power. The blue curve on the left represents the mean and SD of a variable of interest based on the null hypothesis of no difference ($\mu = 0$); and the red curve on the right represents the distribution of a sample mean with standard deviation SD based on the alternative hypothesis of 4-unit difference in the mean from the null.

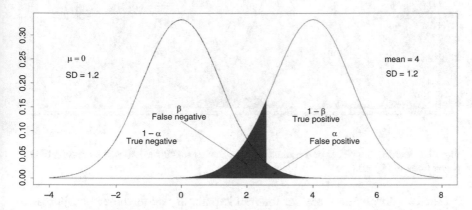

Fig. 10.1 Geometric presentation of statistical power (1-β), type I error α, type II error β, true positive and true negative, false positive and false negative

Despite much difference between the null hypothesis ($\mu = 0$) and the alternative hypothesis (mean = 4), the two distributions overlap with each other. When making a statistical decision using a statistic (i.e., Z value, t value, chi-square value) and an acceptable type I error, mistakes or misclassification cannot be avoided, no matter if type I error α is set at $p < 0.05$ or at $p < 0.01$. The goal for power analysis is to see if the power ($1 - \beta$) is adequate (80% or greater), given a sample size and a type I error.

10.2   Factors Related to Statistical Power

From the description in Sect. 10.1 above, we can see that many factors can change statistical power. Adequate knowledge of these factors is important for power analysis. Knowing the influential factors enables researchers to conduct power analysis and to determine sample size in planning a new research project. In this section, we will discuss four factors: type I error, between-group difference, standard deviation and sample size (Cohen 1988).

10.2.1   Type I error Reduces Statistical Power

For a given study project, increasing Type I error α increases the statistical power $(1 - \beta)$ while reducing type I error reduces the statistical power, keep all conditions unchanged. This relation can be illustrated by comparing Fig. 10.1 in the previous section with Fig. 10.2 below.

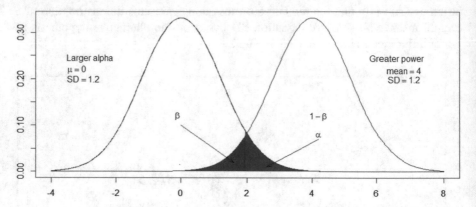

Fig. 10.2 Increasing type I error α (extend the blue-shaded area to the left) will increase statistical power (refer to Fig. 10.1)

The two distributions, one for the null hypothesis and the other for alternative hypothesis in Fig. 10.2 are identical to those in Fig. 10.1 ($\mu = 0$ for null hypothesis and mean = 4 for alternative hypothesis, and SD=1.2 for both). However, type I error α, the blue-shaded area is larger in Fig. 10.2 than in Fig. 10.1. As a result, statistical power $(1 - \beta)$ is greater for the project described by Fig. 10.2 than that by Fig. 10.1.

The relationship between type I error and statistical power has clear implications in power analysis. Type I error $\alpha = 0.05$ or $\alpha = 0.01$ are commonly accepted when designing a research project. Given the same research design, you will have a smaller power if you attempt to obtain results with a smaller type I error (reduce the chance to reject true null hypothesis or to avoid false positive); and vise versa.

10.2.2   Increasing the Between-Group Difference Increases Statistical Power

The whole idea of statistical power is to deal with the overlap between a real distribution and a hypothetic distribution or the distribution of two comparison groups (i.e., the distribution of a sample mean or sample proportion). Given the distribution of the two groups with the same SD, and assuming the same level of type I error, the overlap between the two distributions will decline as the between-group difference

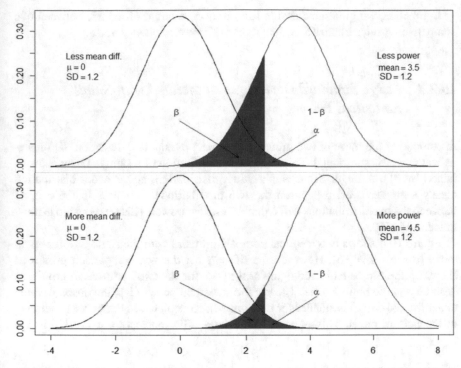

Fig. 10.3 Larger Differences in the Mean between the Two Comparison Groups Equal Greater Statistical Powers

increases, resulting in an increase in statistical power. This relation is illustrated with Fig. 10.3.

Figure 10.3 contrasts two identical distributions with the same SD but different differences in the mean between the two comparison groups. The top panel of Fig. 10.3 shows two distributions with $\mu = 0$ for the null hypothesis and mean = 3.5 for the alternative hypothesis with the difference in the mean = 3.5 (3.5-0.0). Two distributions in the bottom panel are identical to those in the top panel except that that mean = 4.5 for the alternative hypothesis with the group difference increased from 3.5 to 4.5.

From Fig. 10.3, it can be seen clearly, relative to the top panel, the power (1-β, as shown by the unshaded area under the red curve) is much greater for the case presented in the bottom panel. The increase in power is due to reductions in the overlap between the two distributions.

From Fig. 10.3, we can derive that the statistical power will increase as the between-group difference increases because increasing between-group difference will reduce the overlap between the two distributions. Therefore, in theory, statistical power can reach 100% if the between-group difference is so large that distributions of two comparison groups are completely separated from each other.

In practice, with the same design for a project, a larger difference between two comparison groups implies a greater statistical power; and vice versa.

10.2.3   Large Standard Deviations Associated with Small Statistical Powers

In comparing the mean of two groups, the impact of standard deviation SD on statistical power is substantial. This is because distribution of a sample mean is determined by SD. A larger SD means a wider distribution, and a wider distribution means a greater overlap between the two distributions. Increases in the overlap between the two distributions will reduce statistical power. This relationship is illustrated in Fig. 10.4.

Figure 10.4 shows two identical comparison pairs with the same differences in mean (mean - μ = 3.5). However, the SD = 2 for the two comparison groups as shown in the top panel of the figure and SD=1 for the two comparison groups as described in the bottom panel. Clearly the statistical power (1-β, the unshaded area under the red curve) is smaller for the comparison depicted in the upper panel than in the bottom panel. This is because the larger SD increases the overlap in the

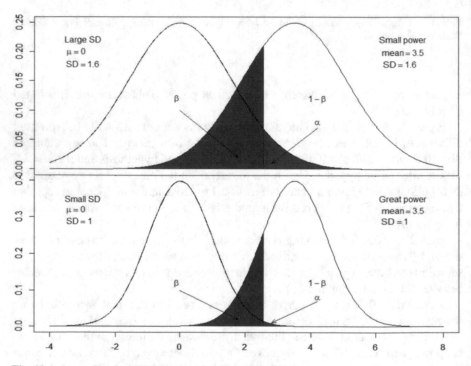

Fig. 10.4 Large Standard Deviation and Small Statistical Power

distributions between the two comparison groups, therefore reducing statistical power.

In planning a research project, we must be aware that an observed SD of a variable may contain data errors (see Chap. 2). Such error can be very large if tools used for data collection are poor and/or standard protocol for data collection cannot be implemented. In other words, *poor data quality will reduce statistical power while improving data quality can increase statistical power*.

10.2.4   Large Samples Associated with Great Statistical Powers

Statistically, large sample sizes are always positively associated with statistical powers given other conditions unchanged. Thus, for a given study project, a large sample size always means a great statistical power. However, increasing sample size will cost a project more to implement. A primary goal of power analysis is to determine the best sample size to adequately power a research project within the budget limit.

Why is increasing sample size associated with greater statistical power? This can be illustrated with Fig. 10.5. The figure depicts three Student t distributions with degree of freedom DF = 2, 5, and 100, with corresponding sample sizes of 3, 6 and 101 (DF = sample size n-1). From Fig. 10.5 it can be seen that as sample size increases, the distribution becomes narrower. As we discussed in previous sections, when a distribution becomes narrow, the overlap of the distributions between two comparison groups will be reduced, leading to greater statistical power.

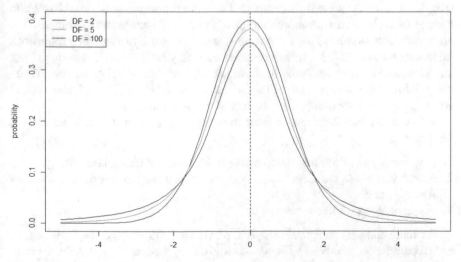

Fig. 10.5 Sample mean distribution becomes narrow as the sample size (degree of freedom DF) increases

It is worth noting that the relationship between sample size and statistical power is nonlinear. This relationship makes it hard to determine sample size to achieve a pre-determined statistical power without detailed power analysis. For example, a 10% increase in sample size will not result in a 10% increase in statistical power; it may result in little increase in power at one condition but great increase in another condition. This is the challenge to determine sample size and statistical power. The purpose of this chapter is to introduce methods to assist in determining the optimal sample size and statistical power based on the nonlinear relationship between the two.

10.3   Strategy for Power Analysis

With the introduction in the previous sections on the concepts of statistical power and its relationship with null and alternative hypotheses, related sample distribution, and type I and type II errors for statistical decision making, we should now be ready to learn how to conduct power analysis. Three strategies are often used in statistical power analysis: (i) determine the sample size, given statistical power; (ii) determine the statistical power given sample size, and (iii) create a sample size – statistical power curve to jointly determine the sample size and power.

10.3.1   Methods for Power Analysis

Methods for power analysis have been well developed for *bivariate statistical analyses*, such as Student t-test to compare two sample means, one-way ANOVA to compare sample means for more than two groups, chi-square test to compare the proportion of a sample with the population and to compare two sample proportions (including prevalence rates, incidence rates, mortality rates, rates of substance use); and simple correlation analysis. In these settings, mathematical equations can be derived for power analysis based on the relationship between type I and type II errors, sample distribution (i.e., mean and SD), and sample size.

In this book, we will introduce three methods to determine statistical power and sample size:

1. Power analysis to compare sample proportions using a chi-square test;
2. Power analysis to compare sample means using a Student t-test, and one-way ANOVA; and
3. Power analysis for linear correlation.

For more complex statistical analyses, power analysis methods are available for partial correlation, multivariate linear and logistic regression. However, these methods are often too complex for investigators with no adequate mathematical and statistical training. In this case, statisticians can be consulted for assistance.

For new statistical analysis methods or methods that are more complex than multivariate regression (i.e., cusp catastrophe models), an approximation method for power analysis can be used, such as Monte Carlo simulation (Chen et al. 2014).

10.3.2 Determine the Sample Size Given Statistical Power

This is often the first strategy for power analysis supporting a research project. At the beginning when conceiving a project, investigators all want to have an adequate statistical power, say 80% to find the true results if they exist. To achieve this statistical power, investigators want to know the number of subjects, i.e., the sample size to be included for the project. With information on sample size for a pre-determined statistical power, investigators can then estimate budget and make personal arrangements for a research project.

To use this power analysis strategy, the following data must be provided: Type I error (both 0.01 and 0.05 can be used) and statistics (i.e., mean, standard deviation, rate, proportion, correlation coefficients) for the study hypothesis-related variables. Given such information, a sample size can be estimated to ensure the specified statistical power and the type I error for statistical inference.

10.3.3 Determine the Statistical Power Given a Sample Size

With information about the sample size and statistical power derived using the power analysis strategy just described above, an investigator may start thinking of alternative research plans. For example, if power analysis using the previous strategy suggests that a sample size of 400 can achieve 80% statistical power with 5% type I error to test if using preventive aspirin is associated with 25% reduction in heart attack. After some assessment of the result, the investigator wants to see what the result would be if the sample size were to be reduced to 350 (considering cost) or increased to 500 (if more funding is available). To provide an answer to this type of questions, we power analysis will be conducted to determine the statistical power given different sample sizes.

Data needed for power analysis using this approach is the same as in the first methods with one exception: Replace the statistical power with sample size. For each sample size, a statistical power will be computed.

10.3.4 Using Sample Size-Statistical Power Curve

With the two methods described above, one can only obtain one estimate at a time, no matter if it is for statistical power or sample size. It would be ideal for research decision-making if *a series of sample size and statistical power* could be obtained given the same setting (i.e., statistics for the study variable, type I and type II errors). This approach is available, and it is termed as the *sample size – statistical power curve* method. This method has often been used in power analysis for research because of its strengths.

10.3.5   Software Packages for Power Analysis

Software for power analysis can be found in three different sources: (1) Online power calculators (e.g., Sample Size Calculator), (2) standalone packages for power analysis (e.g., PASS for power and sample size; and r package "pwr"); and (3) procedures for power analysis within a statistical software package (i.e., SamplePower in SPSS and **PROC POWER** in SAS).

We use the procedure **PROC POWER** from SAS in this book. We select this method not because we want to promote it but because the author of this book used SAS for most parts of his previous research. There is no need to purchase an extra piece of SAS software for power analysis, and all what we need to know is one more SAS procedure, **PROC POWER**.

10.4   Power Analysis to Compare Sample Proportions

In quantitative epidemiology, proportion-related indicators are used very often, including prevalence rate (proportion of persons with a health event in a total population), incidence rate (proportion of persons with a new event in a total population), death rate (proportion of deaths in a total population), smoking rate (proportion of smokers in the total population), rate of suicide (proportion of deaths due to suicide in a total population), and etc. Therefore, comparison of two sample proportions is common in research.

Let us start with an example: assuming data from a reported study had a sample of 890 school students with 429 female and 461 male, and the results indicated that 15.2% girls and 19.2% boys smoked cigarettes during the past 30 days. However, the authors concluded no gender differences in the smoking rates since the difference was not statistically significant at $p < 0.05$ level (Croisant et al. 2013). If you plan to conduct a research project to confirm the results, a power analysis is needed to make sure your study is adequately powered. Lack of statistical power could be one reason the reported study failed to confirm the observed gender difference in the prevalence rate from the study sample.

10.4.1   Basic Steps for the Power Analysis

Power analysis to compare two sample proportions using the **PROC POWER** is efficient. Suppose you plan to conduct a study to compare the difference in HPV vaccination against human papillomavirus infections among youth. Data from literature indicates approximately 40% of US youth received the vaccination; and receiving an educational program may be able to increase the rate to 50%. In planning the project, power analysis must be conducted to determine sample size and statistical power.

SAS Program 10.1 shows how to conduct the power analysis using the example question. The program contains three parts: Part 1 is descriptive, including title of the analysis and other information, Part 2 is for power analysis, and Part 3 plots the result.

In part 1 of the SAS program, a title for the power analysis is specified after the keyword TITLE. Other information can also be added. This part is for documentation purposes.

Part 2 starts with the key word **PROC POWER**, asking SAS to conduct power analysis. The option PLOTONLY after **PROC POWER** tells SAS to output only plot. After activating the power analysis procedure, the rest of the options tell SAS what to do: TWOSAMPLEFREQ TEST = PCHI (Pearson chi-square test); GROUPPROPORTIONS for specifying the two proportions 0.45 and 0.55 to be compared; NPERGROUP for specifying sample size per group; and last, specify type I error alpha (here alpha is set to 0.05; this value can be changed, such as 0.01, 0.1, etc. to test how sample size and power changes).

```
*******************************************************************************
*** SAS PROGRAM 10.1. POWER ANALYSIS FOR COMPARING TWO PROPORTIONS
*******************************************************************************;
**  1. DOCUMENTATION: TITLE AND OTHER INFORMATION;
TITLE "POWER FOR COMPARING TWO PROPORTIONS 0.40 VS 0.50";
**  2. POWSER ANALYSIS;
PROC POWER PLOTONLY;
* SET UP THE CONDITIONS FOR POWER ANALYSIS;
  TWOSAMPLEFREQ TEST = PCHI
  GROUPPROPORTIONS   = (0.4 0.5)
  NPERGROUP          = 270
  ALPHA              = 0.05
  POWER              =.;
**  3. PLOTTING RESULTS: SAMPLE SIZE AND STATISTICAL POWER CURVE;
  PLOT X = N MIN=100 MAX=800 NPOINTS=30
  YOPTS = (REF=0.8 0.9 CROSSREF=YES);
RUN;
*******************************************************************************;
```

In part 3 of the program, the PLOT function is activated to present the results from Part 2. It will produce the so-called sample size – statistical power curve, which is very useful for decision-making. In this part, the keyword PLOT is used to activate the plotting process first; then define x-axis – sample size with the key SAS program letter **X** and then y-axis – statistical power. In the program, the range of x-axis (sample size) is set to vary from 100 to 800. The NPOINTS tells SAS the number of data points (we used 30) to be plotted on the curve. YOPTS asks the SAS program to draw a vertical line as y-axis and label it as Power. Since power is computed, there is no need to set any range. However, the parameters in the parentheses ask SAS to label the 80% and 90% power respectively in the plot.

In practice for different data, the parameters for X and Y plots can be modified, particularly the range for X and the number of data points to obtain best visual presentation of the analytical results. The range varies depending on the difference between the two sample proportions. This can be determined through repeated test-runs such that *the sample sizes corresponding to the 80% and 90% power are located at the left central region of the plot.*

10.4.2 Results of Power Analysis and Interpretation

Figure 10.6 presents the output by executing SAS Program 10.1 above. All information entered in Part 1 of SAS Program 10.1 is presented on the top of the SAS output.

After the title, the sample size - statistical power curve is plotted with exactly 30 data points on the curve, presenting an eye-friendly curve. The figure indicates a curvilinear relationship between sample size (X-axis) and statistical power (Y-axis) to compare the rate of 0.40 (a proportion) with the rate of 0.55 (another proportion). The statistical power increases rapidly as sample size increases from 100 to 400, followed by a slowing down as sample size increases further, and the power reaches 100% after the sample size becomes 700 and greater.

Based on the power analysis, results in the figure clearly indicate that to achieve 80% statistical power, a sample size of 387 (round down from 387.42) per group or a total of 774 subjects is needed. Furthermore, if sample size increases from 387 per group to 518 or 1036 in total, the statistical power will increase to 90%. This part of the result is very useful for decision-making to plan a research project. If funding is a major factor, a sample of say 400 subjects per group or 800 in total to start with would be adequate for a project to ensure at least 80% statistical power, considering potential refusals and missing data. If budget allows (often the case for federally supported projects), it would be great to have a more powerful project with a sample size of 520 per group for a total sample of 1040 to achieve 90% statistical power.

It is worth noting that results in Fig. 10.6 used NPERGROUP in SAS Program 10.1. N = 270 is one point on the x-axis. Numbers different from 270 can be used to obtain the same results as along as it is located within the 100-800 range.

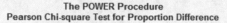

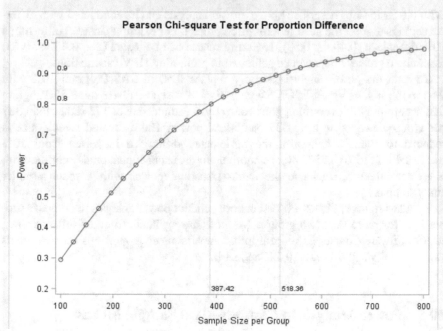

Fig. 10.6 Power analysis results using SAS Program 10.1 for Comparisons of two sample proportions

10.4.3   *Reporting Power Analysis Results*

It can be challenging to reporting power analysis results the first time. We present the following write up as an example.

"By setting the Type I error alpha at p<0.05 level (two-sided), detailed power analysis using PROC POWER in SAS version 9.4 indicated that a sample of 387 subjects per group will warrant 80% statistical power to test a 10% increase (from 40% to 50%) in the rate of HPV vaccination through the educational program. We plan to recruit 400 participants per group for a total of 800 subjects for the project. If more founds are available, we can increase the sample size to 520 per group for a total of 1040 subjects for 90% statistical power."

10.4.4 Alterative Analyses to Determine Sample Size and Power

With the basic steps described above, power analysis can be conducted with different settings to meet the need of a research project. For example, instead of testing a 10% difference (0.40 vs. 0.50), 15% differences can be tested (i.e., 0.40 vs. 0.55) assuming a greater effect can be achieved in promoting HPV vaccination.

To redo the power analysis, simply replace 0.50 in SAS Program 10.1 with 0.55 in the `GROUPPROPORTIONS = (0.4 0.5)` and revise the SAS Program title accordingly. If everything goes correctly, a sample size of 173 rather than 387 per group is needed to have 80% statistical power. The estimated sample size is reduced to about a half with the anticipated difference increased from 10% (0.50–0.40) to 15% (0.55–0.40). In another words, using educational programs with a greater effect can achieve the same statistical power with a much smaller study sample.

As a last remark, **PROC POWER** cannot conduct power analysis to compare proportions for more than two groups. Methods are available in other software (i.e., PASS Software Chapter 256 – Multiple comparisons of proportions for treatments vs. a control, pp.256.1–256.10, NCSS, Ltd).

10.5 Power Analysis to Compare Two Sample Means

Comparing sample means is needed for almost all quantitative epidemiological studies. Student t-test is used to compare two sample means and one-way ANOVA is used to compare sample means of more than two groups. In quantitative epidemiology, the comparison of two or more sample means is a bivariate approach to test possible relationships between a continuous (e.g., age, physical activity level, blood pressure, viral load) and a categorical variable (e.g., gender, with/without a disease, survival/death).

10.5.1 Steps for Basic Power Analysis

The steps for power analysis to compare two sample means are similar to those described in Sect. 10.4 to compare two sample proportions. We use a hypothetical example to demonstrate the method.

Assuming an investigator plans to examine the relationship between the thickness of coronary artery calcium plaque and heart attack. Reported data from comprehensive literature indicates that the mean thickness is 2.5 mm for patients with a heart attack and 1.25 mm for patients without a heart attack; and the standard deviation SD of the thickness is 0.8. SAS Program 10.2 shows how to conduct power analysis supporting the project to make decisions on the sample size and statistical power.

```
**************************************************************************************
*** SAS PROGRAM 10.2.POWER ANALYSIS COMPARING TWO SAMPLE MEANS
**************************************************************************************;
**  1. DOCUMENTATION: TITLE AND OTHER INFORMATION;
TITLE "POWER ANALYSIS FOR COMPARING TWO MEANS 1.25 2.50, SD=0.8";
**  2. POWER ANALYSIS;
PROC POWER PLOTONLY;
* SET UP FOR POWER ANALYSIS;
TWOSAMPLEMEANS TEST=DIFF
   GROUPMEANS = 2.50 | 1.25
   STDDEV     = 0.8
   NTOTAL     = 20
   ALPHA      = 0.05
   POWER      =.;
** 3 PLOTTING RESULTS: SAMPLE SIZE AND STATISTICAL POWER CURVE;
   PLOT X=N MIN=5 MAX=35 NPOINTS=20
   YOPTS = (REF=0.8 0.9 CROSSREF=YES);
RUN;
**************************************************************************************;
```

SAS Program 10.2 is very similar to SAS Program 10.1 except Part 2, the settings for power analysis. Specifically, the statement TWOSAMPLEMEANS TEST=DIFF is used to ask SAS to conduct power analysis for a study to compare two means with Student t-test; the statement GROUPMEANS = 2.50 | 1.25 is used to specify the mean of the two comparison groups from the literature (or pilot studies); the statement STDDEV = 0.8 is used to specify the SD also from literature (or pilot studies); and the statement NTOTAL = 20 is used to specify a tentative sample size of 20 to set up the power analysis. (It is worth noting that this tentative sample size of 20 is much smaller than 270, the value used in SAS Program 10.1 for proportion comparisons). Lastly, adjustments are also made in the plotting part to obtain a better visual presentation of the results. **NPOINT** = 20 rather than 30 is used considering the smaller sample size for comparison of means than proportions.

It must be pointed out that NTOTAL = in this program is referred to the total sample size N, different from SAS Program 10.1 for comparing two proportions. With an estimate of N in this program, N/2 will be the sample per group to compare two sample means.

10.5.2   Results of Power Analysis and Interpretation

Figure 10.7 presents the output from executing SAS Program 10.2. First of all, the output includes all the documentation information, including project title, two comparison means and SD, and a nice sample size-statistical power curve.

From the estimated sample size – power curve, we can see that the statistical power increases as sample size increases. Starting at a very low level when the sample size N < 5, the power increases rapidly as sample size N increases from 5 to

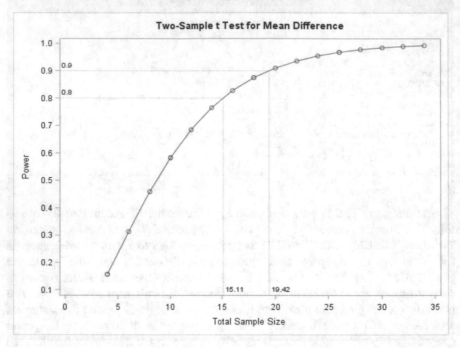

Fig. 10.7 Power analysis results using SAS Program 10.2 for comparisons of two sample means

15, the speed of increase slowed down as N increased from 15 to 30, and leveled off after sample size N increased from 30 to 35 with the power approaching 100%.

Lastly, results in the figure indicate that inclusion of a total sample of 16 subjects or 8 subjects per group will ensure 80% statistical power to test if the difference between 2.50 and 1.25 (SD=0.8) in the thickness of coronary artery calcium plaque and heart attack with type I error set at $p < 0.05$ level. The statistical power will increase to 90% by adding 4 more subjects to the sample in total or 2 more subjects per group.

10.5.3   More Complex Power Analysis for Group Mean Comparisons

SAS Power provides capacity to conduct power analysis for more complex comparison combinations in one program. For example, in practice, an investigator may consider different scenarios in decision-making rather than a simple comparison as shown in SAS Program 10.2. For example, for the same study in the basic analysis above, what would be the results if SD is set at 0.75 or 0.90, rather than 0.80? Also, how many more subjects are needed if the difference in the mean thickness of coronary artery plaque between the two comparison groups is not 1.25 (0.25–1.25), but 1.8, 2.0 or 2.2?

To demonstrate this method, SAS Program 10.3 presents an example to conduct power analysis with four scenarios using hypothetical data. In the program, two potential differences are considered: 4.5 vs. 4.3, 4.0 with two different SD: 1.0 and 1.5 for each.

```
*****************************************************************************************
** SAS PROGRAM 10.3.POWER ANALYSIS MORE COMPLEX SETTINGS
*****************************************************************************************;
** 1. DOCUMENTATION: TITLE AND OTHER INFORMATION;
TITLE "POWER FOR FOUR MEAN-SD COMBINATIONS MEAN=4.5, 4.2, 4.0, SD=1.0 1.2";
** 2. POWER ANALYSIS;
PROC POWER PLOTONLY;
* SET UP FOR POWER ANALYSIS;
TWOSAMPLEMEANS TEST=DIFF
  GROUPMEANS = 4.5 | 4.2 4.0
  STDDEV     = 1.0 1.2
  NTOTAL     = 30
  ALPHA      = 0.05
  POWER      =.;
** 3 PLOTTING RESULTS: SAMPLE SIZE AND STATISTICAL POWER CURVE;
  PLOT X=N MIN=0 MAX=400 NPOINTS=30
  YOPTS = (REF=0.8 CROSSREF=YES);
RUN;
*****************************************************************************************;
```

The program codes in SAS Program 10.3 are very similar to those in SAS Program 10.2 with a few exceptions. In the program, statement GROUPMEANS = 4.5 | 4.2 4.0 is used to specify comparison of 4.0 and 4.2 with 4.5 respectively; statement STDDEV = 1.0 1.2 requests power analysis using SD=1.0 and SD=1.2 for the same power analysis separately. With the specification, information for the following four scenarios can be assessed:

1. Power and sample size for comparing two group means 4.5 and 4.2 with SD = 1.0;
2. Power and sample size for the same comparison with SD = 1.5;
3. Power and sample size for comparing two group means 4.5 and 4.0 with SD = 10; and
4. Power and sample size for the same comparison with SD = 1.5.

As expected, parameters for plotting are adjusted to accommodate the new comparison conditions, including the MIN and MAX for x-axis of sample size, and increased NPOINTS from 20 to 30 for a more detailed plot.

10.5.4   Results of Power Analysis and Interpretation

Figure 10.8 presents the SAS output from Program 10.3. Results in this plot are more complex but better for comparison. The plot consists of four sample size – statistical power curves. Each represents a different design that can be used to support decision-making. Putting all four together makes it easy to interpret the results and make a decision.

From bottom up, the two solid lines in the figure depict two scenarios: (i) A 0.3-unit difference in the sample mean (4.5 vs. 4.2) and SD = 1.2; and (ii) the same difference but SD = 1.0. As SD declines, the sample size-power curve moves up. With mean difference of 0.3, 80% statistical power can be achieved with total sample of 351 subjects or roughly a sample size of 175 to 176 subjects per group. If SD=1.2, 80% statistical power cannot be achieved even with sample size N = 400.

From top down, the two dashed lines in the figure depicts two different scenarios: (i) A 0.5-unit difference in the sample mean (4.5 vs. 4.0) with SD = 1.0 and (ii) the same difference with SD=1.2. In the first scenario, 80% statistical power can be

POWER FOR 4 MEAN-SD COMBS, MEAN=4.5, 4.2, 4.0, SD=1.0 1.2

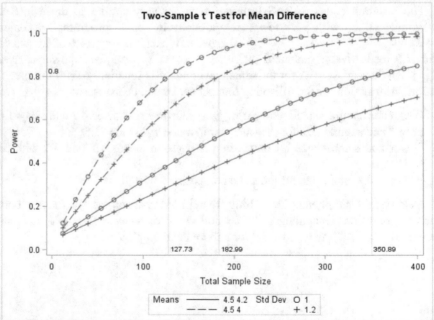

Fig. 10.8 Power analysis results using SAS Program 10.3 for different scenarios in comparing two sample means

achieved with total sample size N = 128 (64 per group); while in the second scenario; 80% statistical power can be achieved with N = 183 (91 to 92 per group).

10.5.5   Reporting Power Analysis Results

By setting type I error at $p < 0.05$, results from PROC POWER analysis indicate that (i) statistical power is sensitive to differences in group means. A statistical power of 80% cannot be achieved even with N = 400 if the between group differences in the sample mean is 0.3 and SD=1.2. If the between-group differences in sample mean increased from 0.3 to 0.5, 80% statistical power can be achieved with N = 128 if SD=1.0 or N = 183 when SD increases to 1.2; and (ii) relative to the mean differences between the two comparison groups, the sample size and power are less sensitive to SD.

   With these results, to design an observational study, more effort should be devoted to select variables with large between-group differences to ensure statistical power. To design intervention studies, smaller sample sizes can warrant 80% statistical power for more effective interventions (i.e., with large mean differences and small SDs).

10.6   Power Analysis to Compare Multi-Group Means

It is very common in quantitative epidemiology to compare means for more than two groups. Typical examples include comparisons of body weight, blood pressure and number of cigarettes smoked by educational levels (often 3-5 groups), racial/ethnic groups (up to five groups), and family income (3-5 groups). In this case, power analysis should be conducted using methods different from those for two-group comparison. This is because multi-group comparison of sample means are conducted using one-way ANOVA.

10.6.1   Method for Analysis

With the knowledge from Sects. 10.4, 10.5 and 10.6, it would be very easy to conduct power analysis for studies attempting to compare sample means across 3 or more groups. SAS Program 10.4 presents an example with hypothetical data.

```
*****************************************************************************
*** SAS PROGRAM 10.4. POWER ANALYSIS TO COMPARE MULTIPLE SAMPLE MEANS
*****************************************************************************;
**  1. DOCUMENTATION: TITLE AND OTHER INFORMATION;
TITLE "POWER TO COMPARING SAMPLE MEANS OF 3 GROUPS";
**  2. POWER ANALYSIS;
PROC POWER PLOTONLY;
* SET METHODS AND 3 GROUP MEANS 8 12 AND 15 FOR 2 SDS 3.6 4.8;
   ONEWAYANOVA
   GROUPMEANS = 8 | 12 | 15
   STDDEV     = 3.6 4.8
   NTOTAL     = 30
   ALPHA      = 0.05
   POWER      =.;
** 3 PLOTTING RESULTS: SAMPLE SIZE AND STATISTICAL POWER CURVE;
   PLOT X=N MIN=0 MAX=50 NPOINTS=30
   YOPTS = (REF=0.8 CROSSREF=YES);
RUN;
*****************************************************************************;
```

   This program is rather similar to SAS Program 10.3 except for two statements:
(i) the option ONEWAYANOVA is used to ask for multi-group mean comparison
rather than the statement TWOSAMPLEMEANS TEST=DIFF; and (ii) the state-
ment GROUPMEANS = 8|12|15 is revised with a vertical line to separate the
three means to be compared. This statement asks the program to compute power by
comparing three group means of 8, 12, and 15, respectively. To assess different
scenarios, two SDs for these means are used, one SD = 3.6 and another SD = 4.8.

10.6.2   Results of Power Analysis, Interpretation and Reporting

Figure 10.9 presents the results by executing SAS Program 10.4. The estimated
statistical power increases as sample size increases. The speed of increase is quicker
for SD=3.6 than SD=4.8. When SD = 3.6 is assumed, N=189 (round up from 18.62)
will be adequate to achieve 80% statistical power (solid line with dots). However,
when SD=4.8 is assumed, N = 30 is needed for the same statistical power (dashed
line with dots).

   Results from the power analysis using SAS indicated that by setting the type I
error at $p < 0.05$ (two sided), a total sample of N = 19 subjects or an average
sample of 7 subjects per group would be adequate to have 80% power to test the
overall differences in sample means across groups with SD=3.6 for the means of
all three groups. If SD increased from 3.6 to 4.8, 80% statistical power can be
achieved by increasing sample size to 30 subjects with an average of 10 subjects
per group.

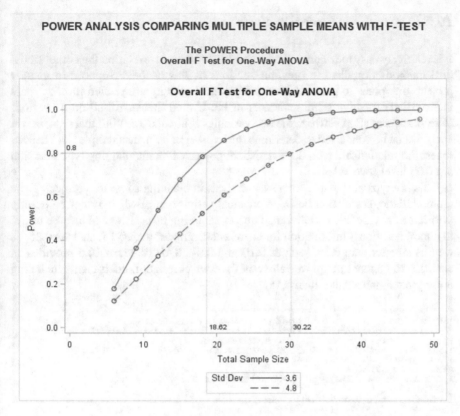

Fig. 10.9 Power analysis results using SAS Program 10.4 for Comparisons of multi-group means using one-way ANOVA

10.7 Power Analysis for Linear Correlation

Linear correlation, also known as Pearson or simple correlation, is a method commonly used in research to quantify the closeness of two continuous variables related with each other. In epidemiology, linear correlation is also used as a bivariate analysis tool to explore and identify candidate variables for further research.

Correlation analysis is also closely related to linear regression. The difference from linear regression is that linear regression directly quantifies changes in the outcome Y associated with changes in the predictor X while correlation analysis cannot tell changes in Y in response to changes in X. Significance of an estimated correlation coefficient is assessed using a Student t-test.

10.7.1   Steps for Power Analysis

It is relatively easy to conduct power analysis for linear correlation than other statistical methods described in previous sections of this chapter. Suppose in a study project, one plans to check if levels of physical activity are related to body mass index (BMI) for high school students in the United States. Based on a previous study, the correlation between the two variables is about 0.15. With that data, power analysis can be conducted to determine the number of subjects (sample size) needed to test the relationship with 80% statistical power while maintaining type I error at $p < 0.05$ level (two-sided).

This is a typical example for power analysis in planning a research project. To be more realistic, correlation between physical activity and BMI may not be exactly 0.15 but may vary in a certain range due to sampling error. It would also be useful to obtain additional information for correlations greater than 0.15, such as 0.25, as well as smaller than 0.15, such as 0.10 and 0.07. SAS Program 10.5 provides an example to conduct the power analysis for four correlation coefficients including those greater and smaller than 0.15.

```
************************************************************************************
*** SAS PROGRAM 10.5 POWER ANALYSIS FOR LINEAR CORRELATION
************************************************************************************;
**  1. DOCUMENTATION: TITLE AND OTHER INFORMATION;
TITLE "POWER ANALYSIS FOR PEARSON CORRELATION (R=0.07 0.10 0.15 0.25)";
**  2. POWER ANALYSIS;
PROC POWER PLOTONLY;
* SETTINGS WITH 4 CORRELATION COEFFICIENTS TESTED AT THE SAME TIME;
   ONECORR DIST = T
   CORR           = 0.07 0.10 0.15 0.25
   NTOTAL         = 500
   ALPHA          = 0.05
   POWER          =.;
** 3 PLOTTING RESULTS: SAMPLE SIZE AND STATISTICAL POWER CURVE;
   PLOT X=N MIN=0 MAX=2000 NPOINTS=25
   YOPTS = (REF=0.8 CROSSREF=YES);
RUN;
************************************************************************************;
```

SAS Program 10.5 is self-explanatory. The statement `ONECORR DIST = T` asks the program to conduct power analysis for linear correlation with t-test to assess significance levels; four correlation coefficients are specified following the statement `CORR = 0.07 0.10 0.15 0.25`. The rest are the same as those detailed in SAS Programs 10.1–10.4.

10.7.2   Results of Power Analysis and Interpretation

Figure 10.10 presents the output from the power analysis using SAS Program 10.5. The plot provides the information about the sample size and statistical power for studies involved in a linear correlation.

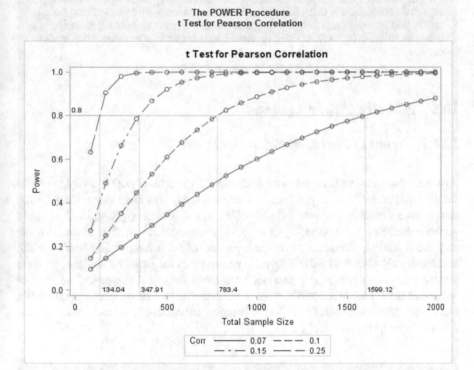

Fig. 10.10 Power analysis results using SAS Program 10.5 - Power and sample size for linear correlation

First, the sample size varies dramatically to achieve 80% statistical power as the r varies from small to large. When r = 0.07, a sample size of 1599 is needed to achieve 80% power; and the sample size reduces to 134 if r is increased to 0.25.

Second, when correlation is rather small (the bottom line with r = 0.07), the statistical power increases rather slowly as sample size increases; however, as the correlation coefficient r increases to 0.25, the power increases rapidly with sample size.

Based on the findings, to achieve 80% statistical power, a sample size N = 134 is needed for a correlation r = 0.25, N = 348 for a correlation r = 0.15, N = 783 for a correlation = 0.10; and N = 1599 for a correlation r = 0.07.

10.7.3   Reporting Results from the Power Analysis

To serve as a template, the following can be used to report results from the power analysis for a research project.

"By setting type I error alpha at p<0.05 (two-sided), power analysis using PROC POWER indicated that a sample size of 348 can power a study with 1-beta > 80% if the expected correlation r = 0.15. Sample size will increase rapidly as r declines. Sample size N will increase from 348 to 783 if r is reduced from 0.15 to 0.10; however, if r increases from 0.15 to 0.25, N=134 would be adequate to provide 80% statistical power."

10.8   Post Hoc Power Analysis

10.8.1   What Is Post Hoc Power Analysis?

Post hoc power analysis, as the name indicates, is to conduct power analysis after a study is completed and/or published. Since the study has been done, data on the sample size and the parameter estimates (i.e., mean, SD, rate, proportion) of study variables are known. Power analysis can then be conducted with data to assess if the completed study is adequately powered, particularly if the reported results are not statistically significant at p<0.05 level. If results from the post hoc analysis indicate that the study is not adequately powered (estimated statistical power <80%), the can be used as the evidence supporting that the conclusion from the reported study is not final, and additional studies with larger samples are needed to ensure adequate statistical power to find the real result.

10.8.2   An Example of Post Hoc Power Analysis

Here an example is provided to demonstrate the procedure for post hoc power analysis. One student in a class conducted a study to examine gender difference in the prevalence of A1c < 53 mmol/ml (7%) among US adults aged 20 and above. With the 2017-18 NHANES data (N = 1340 with A1c results), the estimated prevalence rate was 50.8% for males and 54.1% for females. The difference was not statistically significant.

However, given the sample size and the small differences in the two prevalence rates the student suspects that it could be too early to conclude that the observed gender difference is not true. One way to assess the results is to conduct a post hoc power analysis. SAS Program 10.6 provides an example to conduct post hoc analysis with results of the study conducted by the student.

```
*************************************************************************************
** SAS PROGRAM 10.6 POST HOC POWER ANALYSIS FOR TWO PROPORTIONS
*************************************************************************************;
TITLE "POST HOC POWER ANALYSIS FOR TWO PROPORTIONS 50.8 54.1 IN A1C";
PROC POWER;
* SETTINGS WITH 2 PROPORTIONS 0.508 AND 0.514;
  TWOSAMPLEFREQ TEST= PCHI
  GROUPPROPORTIONS  = (0.508 0.541)
  NPERGROUP         = 670     * SAMPLE SIZE PER GROUP
  ALPHA             = 0.05    * TYPE I ERROR
  POWER             =.;       * ASK TO ESTIMATE STATISTICAL POWER
  RUN;
*************************************************************************************;
```

Program codes in SAS Program 10.6 are similar to Program 10.1 for comparison of two proportions except that no program codes are used to plot the sample size-statistical power curve. The only work is to obtain the number of subjects per group. Since the total sample N = 1340, assuming the same number of subjects by gender, N = 1340/2 = 670 per group is entered to estimated statistical power.

10.8.3   Results of Power Analysis and Interpretation

Figure 10.11 presents the output by executing SAS Program 10.6. Results from the power analysis indicated that the conducted study has only 27% statistical power to detect the gender differences in the prevalence rate of A1c among US adults given

POST HOC POWER ANALYSIS FOR TWO PROPORTIONS 50.8 54.1 IN AIC

The POWER Procedure
Pearson Chi-square Test for Proportion Difference

Fixed Scenario Elements	
Distribution	Asymptotic normal
Method	Normal approximation
Alpha	0.05
Group 1 Proportion	0.508
Group 2 Proportion	0.541
Sample Size per Group	670
Number of Sides	2
Null Proportion Difference	0

Computed Power
Power
0.227

Fig. 10.11 Results from post hoc power analysis using SAS Program 10.6

the sample size with type I error set at p < 0.05 (two sided). Even if the observed difference between 50.8% and 54.1% is statistically significant, we only have a 27% chance to determine that the difference is statistically significant, and a 73% chance to miss it given the sample size and the type I error.

10.8.4   When to Use Post Hoc Power Analysis?

Post hoc power analysis should be conducted after completion of a research study with an unexpected negative result (p > 0.05). A very careful check of all steps of the research revealed no errors, including the theory-based hypothesis, quality of the data, variable recoding, statistical methods and software programing, missing data imputing, sample weights and sampling design. One last issue will be: Is the study adequately powered?

If the study is underpowered, it would be too soon to draw a statistical conclusion. An immediate approach would be to conduct a post hoc power analysis to check the power given the sample size. If post hoc power analysis indicates that the study is adequately powered, it will provide more evidence supporting the negative findings. However, if results from post hoc power analysis indicate the lack of statistical power as shown in the example in the previous section, the result can be used as evidence supporting additional studies to further test the study hypothesis by increasing sample size.

In addition to planning research, post hoc power analysis can be used for research training. It represents a powerful approach for students to understand the importance of statistical power in planning a study, to avoid underpowered studies, and to take caution in drawing statistical conclusions in the cases when p > 0.05 from a significance test.

10.8.5   Cautions in Post Hoc Power Analysis

Post hoc power analysis was not recommended by statisticians when the method was first proposed (Hoenig and Heisey 2001; Levine and Ensom 2001). This was because the statistical power is directly related to the type I error (or p values). Therefore, post hoc power analysis does not add new evidence to a completed study. It is also logically flawed, and suggests the lack of confidence in a completed study. In recent years, some journal editors even ask authors to report results from a post hoc power analysis, particularly if the research involves a chart review of patient data or a secondary analysis of data collected by others.

10.9   Practice

10.9.1   Power Analysis Methods

1. Conduct power analysis to compare two sample proportions.

Proportion		Sample size/group for 80% power	Sample size/group for 90% power
Group 1	Group 2		
0.30	0.40		
0.20	0.30		
0.20	0.32		
0.20	0.35		
0.20	0.38		
0.20	0.40		

2. Conduct power analysis to compare two sample means.

Mean		Standard deviation (SD)	Sample size/group for 80% power	Sample size/group for 80% power
Group 1	Group 2			
1.25	2.50	0.60		
1.25	2.50	0.90		
1.25	2.50	1.10		
1.25	2.60	0.90		
1.25	2.40	0.90		
2.25	3.40	0.90		

10.9.2   Application of Power Analysis in Planning a Research Project of Your Own

Plan a research project of your own, (i) select variables and form study hypothesis, (ii) obtain the data from literature about the sample statistics (i.e., mean and SD, or correlation for continuous variables, proportion, rate and ratio for binary or categorical variables), (iii) conduct power analysis, and (iv) report the analytical results to support your project.

10.9.3   Practice the Methods for Post Hoc Power Analysis

Conduct post hoc power analysis using results from your own study or studies by others in the literature and learn to draw conclusions with results from post hoc analysis.

10.9.4   Finalize the Research Paper

Conduct post hoc power analysis for your own paper to assess if your hypothesis testing is adequately powered. Update and polish your paper by incorporating results from the post hoc power analysis.

10.9.5   Study Questions

1. What do we mean by statistical power? Use epidemiological and statistical language to present your answer.
2. Name the computer software packages available for power analysis and their applications.
3. Indicated if the following statements are right or wrong, and interpret *why* with your own words?

   1. When comparing two sample means, the smaller the standard deviation SD, the smaller the statistical power.
   2. More statistical power is needed to detect a larger difference between two sample means or sample proportions.
   3. Statistical power cannot be changed after a study is completed.
   4. To ensure 80% statistical power, assessing a small correlation (say r = 0.01) requires a large sample while assessing a large correlation (say r = 0.35) requires a smaller sample.
   5. Post hoc power analysis must be conducted for all reported studies.

References

Chen, D., Chen, X., Tang, W., Lin, F.: Sample size determination to detect cusp catastrophe in stochastic cusp catastrophe model: a Monte-Carlo simulation-based approach. Lect. Notes Comput. Sci. **8393**, 35–41 (2014)

Cohen, J.: Statistical Power Analysis for the Behavioral Sciences, 2nd edn. Routledge, New York (1988)

Crosant, S.P., Iaz, T.H., Rahman, M., Berenson, A.B.: Gender differences in risk behaviors among high school youth. Global advances in health and medicine. **2**(5), 16–22 (2013)

Hoenig, J.M., Heisey, D.M.: The abuse of power: the pervasive fallacy of power calculations for data analysis. Am. Stat. **55**(1), 19–24 (2001)

Levine, M., Ensom, M.H.H.: Post hoc power analysis: an idea whose time has passed? Pharmacotherapy. **21**(4), 405–409 (2001)

Ott, R.L., Longnecker, M.T.: An Introduction to Statistical Methods and Data Analysis, 7th edn. Brooks/Cole, Cengage Learning, Australia, Brazil, Korea, Mexico, Singapore, Spain, UK and USA (2015)

Index

Printed in the United States
by Baker & Taylor Publisher Services